Outdoor Play
"Fun 4 4 Seasons"

By

Stephen L. Priest

Also by Stephen L. Priest

- *Outdoor Enthusiast: Never Say, "I Wish I Had ..."*
  ISBN - 1440438404

- *Avoiding Injuries: Tips from Master Outdoorsman Steve Priest*
  ISBN 9781440438455

- *Outdoor Enthusiast: Never Say, "I wish I had ..." e-book*
  ISBN – 13: 9780615225050

Cover Design by LoonsNest.biz

Preface

Outdoor Play "Fun 4 4 Seasons"

by

Stephen L. Priest

Steve's mission is to motivate and encourage families and individuals to make the outdoors a key component of their daily life. Outdoor Play "Fun 4 4 Seasons" describes the insights and healthy lifestyle of outdoor activities. Steve's stories and lessons make you want to put on your backpack, find your running shoes, borrow a canoe from the neighbor, tune-up the bike, and get ready for cross country skiing!

Some folks call outdoor experiences 'play'. If play is defined as the choice made to take a course of action based on the rewards of participation, and getting a perspective that can only come from 'doing', then indeed outdoor adventures are play. In fact, many adults and children do not play enough.

Outdoor exercise has proven to make you healthier both physically and mentally. Your mind gets relieved of personal and business stress and the result is a positive outlook on life. Your body gets stronger with outdoor movement and presence and the breathing of fresh air. All this helps to avoid injuries.

We began by looking in our own backyard where we saw animals, flora, rivers and ponds – and then within a few hours of our homes. Paddling amongst the foliage of October in northern New England all I could think of was a Michelangelo painting. We visited the coast of Maine, and then we were off paddling among its coastal islands. The boundary waters of Minnesota and Ontario summoned us. Florida offered unique ecological perspectives. The Grand Canyon gave us beauty beyond verbal description.

Each outdoor experience and each season and each year brought an expanded opportunity for my outdoor universe.

With each outing, I brought my camera, and when the time came to select pictures for the book, the memories they conveyed made it difficult to limit myself to only a few.

The beginning of *Outdoor Play "Fun 4 4 Seasons* offers a process to be an outdoor enthusiast for those who hesitate because of age, limited time, family commitments, or knowledge of an activity.

The middle sections are divided into the seasons of the year, **Spring, Summer, Fall** and **Winter** with glimpses of Steve's own outdoor undertakings. These sections are taken from the last four years of Steve's blog – **Outdoor Adventurers**. Steve provides a peek into outdoor places and Internet sites to assist you in your research and preparation.

The next to last section, **Places to Play in Northern New England**, provides web references to local activities and clubs to join as incentives to learn and participate – if indeed you need these supports.

The last section, **The Beginning**, is Steve's own personal story of how he went from a couch potato to a daily outdoor enthusiast.

"Everyone must believe in something. I believe I'll go canoeing." - Henry David Thoreau

Dedication

To Cathy, Tim, Shaun, Christine, Madison and Carson

Acknowledgements

My wife Cathy has been steadfast in her encouragement of my daily outdoor commitment. Amongst many of my outdoor activities, Cathy and I have swam, hiked, camped, paddled, walked, and run together. She has been my support team throughout my life.

My sons Tim and Shaun, and friends John Kerrigan, and Dundee Nestler have been my consistent outdoor enthusiast partners. Shaun, Tim and my cousin Linwood Parsons have been my confidants and proof readers throughout the preparation of this book. Without their encouragement this book could not have been.

My outdoor enthusiast friends encouraged me to go to the woods, lakes and rivers of northern New Hampshire, and before we realized it, we had regular outdoor excursions. My cousin Linwood took us to the Allagash Wilderness Waterway in Maine – three times in fact! Other friends heard our wilderness stories and read my Outdoor Enthusiast blog, and then, all of a sudden, we had yearly outdoor commitments.

I thank George Potter for encouraging me to start my Outdoor Enthusiast Blog http://outdooradventurers.blogspot.com/. This blog has provided most of the material in **Outdoor Play.**

My earlier books were arranged by chapters of outdoor activities (e.g. running, hiking, canoeing, skiing, triathlons) – whereas this book is arranged by the seasons of the activities presented (e.g. **Spring, Summer, Fall** and **Winter**).

John Kerrigan, besides being a participant in most of the activities presented in this text, encouraged me to create videos of our adventures. He introduced me to Microsoft Movie Maker from whence I learned to incorporate my videos into my Outdoor Enthusiast Blog. I then became an Outdoor TV show volunteer producer at Bedford Community Television.

Jefferson Nunn was bold enough to see visions of sharing my stories with other outdoor enthusiasts, as well as those wanting to be.

Linwood Parsons and Dundee Nestler both contributed significantly to my outdoor know-how with their unique outdoor perspectives and skills of which I am indebted.

Linwood did substantial editing on this book and did all the graphic design for the cover. He also had the patience to teach me Corel. Indeed, without Linwood this book may not have been.

Dick Satter continually calls me to go bike riding and running –and to get therapy to mend my injuries. He has been my pusher whom I admire for his own commitment to outdoor activities. I thank him for his concern and his friendship.

My Dad had a great love of Maine, and my Mom saw that we — seven children and all the grandchildren — were encouraged in our outdoor endeavors. One of my favorite memories of Mom is when in my first road race she would not let the race timer leave until I had crossed the finish line — in last place and all by myself!

My granddaughter, Madison, was my support team in one of my triathlons and my grandson Carson is featured in the canoe rescue training in the **Summer** section. As a family we hike, swim, paddle, and ski.

The book you are about to read is not about me. I certainly may be the central character in the stories, but in addition to the aforementioned, Tom Austin, Lennie Carroll, Ron Millett, Linda Nestler, Paul Nestler, Betty Parsons, Austin Priest, Braden Priest, David Priest, Dennis Priest, Helen Priest, Leanne Priest, Marlene Priest and Joe Ryan have all been part of my outdoor life.

For those friends I have inadvertently left out, 'thank you.'

Contents

How to Become an Outdoor Enthusiast

"Everyone must believe in something. I believe I'll go outdoors." – S. Priest

Outdoor Play "Fun 4 4 Seasons" enthusiastically portrays a daily commitment to the outdoors for health and fitness. This book is full of short story adventures that give the reader an overview of multiple outdoor things to do. The message is to get outdoors and do something. The only competition you have is the task at hand. Do not worry about reaching the top of the mountain - just concern yourself with staying on the path.

Some folks call being outdoor 'play'. If play is defined as the choice made to take a course of action based on the rewards of participation, and getting a perspective that can only come from 'doing', then indeed outdoor adventures are play. In fact, many adults and children do not play enough.

Exercise has proven to make you healthier both physically and mentally. Making a commitment to daily outdoor activities, such as walking and running, add to your endurance for all outdoor activities. Best yet, your body will be stronger with exercise, thus avoiding many injuries. So how do you get started being an outdoor enthusiast?

Some people can be discouraged from exercising by not knowing what to do or how to do it. Those who were athletic in childhood may be frustrated by how their abilities have deteriorated over time. Certain individuals need to try new activities so they won't be comparing themselves to others or earlier performances.

This first section is an introduction to the major intent of this book - to promote the outdoors as a component of one's daily life. I will suggest a process to become an outdoor enthusiast for those who hesitate because of age, limited time, family commitments, or knowledge of an activity. I have used this process to get where I am today.

The middle sections are divided into the seasons of the year: **Spring**, **Summer**, **Fall** and **Winter** with glimpses into my own outdoor feelings and shared learning with supporting web references and videos. These sections are taken from the last four years of my blog – **Outdoor Enthusiast**. These posts provide a peek into outdoor places and Internet sites for additional research and preparation.

The **Places to Play in Northern New England** section provides web references to local activities and clubs to join as incentives to learn and participate.

The last section, **The Beginning**, is my personal story of how I went from a couch potato with a limp from a torn Achilles tendon injury to a daily outdoor enthusiast.

You are only limited to an outdoor activity by boundaries set by yourself. Just by following simple steps, you will be well on your way to expanding your horizons and removing barriers and boundaries to enjoying the outdoors and a healthier you.

In my case I will start the "beginner" reader with walking outdoors or on a treadmill. Progression to outside exercise is presented as distances between telephone poles. I will explain "telephone poles" later.

First, like all advice on exercise, it is strongly recommended you get your physician's approval.

Second, it is OK for a family member or friend to join you in this endeavor, BUT DO NOT WAIT because of their schedule. Rely on no one but yourself. No excuses.

No matter which outdoor excises you choose, you need to get your cardio system in shape. Your heart is the engine that needs preparation and tuning. You can do this with both exercise and proper eating habits.

Frankly, in my case, the key is exercise and the eating habits will follow naturally. The more exercise I did, the better my eating awareness and habits became. This chapter does not focus on food. It addresses exercise, and in particular talks about gradually working up from simple and short walks, and the intensity and duration of the exercises will be determined over time.

Start Right Outside Your Home

What is great is you can start right outside your home! For safety's sake, remember to ALWAYS walk and run on the sidewalk, or on the side of the road facing oncoming traffic.

Keeping a diary of each day's progression, including how far you went, the method of exercise (walk, run/walk, run) will help motivate you when you see the progress you are making.

Next, RESIST TEMPTATION TO GO FASTER AND FURTHER. If you do, you will most assuredly be injured.

Okay, let's get started.

> **Day 1**: Go outside and walk the distance between two telephone poles, then walk back home.
> **Day 2**: Go outside and walk the distance between three telephone poles, then walk back home.
> **Day 3**: Go outside and walk the distance between four telephone poles, then walk back home.
>
> Continue this progressive program for days 4 and 5. If you have breathing problems, or get exhausted, do not add the extra distance.
>
> **Day 6 and 7**: Rest. Skip only two days a week. Light rain is no excuse for not accomplishing your day's goal.
> **Day 8**: Go outside and run the distance between two telephone poles, then walk back home.
> **Day 9**: Go outside and run the distance between four

3

telephone poles, then walk back home.

Day 10, 11, 12: Run six, eight and ten telephone poles respectively (yes, you have increased the number of poles).

If you have followed this fixed schedule, you will feel the urge to get into your car and measure your distance. Do it!

Now develop your own plan to reach one mile in six weeks.

Some frequently asked questions on getting started:

- How far is the distance between two telephone poles? ANSWER: Well, I have 60 paces (about 60 yards) between the poles on my street. No telephone poles? ANSWER: I just gave you a distance.

- What if I feel good and want to go further and faster? ANSWER: DO NOT, I repeat, DO NOT try walking or running beyond the specified distances. People, feeling good, try to go further and faster, THEY GET INJURED, and then they are set back for months. DO NOT, I repeat, DO NOT try to get ahead of this schedule.

- What if I am injured, such as with shin splints or a sore knee? ANSWER: Then back off a bit from your running distance and do more walking. As your injury pain subsides, return to an increased schedule. Try not to skip a daily run or walk, unless you feel the pain is causing the injury to worsen.

- Do I need a particular shoe or sneaker to start? ANSWER: Nope - no excuses. Get outside. When you reach day twelve, you are now ready to buy sneakers or running shoes.

- Do I need sweat pants, shorts, or polypropylene clothing? ANSWER: Nope, again no excuses. Get outside. When you reach day twelve, you are now ready to look like a runner –

4

buy yourself some running shorts, light jacket and long lightweight pants.

- Do I need a hat? ANSWER: Yes. Old, new, torn or whatever. You need a hat to protect you from the sun and rain. Get outside.

Four reminders to becoming an outdoor enthusiast:

1. Be sure to follow the schedule of this program.

2. RESIST TEMPTATIONS TO GO FASTER AND FURTHER, or else, guaranteed, YOU WILL GET INJURED.

3. Be consistent in doing your walking and running. NO excuse to missing a day.

4. Do not let weather, lack of an outdoor companion, or fancy clothing deter you.

To get a sense of how another person did with this program, it took Outdoor Steve six weeks before he ran one mile without stopping to walk. Thereafter, he never exceeded one mile for the next year. After a year, he began to increase his distance. As he gained confidence in his physical conditioning, he complemented his running with other outdoor challenges. His accomplishments have included cycling, hiking, swimming, canoeing, kayaking, triathlons, biathlons, cross-country skiing, and marathons.

When presented with an outdoor opportunity, such as a one-week paddle on the one-hundred and seven-mile Allagash Wilderness Waterway, do I say, "I have too many things to do?" Or do I say, "Yes!" because this is a great opportunity to enjoy my sons and friends? The work and home chores will be there when I get back.

As you read the short stories in this book, let your body and mind experience the wonderment of personal enlightenment and outdoor play.

Most of these short scenarios are taken from my **Outdoor Enthusiast** blog (http://outdooradventurers.blogspot.com/). Each post has Internet references "what, where, why and how" so the reader can do much more than simply learn about one person's outdoor quests. These stories are intended to both motivate and instruct the reader by providing outdoor places to go and things to do.

My mission is to motivate and encourage families and individuals to make the outdoors a key component of their daily life.

Get on your bike. Go hiking with your family. Run with a neighbor. Take telemark ski lessons. Try an Ottertail paddle. Take swimming lessons. Go spinning on your bike. Visit a museum. Go to an Audubon seminar.

Never say, "I wish I had gone outdoors".

Spring

Two roads diverged in a wood and I – I took the one less traveled by, and that has made all the difference – Robert Frost

A Mid-week Trek to Tuckerman Ravine

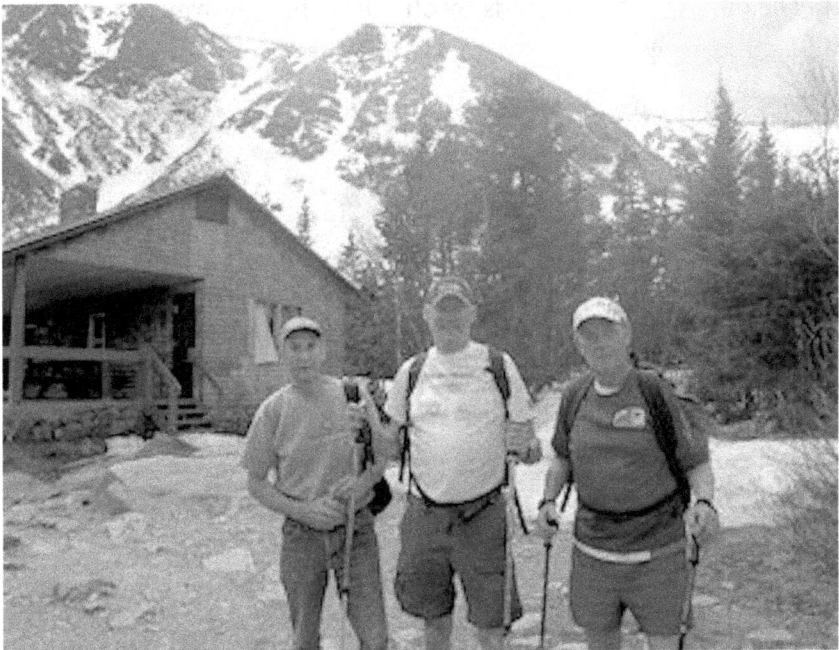

Tuckerman Ravine Overlooking Hermit Hut

Today was a perfect time to hike to Tuckerman Ravine. In two hours Dundee, Dick and I made the three-mile uphill trip via Tuckerman Ravine Trail to Hermit Lake. The summer-like day was emphasized by Dick and I wearing t-shirts and shorts (we did have warm clothes in our backpacks for any change in weather.)

Tuckerman Ravine

Tuckerman Ravine, isolated on the east side of Mt. Washington in the White Mountain National Forest, is famous for its daredevil spring skiing, snowboarding, mountaineering, ice climbing and hiking. Moreover, Tuckerman's remoteness and its ever changing weather conditions and terrain can be dangerous – and even fatal. (http://www.tuckerman.org/tuckerman/tuckerman.htm)

If you are thinking of skiing Tuckerman, you should be an expert skier in good physical condition. The headwall at Tuckerman is between 45-55 degrees and the vertical drop is approximately 1200 ft. The only way to the top is by climbing the headwall. (http://www.out-there.com/tuckerman.htm).

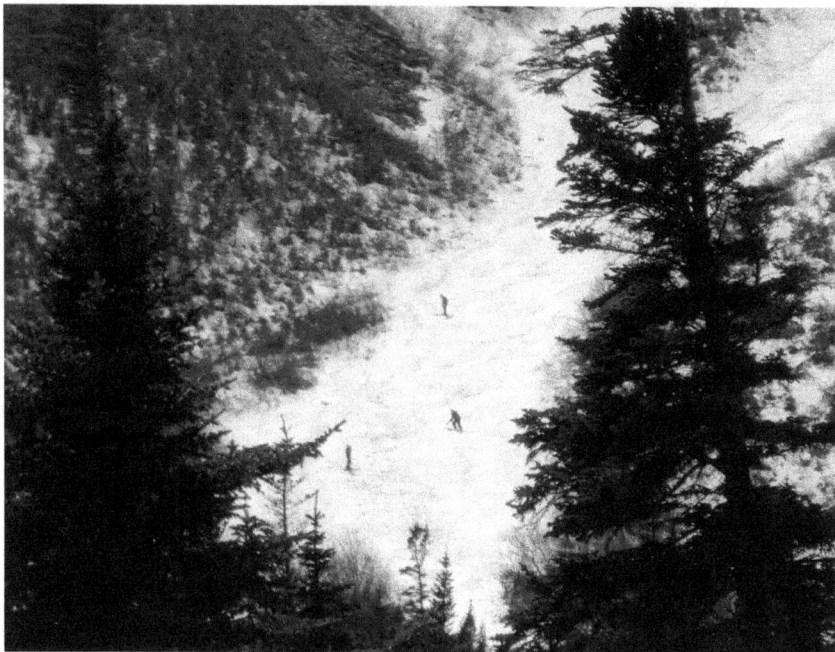

Skiers on Tuckerman

The hike started on a dry and bare rocky Tuckerman Ravine Trail. As we ascended to the middle section, we encountered snowmelt small streams crossing the trail, and we gingerly traversed slippery ice. The upper part of the trail was snow covered, and we could hear and see water flowing underneath our feet.

Fellow outdoor enthusiasts, carrying their downhill and telemark skis, boots and gear, passed us. Other hikers, like us, are there for the thrill of the surreal scene of this magnificent beautiful ravine with a reputation for beauty, avalanche danger, and untold climbing challenges.

Shared Thoughts:

• A trek to Tuckerman's is a perfect place to bond with your significant other, family, and friends. My wife Cathy and I have made this trek many times, and years ago, my son Tim and I encountered a sudden storm that nearly put an end to our lives. Memories of love, emotion, and bonding are part of my Tuckerman experience.
• 10:30 am temperature 82 degrees AMC's Pinkham Hut, 12:30 pm temperature 68 at base of Ravine.
• We were aware of an air and ground search for a 17-year-old hiker Eagle Scout who had been missing in this area since Saturday. At around noon we heard from a hiker the scout was found safe and in good condition.
• Camaraderie of all skiers was evident throughout the hike as we shared "where are you from", "conditions of your ski", "which side of the ravine did you ski?", and "Have you heard if they found the scout?"
• We wished a ten-year-old boy "happy birthday" after we learned he and his dad skied Hillman's Highway trail, the longest run in Tuckerman.
• We drank water every ten minutes to not get de-hydrated. My backpack was filled with a quart of water, two peanut butter jelly sandwiches, compass, map, duct tape, ace bandage, contractor trash bags for an emergency overnight, warm clothes, gaiters, winter hat, and gloves. We all wore hiking boots (wearing sneakers on this very rocky hike invites a sprained ankle and wet feet).

• After lunch at the caretaker hut, we started up the right section of the Ravine, but stopped because of rocks covered with slippery ice and brewing dark storm clouds moving swiftly over the headwall. Since storms come up quickly in this area, we did not hesitate to leave when we saw the threatening conditions.

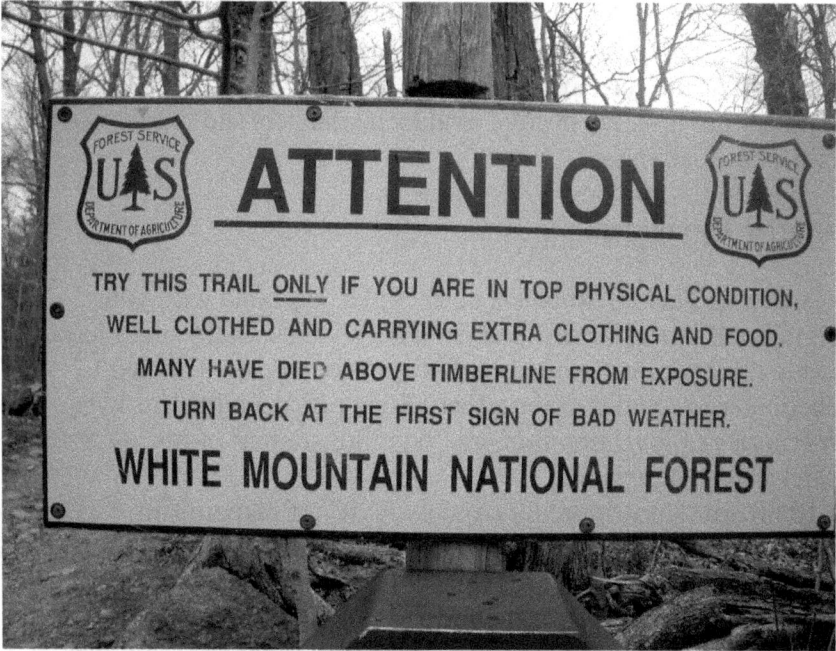

ATTENTION

TRY THIS TRAIL <u>ONLY</u> IF YOU ARE IN TOP PHYSICAL CONDITION, WELL CLOTHED AND CARRYING EXTRA CLOTHING AND FOOD. MANY HAVE DIED ABOVE TIMBERLINE FROM EXPOSURE. TURN BACK AT THE FIRST SIGN OF BAD WEATHER.

WHITE MOUNTAIN NATIONAL FOREST

• Thinking of going to Tuckerman? Great, but before you go be prepared with a review of the HikeSafe program http://www.wildlife.state.nh.us/Outdoor_Recreation/hiking_safety. htm. The N.H. Fish and Game Department and the White Mountain National Forest have partnered up to create a mountain safety education program called "HikeSafe." A large component of the program is the Hiker Responsibility Code. The code applies to all hikers, from beginners on a short hike to experienced outdoor enthusiasts embarking on an expedition. Please practice the elements of the code and help the HikeSafe program spread by sharing the code with fellow trekkers. Creating an awareness of HikeSafe will help increase hiker responsibility and decrease the need for Search and Rescue efforts.

Dick, Dundee and I will never have to say, "We wish we had hiked to Tuckerman's Ravine to watch the skiers and enjoy Tuck's majestic wilderness mountain scenery."

Video Reference Spring Hike to Tuckerman's

- Blog: Fantastic Spring Mid-week Hike to Tuckerman Ravine
  http://outdooradventurers.blogspot.com/2009/04/fantastic-mid-week-trek-to-tuckerman.html

Boston Marathon Day in April on Patriots Day

My friends Ryan and Kevin were running the Boston. Temperature was 45 degrees at race time. Over twenty-six thousand runners. I parked in the EMC lot and took the marathon bus to the center of Hopkinton. I walked around Athlete's Village, but could not find either friend.

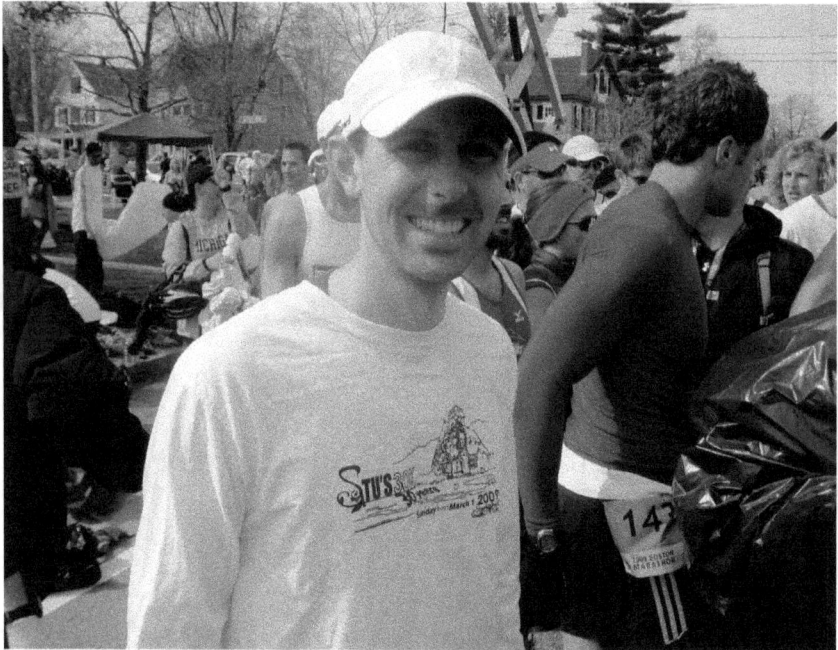

Ryan – Minutes to Go

I kept in cell phone contact with my son Shaun, and friend John Kerrigan – later they would text message me Ryan and Kevin's locations and times on the course.

Four Scheduled Starts

The Boston Marathon has four starts. The Wheelchair competition starts ten minutes before the elite Women scheduled at 9:32 a.m.

After the elite women start, the race features 2 waves, with Wave 1 starting at 10:00 a.m. (blue bibs numbered 1,000 to 13,999), and Wave 2 starting at 10:30 a.m. (yellow bibs numbered 14,000+).

All runners have a timing chip laced into their shoes, so regardless of the runner's starting time or wave, each runner's start time begins only when they cross the starting line.

Finding Ryan and Kevin at the Start

Ryan wore bib 1862, and his corral was right behind the elite runners. This low number means Ryan is an exceptionally good marathoner. I went to the 1000-1999 corral to search for Ryan. It was ten minutes before Ryan's start, so I anxiously kept yelling 'Ryan!' I was determined to find him before he started. Finally, Ryan heard me calling his name – and we excitedly exchanged greetings and I offered my quick words of encouragement and success. It was nearly time for Ryan's 10 am start.

I now had to find Kevin for his 10:30 am Wave 2 start. Trying to spot Kevin in this motley throng of thousands of runners was beginning to seem impossible. It was surreal seeing runners of all shapes dressed in assorted attire.

Everyone was nervous, stretching, chatting, shaking hands - and all this mixed with the smell of liniment and old sweaty clothes. I had a thought that I should be running! It lasted less than a nanosecond, as I realized the training and effort all these athletes did to get to this starting line.

I ran Boston three times – and I knew the pain they were about to endure – especially the back of the packers when in three plus hours they face heartbreak hill with cramps and exhaustion. Moreover, they still have an hour to go before they finish.

The public address system starts a countdown for the 10:30 am start – and nobody moves at the back of the corrals! Yup, it will take nearly ten minutes before Kevin crosses the starting line. No matter, as his microchip will give him an accurate time.

As each corral begins to slow move, forward, my eyes finally spot Kevin – and he is on my side of the corral. I run to him and join his slow shuffle as he and his fellow marathoners edge toward the starting line.

I give three bits of advice to Kevin 1) Drink lots of water, 2) It is OK to pee in your pants, 3) Enjoy the run!!

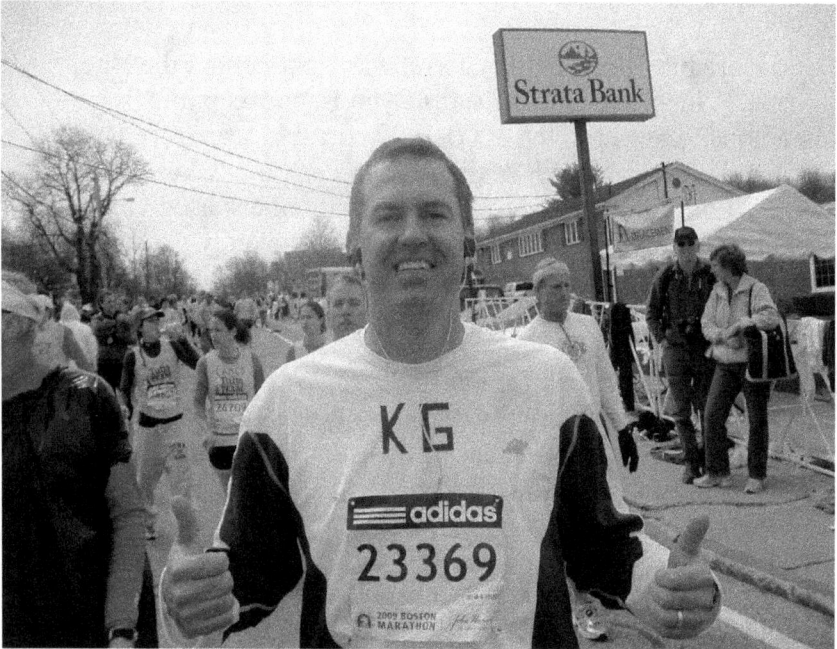

Kevin is Ready

Twenty Mile Mark – Heartbreak Hill

I take the spectator bus back to the parking area, pick up my car, call Ryan's Dad for his location at the 20 mile mark, check my map, set my GPS and I am off to the corner of Commonwealth Ave and Sumner Street where John is standing – the beginning of the famous Heartbreak Hill.

My twenty minute trip down the Mass Pike is passed listening to the marathon on the radio. I exit at Center Street Exit 17 in Newton, pull off the side of the road, and set my GPS to the 536

Sumner Street address John gave me. I was only 1.5 miles away. I found Sumner Street, and a side street to squeeze my Jeep in with dozens of other illegally parked cars. No doubt, there were too many cars to tag or tow!

Ten minutes after exiting from the Pike, I was standing next to John at the twenty-mile mark of the course. John's son-in-law had text messaged John that his smart phone app showed Ryan would be reaching our area within the next ten minutes.

We see Ryan! His six plus minute pace looks smooth - he smiles as he sees us, and I fumble my camera! Gosh!! I manage only one good video – of him running away from us.

John leaves and heads to the finish to greet Ryan.

Bill Rogers runs by me – I wish I had my camera ready. He won the Boston in two of the years I ran the Boston. What a great athlete and representative of the Boston Marathon.

I now await Kevin. I had set my watch when Kevin started to run at Hopkinson, and my best guess was he would do a nine-minute mile pace.

It was about 1:30 pm, and the temperature was beginning to drop. It was getting windy. I zipped up both my sweater and jacket. I was thinking Kevin is getting dehydrated, and when he reaches me, will be cold and shivering. I will offer him my sweater and windbreaker. I watch the bib numbers of the runners. Kevin's bib is 23369. The runners passing by me have not yet reached the 20,000 series bib numbers, which means runners that started in Kevin's corral have not yet reached me.

It is now close to 3:25 on my watch and by my calculation, Kevin should be here. Did I miss him? I was sure he was going to finish, but how long should I wait here before I leave? I called my son, Shaun, and his last checkpoint for Kevin was at the 30K (about 18 miles).

I see Kevin!! I start jumping, yelling and waving for him to see me. I have his water and orange ready. He says his stomach has been bothering him for some time – and he does not want anything. I walk with him listening to his thoughts about "I never knew it would hurt this much." What do I say to him to encourage him in a quest he started six months ago. Since I had been in his position three times, I knew that plain words were not enough. Out of my mouth came "You are at the twenty mile point. You are now in a 10K race!"

He picked up his running pace and away he went!

I headed home to watch the marathon I had recorded on my DVR.

Ryan finished in 2: 48.26. Kevin finished in 4:44:08. Great accomplishments for two highly trained athletes!

I will never have to say, "I wish I had been at the Boston Marathon to root and support Ryan and Kevin."

Video References
- Blog: Boston Marathon 2009
  http://outdooradventurers.blogspot.com/2009 /04/boston-marathon-day-april-20-2009.html

Paddle Florida - Get Down on the Suwannee River, and Go with the Flow!

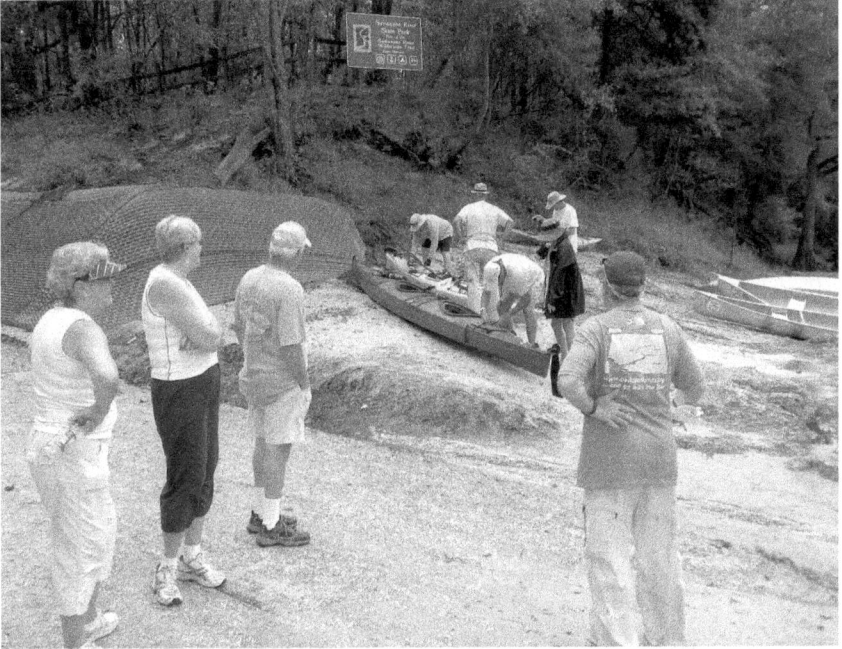

Suwannee River State Park Take-out - Paddle Florida Group

My sister Barb and her husband Larry, took my wife Cathy and I hiking at the Suwannee River State Park in Live Oak, Florida. Unexpectedly, we came upon a group known as Paddle Florida . Twenty kayakers were making a 123-mile eight-day trip from the Spirit of the Suwannee Music Park in Live Oak, Florida to beautiful Manatee Springs State Park. We greeted them as they pulled ashore to prepare for a night of tenting.

We met Bill Richards, leader of the group. Bill enthusiastically answered my many questions about **Paddle Florida**. Moreover, Larry had just seen a huge fish jump in the middle of the river, and Bill identified the fish as the prehistoric Gulf Sturgeon.

Paddle Florida is held in cooperation with the Florida Park Service and the Suwannee River Water Management District. These two organizations have created the 171-mile Suwannee River Wilderness Trail. The Trail makes the Suwannee River accessible to paddlers, hikers, bikers, equestrian enthusiasts and other outdoor groups.

The Suwannee River trek sounds similar to the NH/ME Androscoggin River Trek to the Sea where participants can join the moving river celebration as a day trip, do a series of days, or paddle the entire 170 miles.

You can contact Bill Richards at bill@paddleflorida.org to learn more about the Suwannee paddle, as well as other great paddles of Paddle Florida.

Now, I never have to say, "I wish I had been to the Suwannee River, met a member of Paddle Florida, and learned about the ancient Gulf Sturgeon."

Hmm, do you suppose a trek with Paddle Florida is in the future for Outdoor Steve?

Video References
- Blog: Paddle Florida - The Suwannee River, and Go with the Flow
  http://outdooradventurers.blogspot.com/2009/10/paddle-florida-get-down-on-suwannee.html

I Never Have to Say, "I wish I had paddled Florida's Suwannee River"

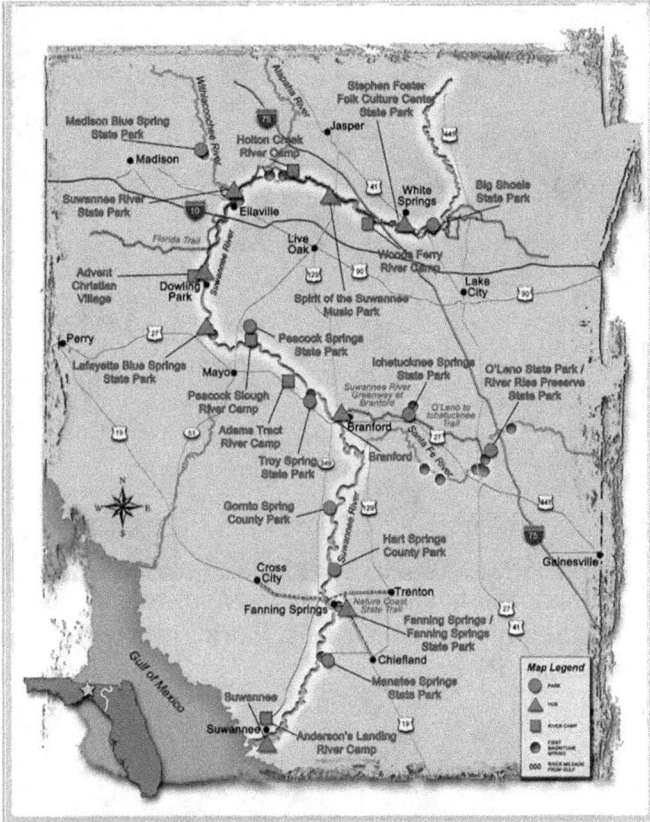

In late March, we spent five days paddling seventy miles of the upper Suwannee River. Dundee paddled his fifteen-foot aluminum Grumman canoe, Shaun was in an eleven-foot Old Town Cayuga kayak, and John and I in my sixteen-foot Old Town Penobscot canoe.

Florida has designated the Suwannee River as an Outstanding Florida Water. The Suwannee flows and winds 265 plus miles from the Okefenokee Swamp in southern Georgia to the Gulf of Mexico in Florida. It has fifty plus springs along the way. The river's limestone outcroppings and a drop in elevation create Florida's only whitewater rapids at Big Shoals and Little Shoals.

Put-In at Cyprus Creek South Tract

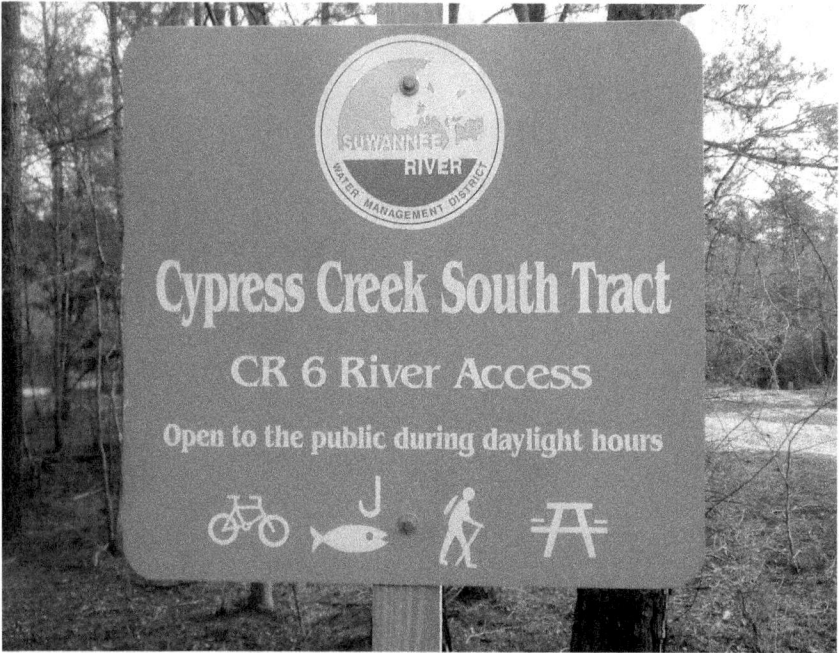

My sister Barbara and husband Larry drove us to our put-in at Cyprus Creek South Tract in northern Florida where CR 6 crossed over the Suwannee River.

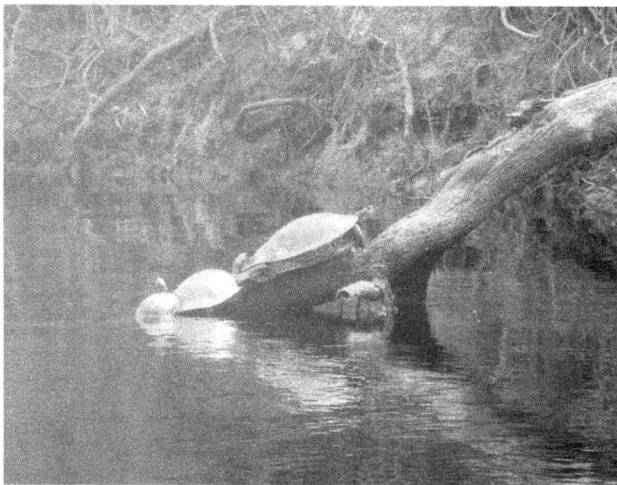

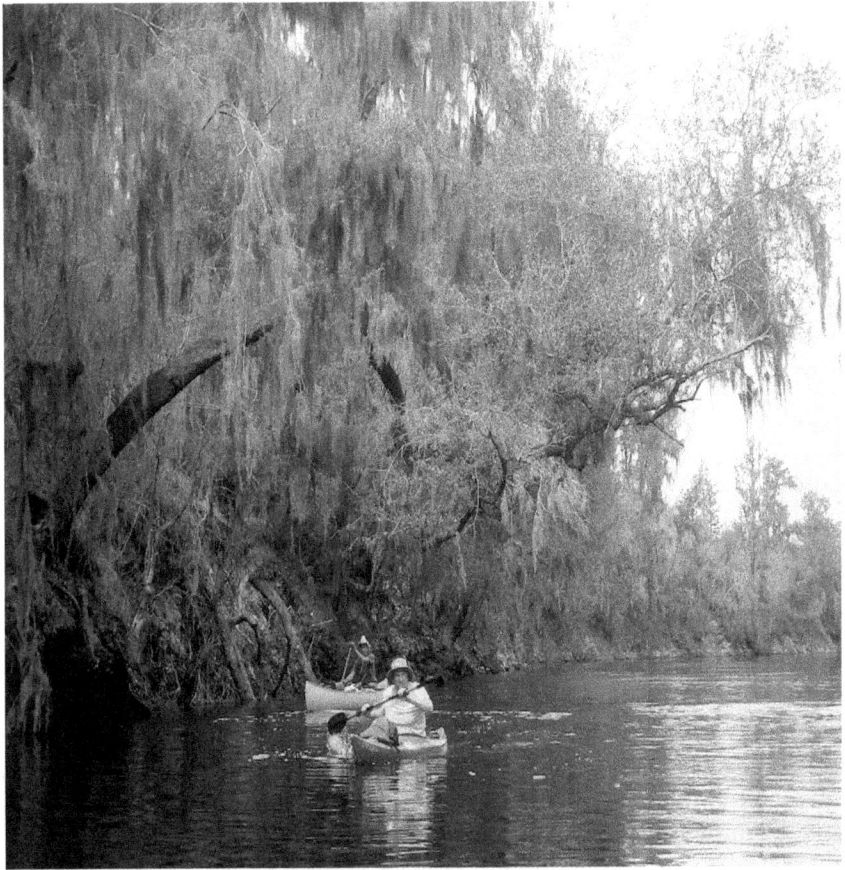

Hanging Spanish Moss

Interestingly as the trip went on, we recognized similarities with our NH/ME/ treks, such as in New Hampshire we kept our eyes open for moose, whereas on the Suwannee we watched for alligators.

In Maine we would admire stands of pine trees, while here in Florida we saw Spanish moss hanging from stately Cyprus and Live Oak trees. Our northern river paddles often passed through ledges and canyon-like sections, whereas in the Suwannee we experienced high bluffs of limestone walls funneling the river.

The river is lined with sandy banks and beaches made from the thick limestone that underlies the entire state. The Suwannee River pulverizes the limestone into white beach sand, and hidden underwater stone formations cause the river to whirl as if there was a spring or a whirlpool waiting to draw us into its black hole. Often, particularly at sharp bends, twisting water would attempt to turn our vessels upstream.

We frequently saw rope swings along the river. Summer had not yet come here, so we could only let our minds wander as to how much fun it would be to swing over the water, release, and drop into the cool Suwannee.

The upper and middle Suwannee is a dark brown-black color. This color is tannic acid released by decaying vegetation.

Our GPS showed the current to be around 3 miles per hour from our put-in through Big Shoals. Thereafter we noticed the current to be around 2 mph.

Day One – A Twenty mile Paddle to Big Shoals

In mid-morning we met two Florida State biologists. They demonstrated their shocking technique to inspect fish. This was particularly interesting, as last spring Dundee and I assisted NH Fish and Game as volunteers stocking salmon fry on the Souhegan River, and we were told about monitoring the fish population with a similar shocking technique. Blog: Stocking Salmon (http://tiny.cc/49mruw)

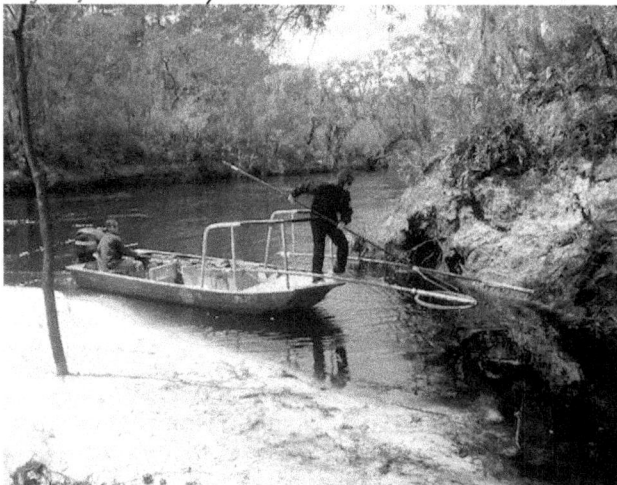

Biologists Inspect Fish

We camped for the night on the bluff overlooking Big Shoals. Big Shoals is the Suwannee's (and Florida's) only set of rapids. Big Shoals rapids were at Class III level, so we decided to portage (about a quarter mile carry).

Below is Shaun eating his breakfast of an orange followed by an egg cooked in the orange peel, all planned by Chef John (we nick-named him, Emeril Lagasse, the famous chef from Massachusetts).

Cook Your Egg in an Orange Over an Open Campfire

1st Eat an Orange for Vitamin C

2nd. Crack & Drop Egg into Eaten Orange Half

3rd. Cover Egg with Other Half of Orange and Cook Over Campfire

The picture below is a fellow named Matt who built his own self-powered sail boat. We briefly shared conversation as we both portaged around Big Shoals rapids. He shared with me he was in a race around Florida with six other custom engineered boats that were powered only by wind and man power. He took a few minutes to describe his most intriguing boat.

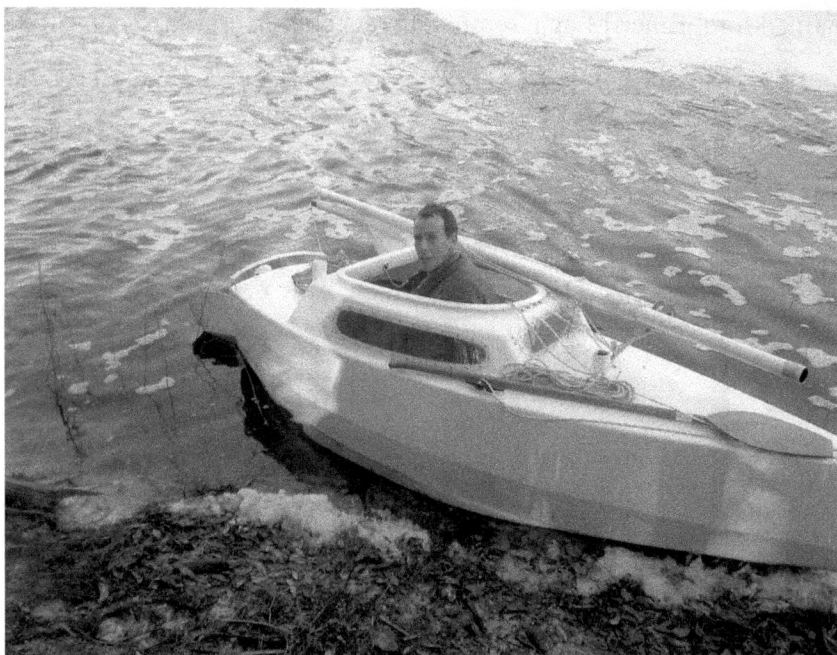

Day Two – sixteen miles to Swift Creek camp

We saw four alligators as they lay on the banks looking like logs, and when they spotted us, they quickly slid into the water before we could get a picture. We spotted many large turtles throughout the trek. I spotted a river otter twice, and again they are quicker than my picture taking finger can react. Hawks, red cardinals, and vultures flew overhead. We heard what sounded like Barred owls at night.

Ogeechee Tupelo Tree

As we paddled we noticed a tall odd-shaped tree that was similar in color and height to the Cyprus, but obviously was a different species. In planning for this trip Dundee and I visited his relative who had worked along the Suwannee, and he told us to be aware of the Ogeechee Tupelo tree near or in the water.

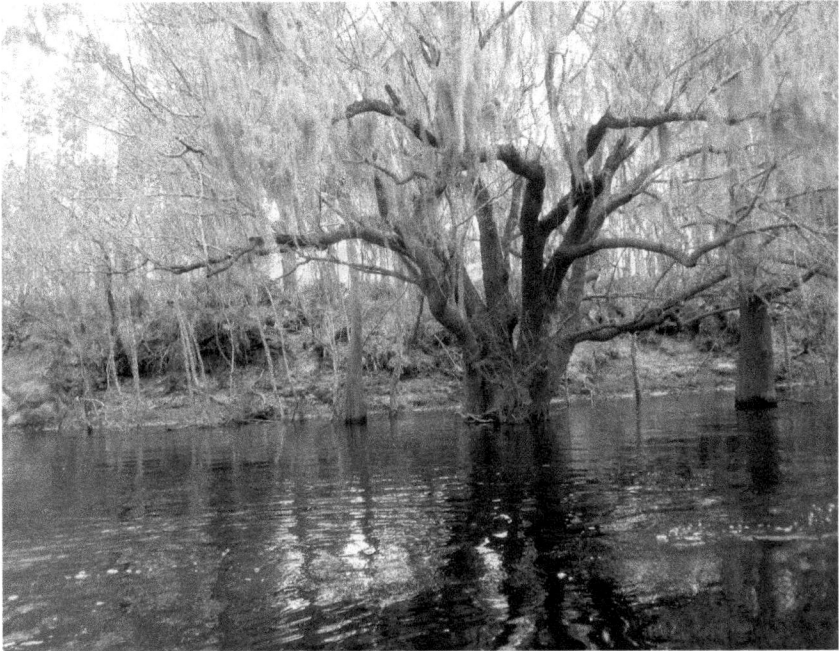

Ogeechee Tupelo Tree

The tree is unique to warm and wet areas in northern Florida, Georgia, South Carolina and North Carolina. The trees we saw were close to 40 feet in height and with a spreading flat-topped crown. Multiple, irregular branches and roots emerged from their trunks. It had dark brown or grey, ridged bark, and the base of the tree had swollen buttress-type roots. We were told that local people often use its fruit to make jelly.

Admittedly, the Ogeechee Tupelo tree looked weird to us, and you can judge for yourself by playing the **Video Reference** at the end of this section.

We noticed as we got closer to Big Shoals, the river bank changed to more rock than sand, and we stopped seeing Ogeechee Tupelo trees.

Day Three to Swift Creek

We generally sought camp on the river between 4 and 5 pm. Edwin McCook, Land Management Specialist for the Suwannee River Water Management District, had given us maps and GPS points of preferred riverside camp sites, and these points came in handy in looking for a good night's accommodation.

I spotted a three foot brown and tan spotted snake, but again no picture.

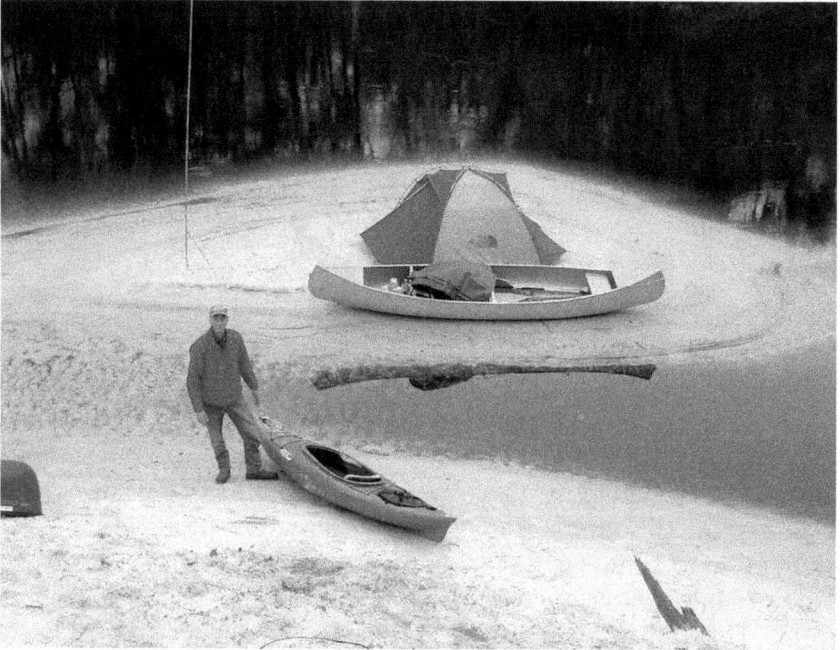

Pitching a Tent on a Sand Island in the Suwanee River

Dundee decided to pitch his tent on a sand island in the river. In the morning he was on a peninsula as the river had dropped a few inches. Think of what might have happened if it had gone up!

Day Four – fifteen miles to Holton Creek River Camp

The Suwannee River Wilderness Trail River Camps (SuwaneeRiver.com), such as Woods Ferry and Holton Creek, are spaced a day's travel apart, and generally accessible only by the river or a hiking trail. We stayed overnight at the Holton Creek River Camp, and its resident host, Ed, made our stay exceptional. We highly recommend these river camps.

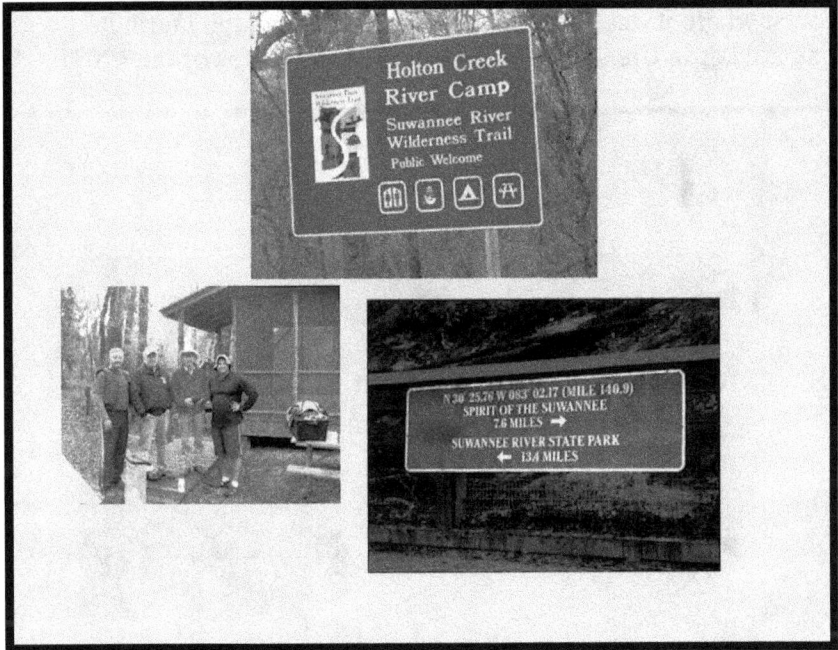

Holton Creek River Camp Signs

The Florida National Scenic Trail

We started noticing orange trail markers, similar to the painted white trail signs on the Appalachian Trail (AT). These markers signify The Florida National Scenic Trail (FNST). The 1400 mile trail comes across from Osceola National Forest to the Suwannee at Big Shoals on the east bank. It follows the east bank to White Springs and crosses the river at SR 136 Bridge and follows the north bank of the river to near Dowling Park in Twin Rivers State Forest where it turns west to the Florida panhandle. During our stay at Holton Creek, Shaun and I hiked two miles of the FNST.

Following the
Suwannee River Wilderness Trail

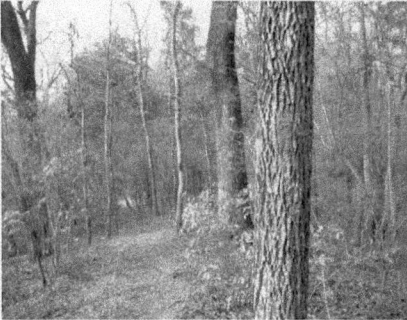

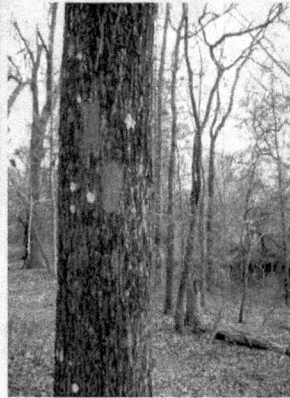

A Junction or major change of the
SRWT is ahead

Following the Suwannee River Wilderness Trail (SRWT)
A Junction of the SRWT is Ahead

Sulphur Springs – a Cure for Your Ailments

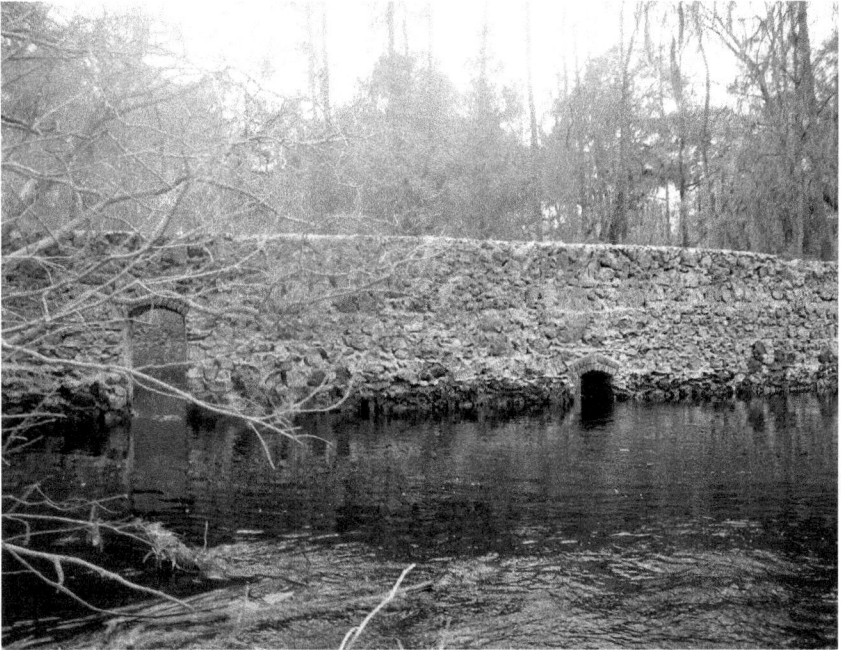

White Sulphur Springs once popular as a health resort.

Sulphur springs on the Suwannee River were once promoted as a cure for almost any ailment. Today these sites are simply places of interest. At Suwannee Springs there is an old pool built out of limestone around a spring that was a resort in the late 1800's and in the early 1900's Folks would come and soak in the sulfur spring water for its healing properties.

Enjoying the Suwannee – and more

This was a fabulous trip. We had only paddled in northern New England, and we were all pleasantly surprised with the ecology, cleanliness of the river shoreline and campsites, and its ecosystem with many birds, trees and animals. As northerners, we were a bit hesitant about being in alligator country, but we quickly learned gators were most likely to disappear when they saw humans.

Before we started our paddle of the Suwannee we checked the water level at the Suwanee River Water Management District

The predicted river water level
was expected to be fine for the days of our riverside camping and
paddling.

When we arrived at the Stephen C. Foster State Park, the White
Spring's water gauge marker it indicated 60 feet above sea level.
Our pre-trip reference of the SRWMD web site was right on.

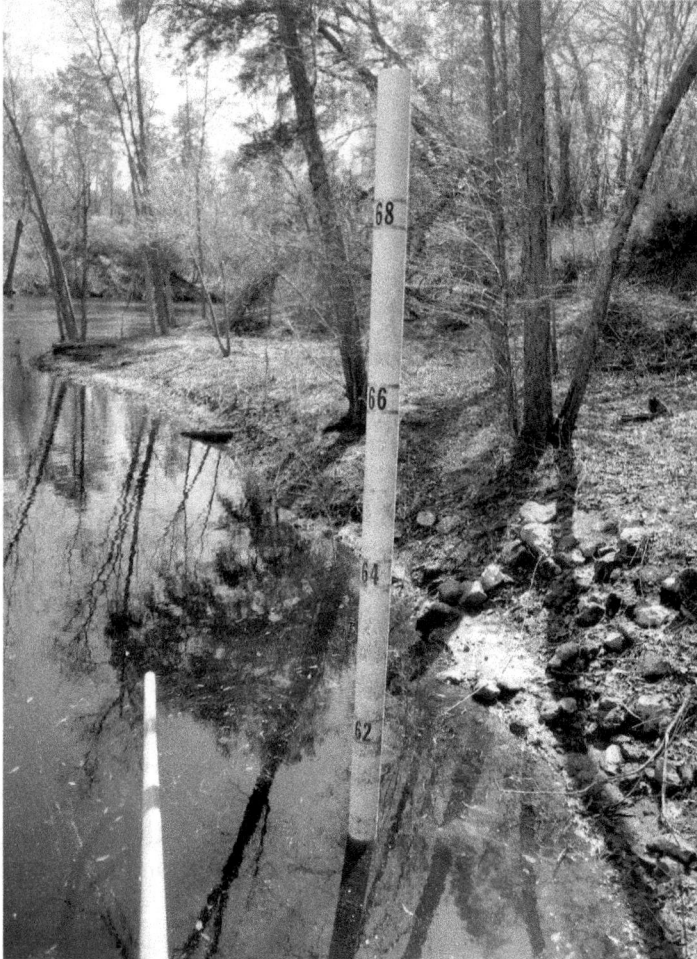

White Spring's Water Gauge at Stephen C. Foster State Park

If one did decide to paddle the Suwannee, based on our seventy mile trek, I would recommend extensive planning with the GPS in anticipation of campsites.

Our late March trek was perfect for minimum bug annoyances, and it rained only one night. We did three nights of primitive camping (read that to mean no showers or toilet facilities) and on the fourth night at Holton Creek river camp the screened shelter, toilets, and showers were divine. If primitive camping is not your forte, then certainly the river camps offer a pleasant alternative.

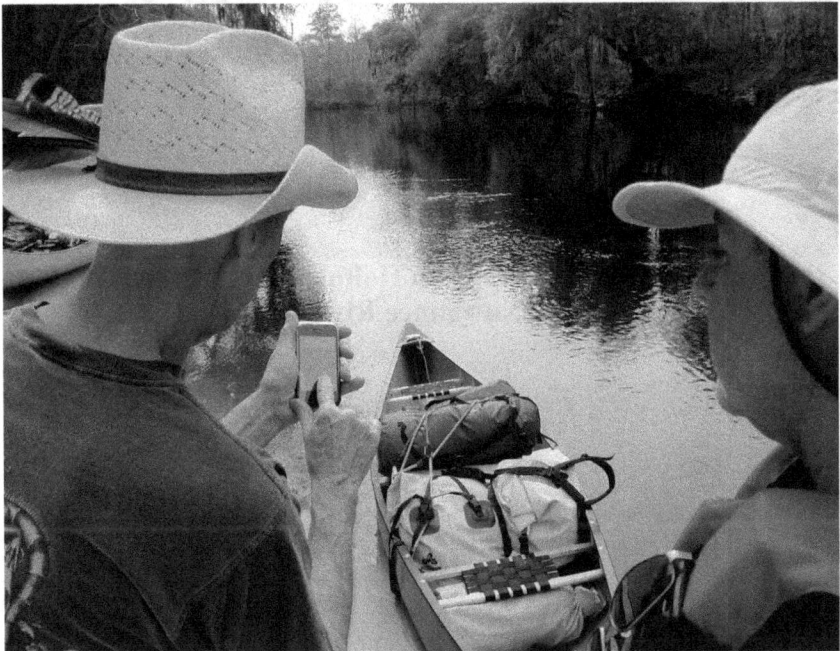
Checking the GPS App

We did have a minor a challenge depending solely on GPS navigation for paddling distance. The GPS app was not oriented for the Suwanee River, and it frequently gave us "as the crow flies" miles to go, whereas, the river twisted and turned many times. For example, the GPS read 8.4 miles from Holton Creek to the Suwannee River Park, whereas, the river sign read 13.4 miles. Our map showed the many U and S turns along the way and John, our navigator, was able to adjust.

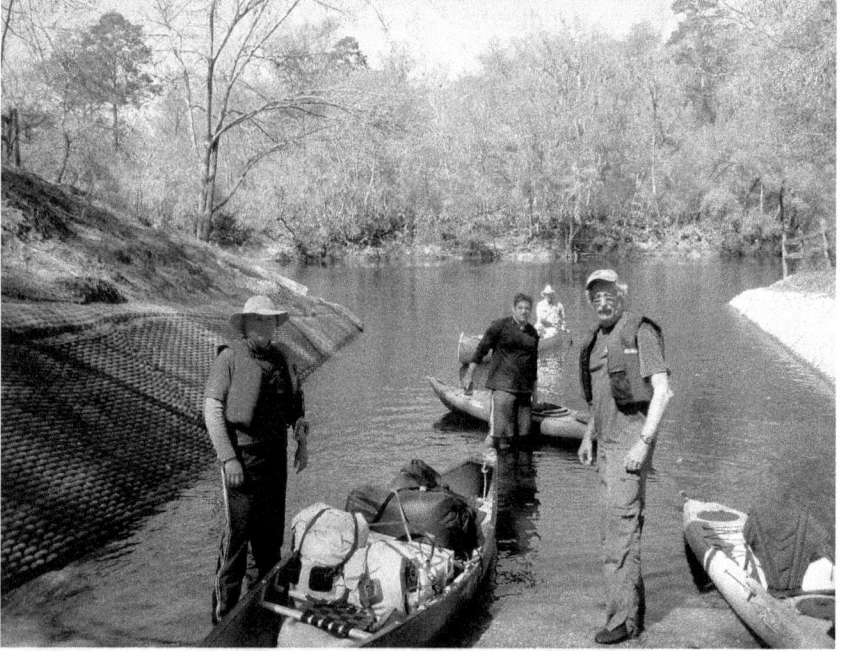

Day Five – Thirteen Miles from Holton Creek River Camp to Take-Out at Suwannee River State Park

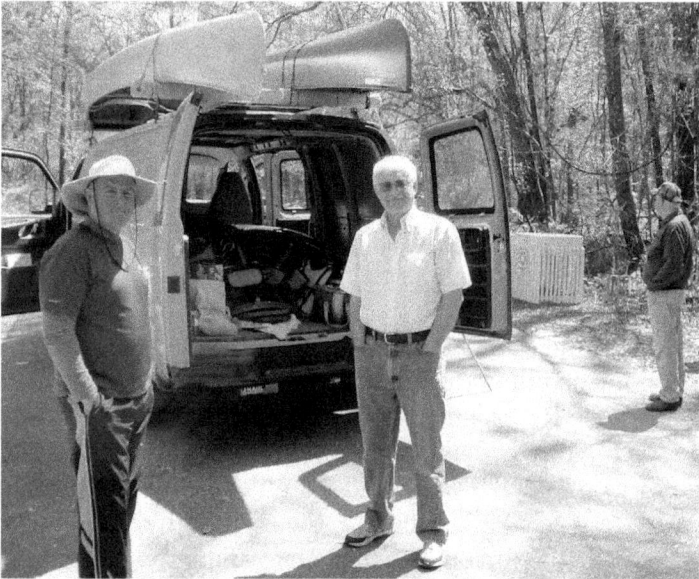

Packed up and Ready to Leave the Suwanee

Never say, "I wish I had …"

I definitely would consider doing the remaining 155 miles to the Gulf of Mexico. The Suwannee is a gem and a paddler's delight.

I never want to say, "I wish I had paddled the Suwanee River to the Gulf of Mexico".

Website References for the Suwannee River

- Suwannee River Water Management District at www.mysuwanneeriver.com/, and Suwannee River Wilderness Trail at www.suwanneeriver.com/.
- Learn about the Ogeechee Tupelo tree at www.audubonguides.com/species/Trees/Ogeechee-Tupelo.html

---

Video References for Suwannee River Paddle

- Blog: Never Have to Say, "I wish I had paddled the Suwannee River http://outdooradventurers.blogspot.com/2010/03/i-never-have-to-say-i-wish-i-had.html
- Video: Big Shoals rapids, our superb breakfast of an egg cooked in an orange followed by a campfire chocolate banana split, and our portage around Big Shoals. http://www.youtube.com/watch?v=7HTqcR2ep4U&feature=player_embedded
- Video: Ogeechee Tupelo tree looked weird to us http://www.youtube.com/watch?v=VDPMowZvvRo&feature=player_embedded

---

Horseshoes at Granite State Senior Games

I was the horseshoe event manager for the Granite State Senior Games (GSSG). Pitchers (as horseshoe throwers are called), all over the age of 50, compete in five-year age/gender categories. I was a pitcher in previous GSSG tournaments, but this was my first as the event manager. Certainly, it was a revelation to me.

While each thrower is only concerned with their own age category, the event manager, in fact, is organizing eight or more separate mini-tournaments. Thus comes the rub. The challenge for the event manager is to give each pitcher an opportunity to compete in their age bracket. However, at times there may be only one person in an age category. Thus finding volunteers from another age group or mixing ages may need to be discussed with a competitor.

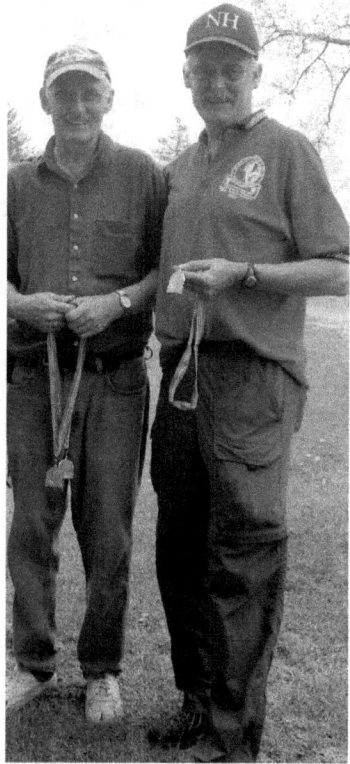

Before the tournament I had registered to participate in the singles and doubles competition in my age category. As I planned the rules and pitcher assignments, it became obvious I may not be able to be both a manager and a pitcher.

The Method of Scoring

I prepared a handout for the pitchers to have the key rules of the GSSG games, as well as to provide me guidelines for instructions to the pitchers. I used the Summer National Senior Games Horseshoe rules (http://www.smaaa.org/documents/2013RuleBook.pdf) and the

National Horseshoe Pitchers Association rules
(http://www.horseshoepitching.com/) supplemented by local rules
to speed up play.

I incorporated two means of scoring. First, was the count-all shoes
method to determine the skill of players and assign them a person
to play. Second was the cancellation scoring method determined
by the "best" pitcher in each category. Although these two
methods are encouraged in the NSGA rules and procedures, I
found using two scoring methods in this GSSG tournament(s) very
confusing to the players, since most had never played in organized
tournaments. Since the purpose of these games is primarily for
"fun", rather than competition, I will suggest next year's manager
consider only the count-all shoes scoring method.

One interesting pitcher was Ron from the state of Washington.
This 65-year young man had a quest to participate in as many state
senior games as he could. The New Hampshire games were his
tenth this year. While not being able to do all of the GSSG sports,
he would do the swimming event the same day as horseshoes.

A special treat for me was my brother David being a pitcher. He
won a silver medal in his singles category. The doubles
competition was at the end of the tournament, and I was able to
join David as his partner. We won Gold in our category!

Surely one person cannot manage this multiple horseshoe event.
Lucille was a tremendous help with set-up, awarding medals, and
record keeping. Jim, Stan, and Hannah assisted with scoring.

I will never have to say, "I wish I had managed a GSSG horseshoe
tournament."

Video References
- Blog: Granite State Senior Games
  Horseshoes
  http://outdooradventurers.blogspot.com/2009/05/horseshoes-at-gssg.html
- Granite State Senior Games
  http://www.nhseniorgames.org

Stocking Salmon for NH Fish and Game

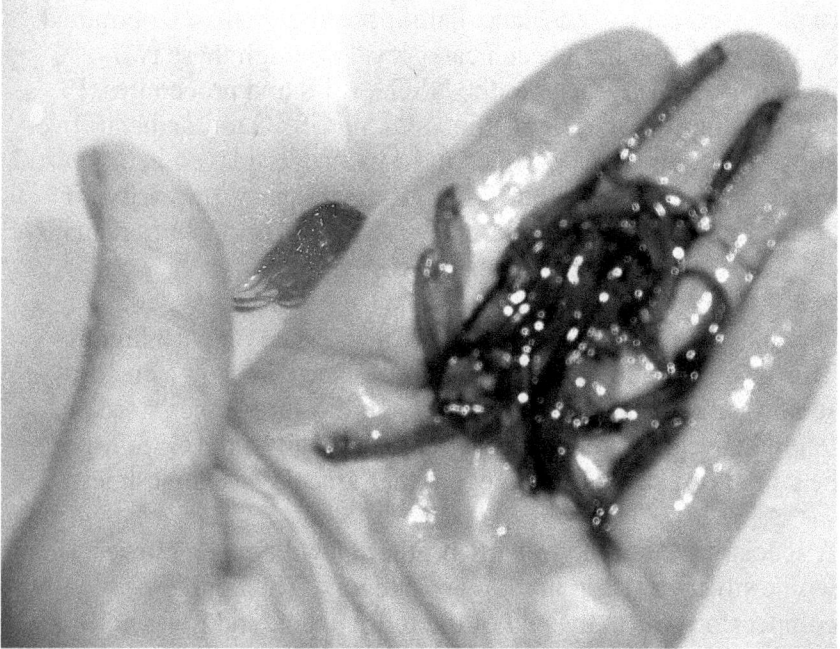

A Handful of Salmon Fry

There was an article in the New Hampshire Sunday News on the NH Fish and Game asking for volunteers to stock Atlantic salmon fry in the waters of NH.

I asked my friends George and Dundee to join me, and we spent the most interesting day learning and stocking salmon fry. See the below article that caught my attention and tells it all.

****

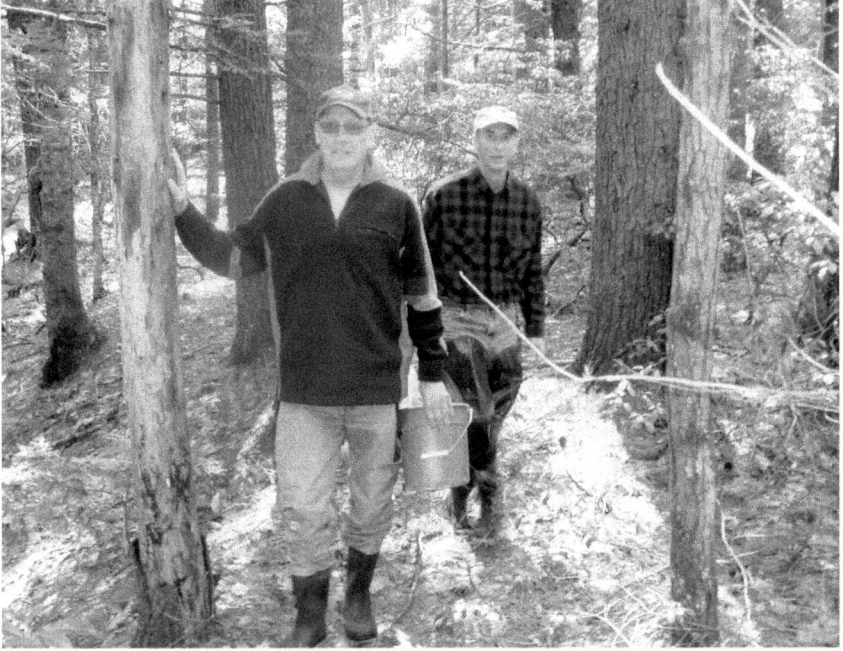
Waders on and a Bucket of Salmon Fry

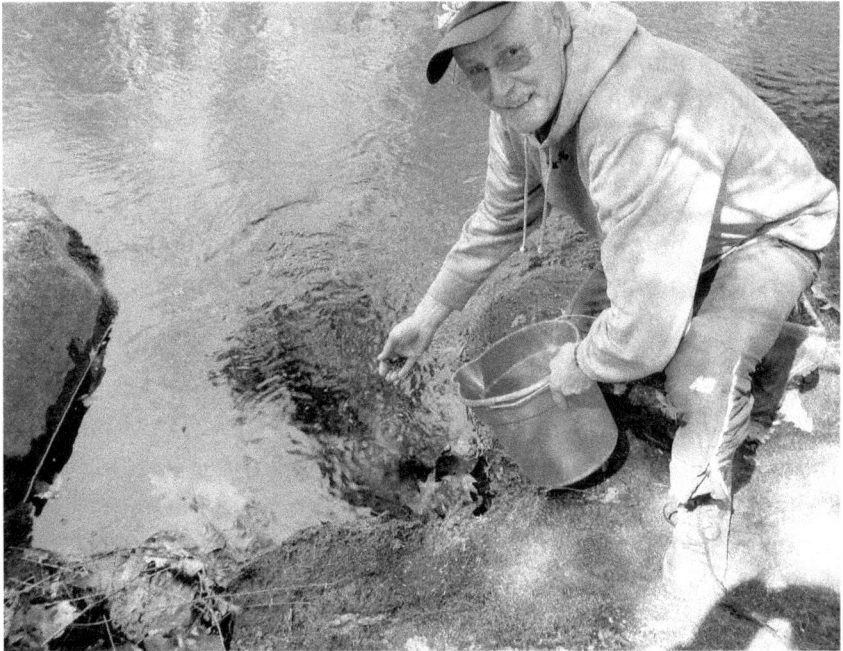
Gently Pour the Fry into the Stream

Volunteers Needed to Help Stock Atlantic Salmon Fry

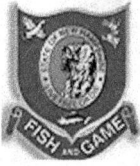

New Hampshire
FISH AND GAME
Connecting you to life outdoors

CONCORD, N.H. -- The New Hampshire Fish and Game Department is looking for volunteers to help stock millions of inch-long salmon fry (young salmon) into the Merrimack River basin, several rivers and streams in the Upper Connecticut River watershed in northern NH, and the Monadnock region of southwestern New Hampshire's Connecticut River watershed.

The stocking plays a vital role in restoring runs of salmon to New Hampshire's waterways. Fry released in these river systems and their tributaries stay and grow in the rivers for about two years before migrating to the ocean. When the salmon are about four years old, they will try to return to these rivers to spawn.

MERRIMACK RIVER: Volunteers will release close to 1.1 million salmon fry in the Merrimack River watershed on April 7, 9, 14, 16, 28 and 30. Another batch of fry will be released in the Merrimack watershed on May 5 and 7. Approximately ten volunteers are needed for each day of stocking.

UPPER CONNECTICUT RIVER WATERSHED: More than half a million salmon fry will be stocked in northern New Hampshire. There will be opportunities for six days of volunteer stocking (including one Saturday) in the Upper Connecticut River watershed during the first two weeks of May. The upper part of the Ammonoosuc River from Bretton Woods down to Littleton will be stocked with salmon fry on Friday, May 1 (meet at Foster's Crossroads Store in Twin Mountain at 10:00 a.m.). The second day of stocking will be Saturday, May 2 (meet at the Wal-Mart parking lot in Littleton at 9:30 a.m. and proceed downriver).

MONADNOCK REGION: Over half a million Atlantic salmon fry are also stocked each spring in the Monadnock region in southwestern New Hampshire's Connecticut River watershed. Additional volunteers are not generally needed for this effort, which involves seven days of stocking in late April and May.

Many individuals and groups take part in the fry stocking effort, including state and federal fisheries personnel, conservation organizations such as Trout Unlimited, and other interested citizens. Volunteers carry the inch-long salmon fry to release points along rivers and streams in the watershed. They should be prepared for an all-day commitment and rigorous walking with heavy buckets of water and fish. Waders, hip boots or old sneakers are recommended footwear for stocking. You may get wet, so bring extra socks and clothing layers, etc. Stocking will take place rain or shine. Pack a lunch and drinking water, waders or hip boots and be prepared to spend the whole day on the river.

The New Hampshire Fish and Game Department is the guardian of the state's fish, wildlife and marine resources and their habitats. Visit **www.fishnh.com**.

Never say, "I wish I had stocked Atlantic salmon in NH streams."

****

References for Stocking Salmon for New Hampshire Fish and Game
- Blog: Stocking Salmon for NH Fish and Game
  http://outdooradventurers.blogspot.com/2009/04/volunteering-for-nh-fish-and-game-to.html
- New Hampshire Fish and Game
  http://www.fishnh.com
- Anadromous Fish Restoration Program in NH
  Http://www.fishnh.com/Fishing/Anadromous_Fish_Program.htm

Summer

I went to the woods because I wished to live deliberately, to front only the essentials of life, and see if I could not learn what it had to teach, and not, when I came to die, discover that I had not lived.
– Henry David Thoreau, Walden

Four Days in Northern New Hampshire Hiking, Paddling, Tenting and Moose Sighting.

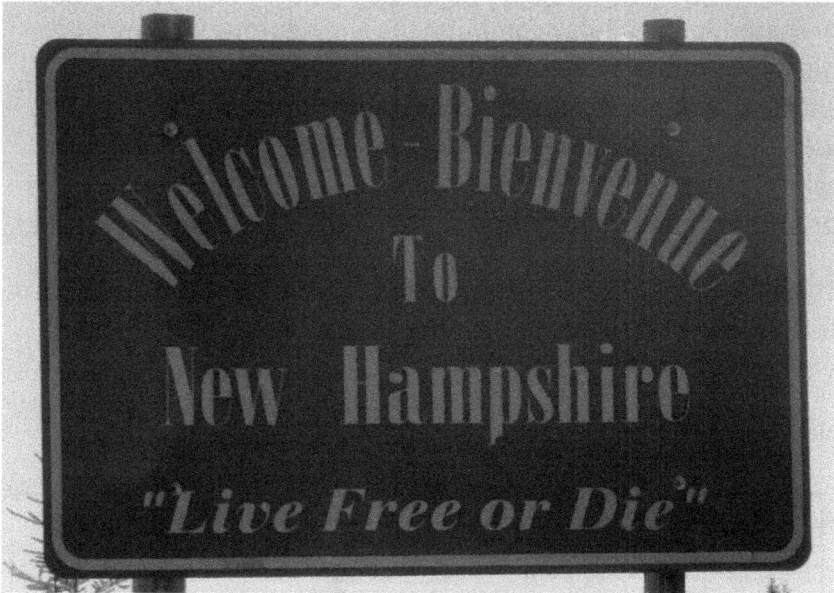

Grab a cup of coffee or another favorite beverage, kick up your feet, and enjoy how a family bonds in the great north woods of New Hampshire. My 18-year-old nephew Austin graduated from his southern California high school. For Austin achieving this educational milestone, my wife, Cathy, and I arranged for him to fly to New Hampshire in July to experience our "Live Free or Die" outdoors.

The four day trip describes:

(1) Hiking Tuckerman Ravine Trail from the Appalachian Mountain Club's (AMC) Pinkham Notch hut to the AMC Lake of the Cloud (LOC) hut for a one night stay.

(2) Hiking from LOC hut to the peak of Mt Washington, the highest mountain in the northeast at 6,288 feet and "Home of the World's Worse Weather".

(3) Tenting for two days at Lake Francis State Park in the Connecticut Lakes area of Pittsburg, NH.

- Hike to and around the 4th Connecticut Lake located on the border of Canada and the United States. The 4th Connecticut Lake is the headwaters of the 410 mile long Connecticut River

- Paddle the Third Connecticut Lake

- Paddle Lake Francis

- Moose sightings on 18 mile Moose Alley

In addition to Austin and me, our fellow trekkers were his father (my brother Dennis), my sons Timothy and Shaun, my two grandchildren 15 year old Madison and 12 year old Carson, Ron my brother-in-law, and invited friends Justin and his 17 year old daughter Sarah. Ten would hike to the Lake of the Clouds (LOC) hut and Mt Washington, and seven of us would continue to the Great North Woods Lake Francis State Park campground.

Preparing the Hike to Lake of the Clouds Hut (LOC) and Mount Washington

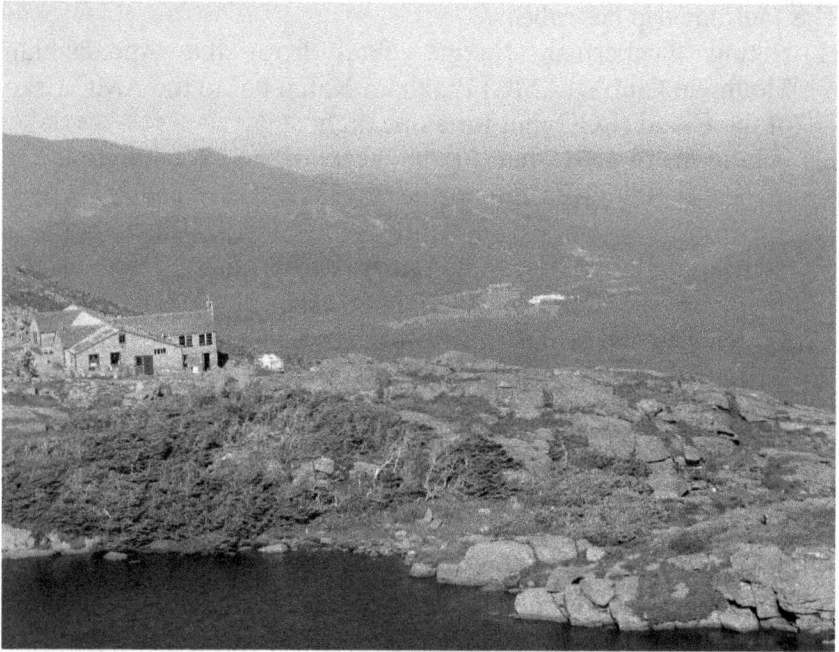

View Overlooking Lake of the Cloud Hut

As the hiking trek leader I had responsibility for the safety of my fellow outdoor enthusiasts:

- Which trail should we take?
  I had hiked Tuckerman's many times, and although Tuckerman's Ravine Trail is one of the most dangerous trails to LOC and Mt Washington, I wanted my group to experience safely the scenery, excitement, and knowledge of hiking this unique trail.

- What time in the morning do we start our hike to LOC?
  LOC serves their family style meals at 6 pm sharp (breakfast at LOC is 7 am sharp). I expected the hike from Pinkham to LOC to be between 4 and 5 hours.

- What kind of clothing, supplies, and food do we need for a one-day overnight hike in the White Mountains?
  Hiking Tuckerman Ravine Trail is not to be taken lightly. Snow, high winds, rain, lightning, and fog can be expected

year round – this means ALWAYS prepare to spend the night on the trail in the mountains.

- What emergency supplies do we need in case of an unanticipated overnight while hiking?

  o AMC's Ten Essentials for a Safe Hike are mandatory. I enforced this by giving each person their own whistle and flashlight.

  o For each person I provided a 3 mil / 30 gallon contractor bag (aka trash bag) in case we had to immediately camp on the trail (or daresay get lost for an overnight). To use this bag we would make holes in the corner of the bag for our eyes and mouth, slip the bag over the head, and have some level of protection.

  o Duct tape. You never know when this can come in handy e.g. broken eye glass frame, sling, strap, etc.

You need to be in good physical shape for a five plus hour hike up Tuckerman's Ravine with sections nearly straight up (no need for climbing ropes), but certainly there are places where you use your hands to assist crawling up rocks. My training schedule included two hikes up Uncanoonuc Mt in Goffstown, NH. Uncanoonuc, combined with two months of four times a week speed walking four miles in my hiking boots, prepared me for Mt Washington, and in particular climbing the headwall of Tuckerman Ravine.

An Educational Dinner
Hmm, how do I emphasize the importance of hiking safety to teenagers? The night before our trip my wife Cathy made a great spaghetti dinner for Austin, Madison and Carson. This dinner was my opportunity to stress safety and necessary items for the hike. Unannounced, I demonstrated my hiking whistle (One toot for, "Where are you?" Two toots, "Come to me", and three toots, "Emergency".) I gifted to each a whistle and asked them to

demonstrate a signal. Yes, they thought I was "loony", but indeed they practiced a lifesaving skill.

We spoke about hiking in groups. My son, Tim, has hiked with me many times and has my confidence in tight situations. He would lead one group up the mountain. Ron was also experienced, and he would lead another group. The sweep group (the slow hikers) would be led by me. Other than the aforementioned, no one was to get ahead of their leader – no matter what. We did not want to experience a lost hiker.

We cautioned about the importance of stopping every 10 to 15 minutes to drink water. An earlier hiking involvement, followed by a wilderness first aid course, made me realize dehydration can cause nausea and headaches and is easily avoided by frequent drinking of water. Mt Washington is a steep, long hike, and hydration is critical for our troop to completing a safe and enjoyable hike.

I emphasized **NO COTTON CLOTHING** – including underwear. I underscored this "strange request" by asking, "How long does it take cotton to dry out after getting wet?" In survival situations, cotton is known as "DEATH CLOTH." Cotton holds moisture instead of wicking it away from the skin, and when wet, cotton has zero insulating properties.

Pinkham Notch to Lake of the Clouds (LOC)

I had concern in guiding my group safely up to Lake of the Clouds. Years before when Tim and I took the Tuckerman Ravine Trail to Lake of the Clouds hut, we faced thick fog and could see only a few feet ahead. On that trek we used cairns, the rock piles used to designate the trail when above tree line, as the means to insure we kept on the trail. On this trip I needed to watch closely the expected Mt Washington area weather to be sure I did not put my party in danger if the weather report indicated severe conditions.

They say a picture is worth a thousand words. Enjoy the short **Video Reference** below of our hike up Tuckerman Ravine Trail to

Lake of the Clouds Hut followed by a next day hike to Mt Washington.

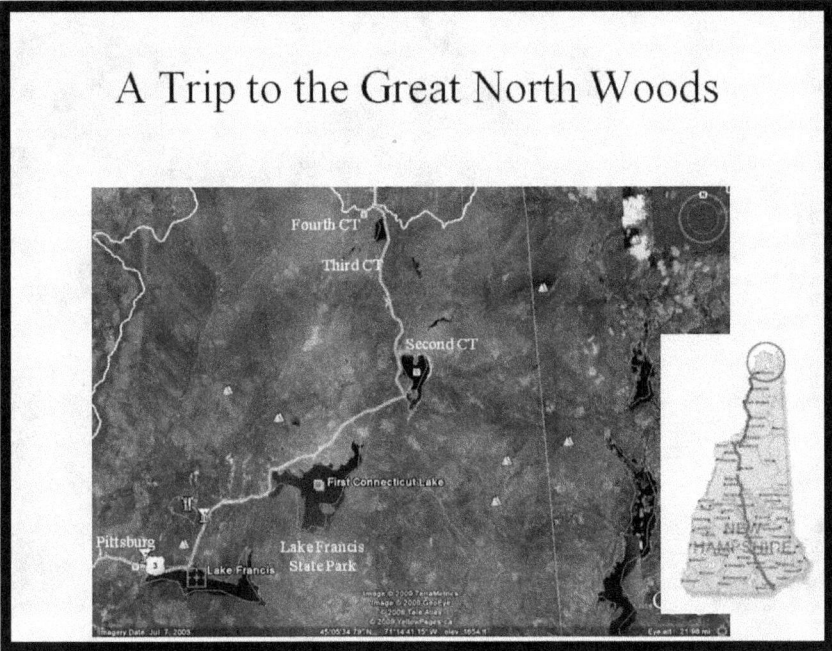

A Trip to the Great North Woods

The northern tip of New Hampshire has a pristine area known as the Great North Woods. I wanted Austin and my grandchildren to enjoy and appreciate this treasure of New Hampshire. Its many summer outdoor opportunities include paddling and fishing the Connecticut (CT) Lakes (Forth CT, Third CT, Second CT, First CT and Lake Francis), hiking around the Fourth CT, and Moose sighting.

Moose Sighting.

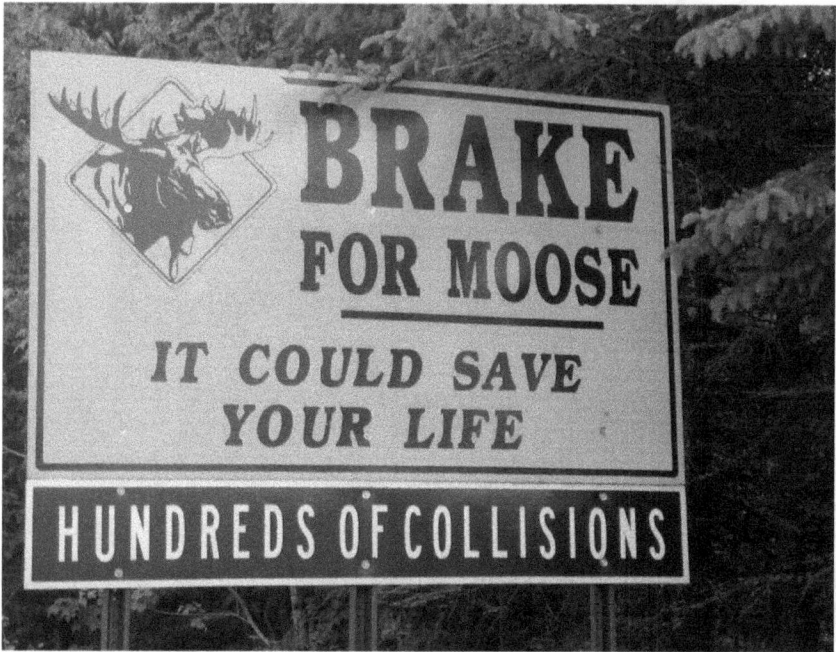

The moose is the biggest and most mysterious and majestic four-legged inhabitant of northern New Hampshire. Seeing a moose is always a thrill for me. Certainly for Austin and my grandkids, the thought of seeing these huge six to seven foot tall and 700 to 1200 pound animals was an expectation like waiting to get a glimpse of Santa Claus! There are 6,000 or so moose in New Hampshire and being in the Connecticut Lakes area in particular enhances the opportunity to see a moose. The last 18 or so miles on route 3 in Pittsburg is designated Moose Alley. Driving slowly on Moose Alley at 5 am also enhances your chance to see a moose. And, dusk is another good time.

What is the best way to find moose? My answer is always simple – look for cars pulled off alongside the road. For two days at dawn and dusk we drove very slowly up Route 3. See our moose sighting success in the below **Video Reference**.

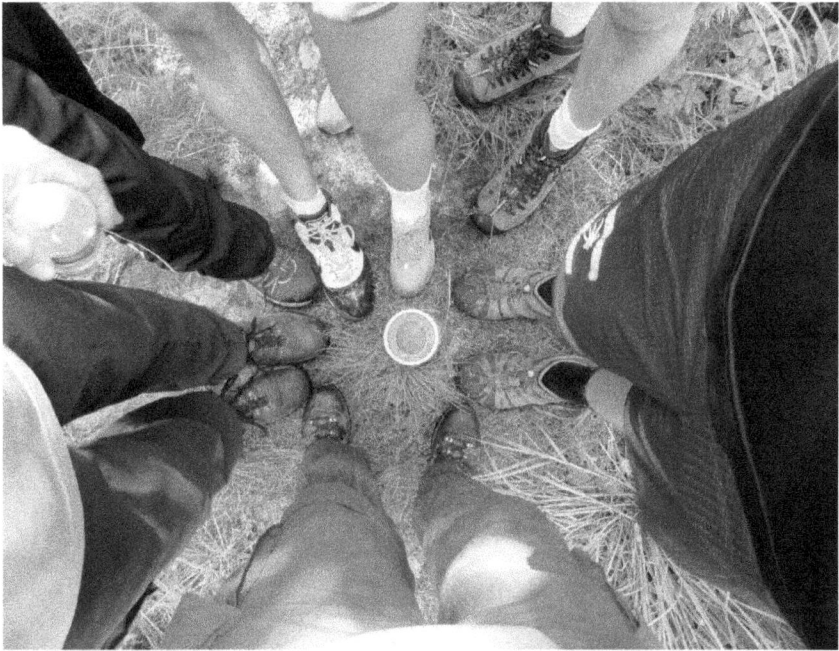

Group Hug Around United States - Canada Boundary Maker

As we hiked to the Fourth Connecticut Lake I shared a history lesson not readily known. For a few years in the 1830s, an area of today's Pittsburg, NH was an independent republic, not part of New Hampshire and not part of the United States. The US attempted to tax the 360 inhabitants, and Canada tried to make them serve in its military, so the people decided to establish their own sovereign nation called, **The Republic of Indian Stream.** The existence of the Republic was ended by New Hampshire in 1835. Later, the Webster -Ashburton Treaty of 1842 established the border between Canada and the United States – the border markers that we would crisscross as we hiked to the Fourth Connecticut Lake.

Hiking the Fourth Connecticut Lake

The 78 acre Fourth Connecticut Lake is located on the USA/Canada border. It is called a "Lake", but in my mind is similar to a small bog or marsh. The narrow swampy walk around the lake took us a half hour. We stopped to take pictures at the outlet stream - the Fourth CT is the headwaters of the 410 mile long Connecticut River that ends in Long Island Sound. The trail to the lake starts at the United States-Canada customs border crossing station in Pittsburg, NH on the international border between the United States and Canada. The whole hike from custom station to lake, walk around the lake, a brief ten minute break, and the hike back, was less than two hours.

Paddle Third Connecticut Lake

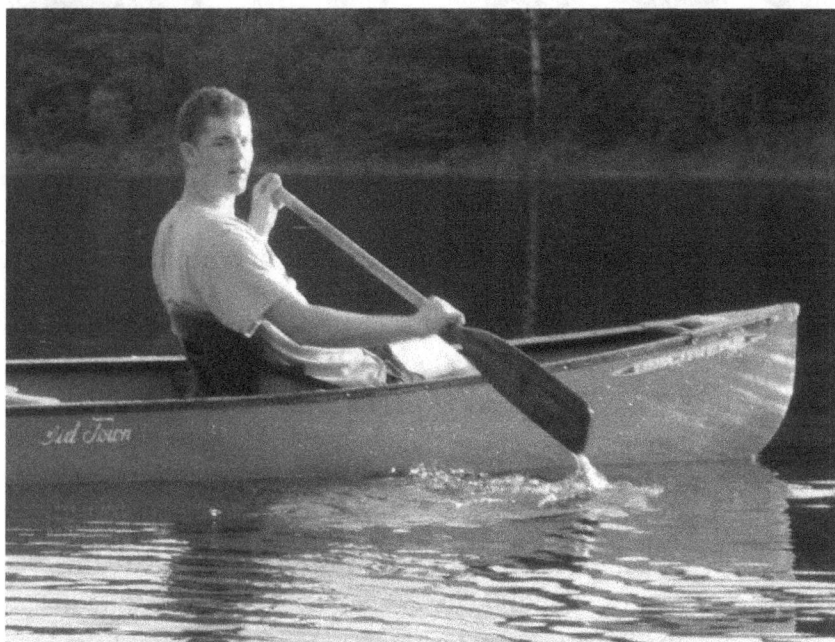

A Canoer on the 3rd Connecticut Lake

The 235 acre Lake is located about a half mile downhill from the Fourth Connecticut. During our paddle on this pristine lake we saw beaver lodges and dams, loons, and the outlet to Second Connecticut Lake. Carson went for a swim. As we paddled around the northern end of the lake, we stopped to see the inlet from Fourth Connecticut Lake.

Video References Hiking, Paddling, Tenting and Moose Sighting in Great North Woods of NH

- Blog: Four Days in Northern New Hampshire with Family and Friends Hiking, Tenting, Paddling, and Moose Sighting
  http://outdooradventurers.blogspot.com/2012/07/four-days-in-new-hampshire-of-family.html
- Hiking Tuckerman Ravine
  http://www.youtube.com/watch?feature=player_embedded&v=AkoJXIqB0kU
- Moose Sightings
  http://www.youtube.com/watch?feature=player_embedded&v=O-P__VJveeo
- Crossing Headwaters of 460 mile long Connecticut River at 4th Connecticut Lake
  http://www.youtube.com/watch?feature=player_embedded&v=dXM42H5KjuA

The Locks of the Trent-Severn Waterway

I found this blog post very difficult to make concise. Our Trent-Severn Waterway trek is so unique - such as experiencing going through fourteen locks and living for eight days in a houseboat moving each day along the Waterway. With so much content, how do I describe all this and keep the videos under a few minutes?

The Trent-Severn Waterway is one of Canada's most spectacular waterways. The Waterway stretches 240 miles from Lake Ontario's Bay of Quinte to Lake Huron's Georgian Bay. My wife and I readily accepted an invitation to join our friends Linda and Dundee for a week on a houseboat on the Trent-Severn Waterway.

Friends have asked many questions such as, "What and where is the Trent-Severn Waterway?", "What was the houseboat like?", "What did it feel like going through a lock?", "How did you navigate?", and "Did you spend all your time on the houseboat?" I finally came to the conclusion I could only do this by breaking the trip into small videos and letting you choose for yourself which ones to view.

The waterway is an impressive chain of lakes and rivers linked by more than 40 locks and some 33 miles of excavated channels. All of the locks are situated in beautiful park-like settings and most are integrated within small and inviting villages. Indeed, the Waterway is a unique gem of Canada.

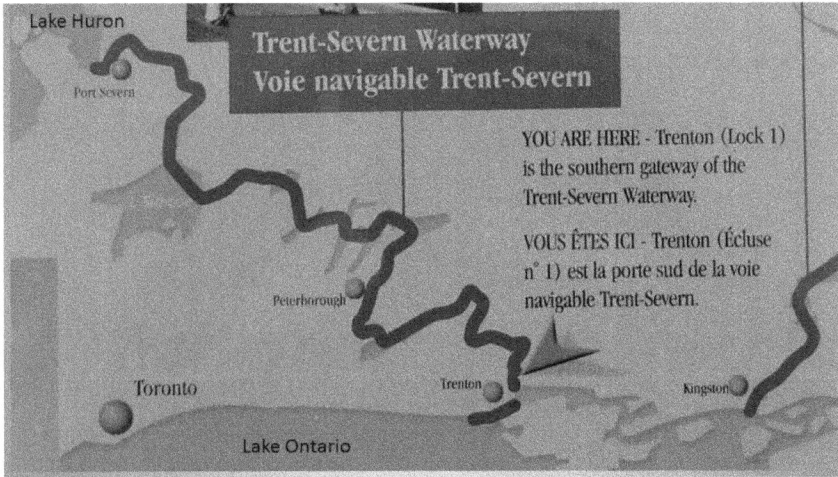

Trent-Severn Map – Lake Ontario to Lake Huron

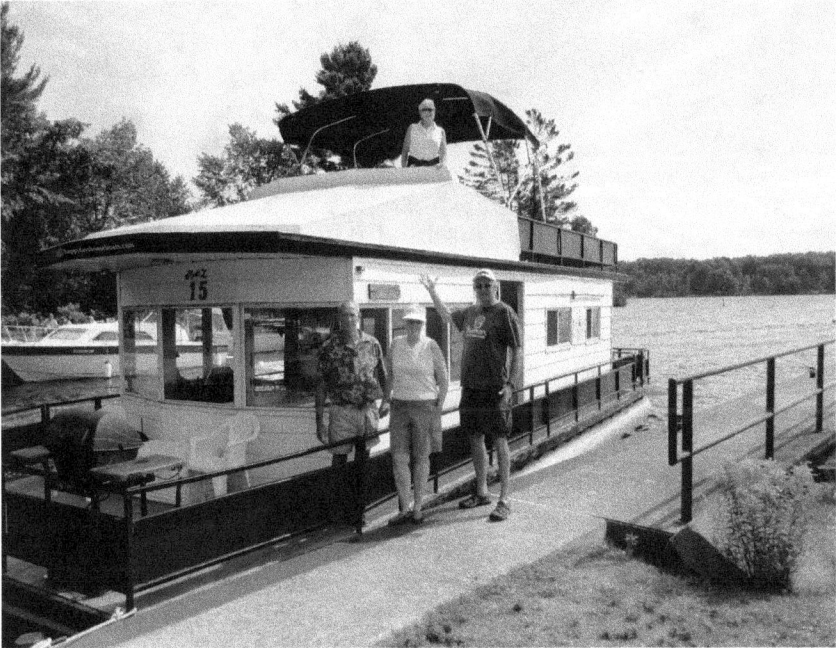

Waiting to Enter a Lock

Given the extensive length of the Waterway, our timeframe of eight days, and the need to return our rented houseboat to where we picked it up at **Happy Days Houseboats** in Bobcaygeon, Ontario, our trip would take us through only seven of the locks as we headed from Lake Ontario and turned around after we locked through Kirkfield Lift Lock. On our return we would repeat each of these seven locks.

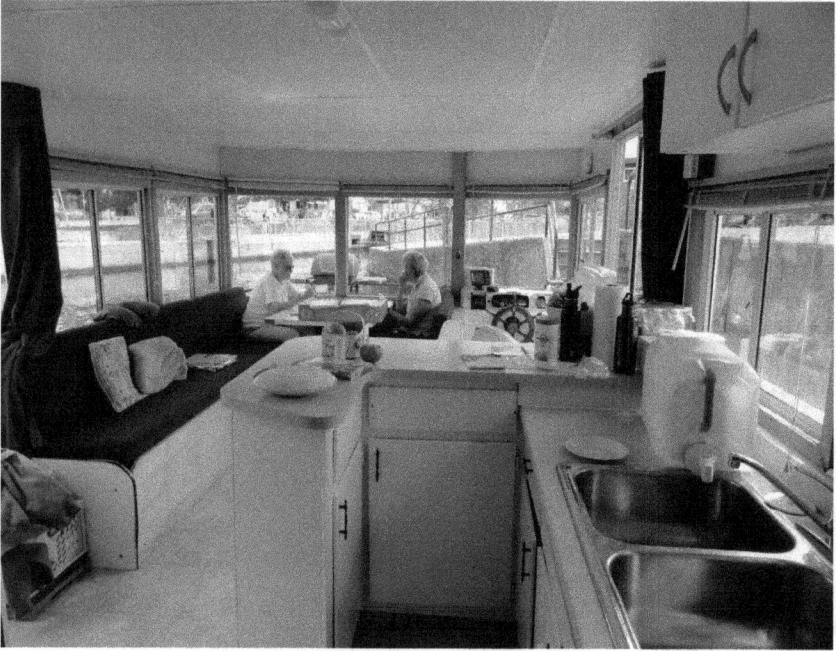

Our Houseboat Kitchen

The Waterway is home to two of the world's highest hydraulic lift locks, located in Peterborough and Kirkfield. Indeed, we locked the Kirkfield lift twice.

In addition, we visited via car four locks (Trenton, Glen Miller, Sydney and Peterborough Lift Lock). These visits gave us another perspective of the locks because at two of these locks the lock master allowed me into their lock houses to be an "associate" to work the controls to "lock in" and "lock out" the boats. I was even told by one lock operator, *"You are the oldest kid whoever assisted us!"* Indeed all the lockmasters and operators were wonderful.

The Lock Operators – Ontario Ambassadors

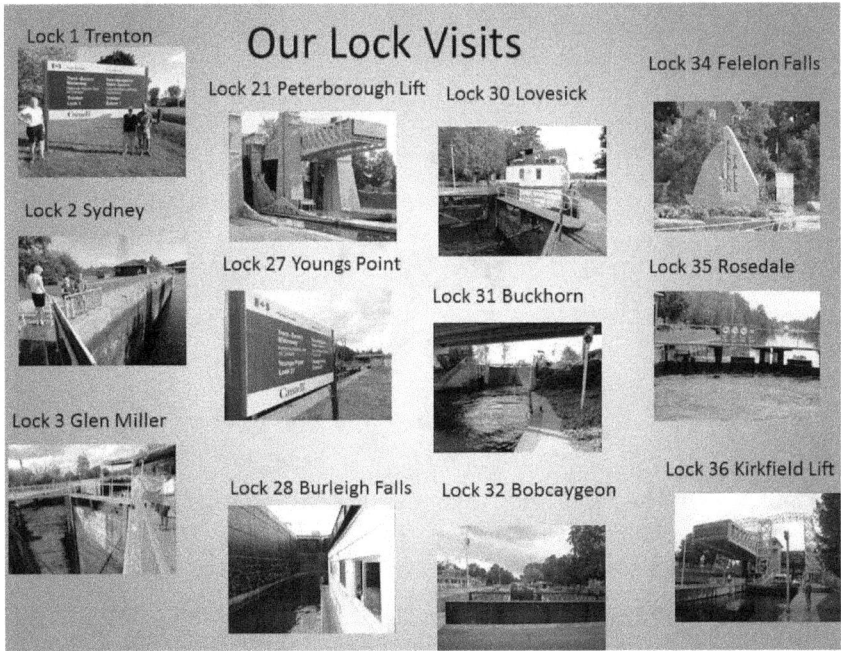

Our Lock Visits

Lock 1 Trenton
Lock 21 Peterborough Lift
Lock 30 Lovesick
Lock 34 Felelon Falls
Lock 2 Sydney
Lock 27 Youngs Point
Lock 31 Buckhorn
Lock 35 Rosedale
Lock 3 Glen Miller
Lock 28 Burleigh Falls
Lock 32 Bobcaygeon
Lock 36 Kirkfield Lift

The lockmasters and operators who guide and oversee the locks as your boat passes through offer extraordinary assistance and indeed are ambassadors to Trent-Severn, Ontario, and certainly Canada. The warm welcome and support we received from them in going through the locks were exceptional.

Each night we slept on the houseboat at designated areas outside the locks. One night we tied to trees on Wolf Island in Lower Buckhorn Lake with the back of the boat anchored in the lake.

The Trent-Severn includes fixed chamber locks and hydraulic lift locks (at Peterborough and Kirkfield, two of the world's highest hydraulic lift locks. Indeed, we locked the Kirkfield lift twice.) A lock is a device for raising and lowering boats between stretches of water of different levels on lake, river and canal waterways. The distinguishing feature of a conventional lock is it has a fixed chamber in which the water level is lowered or raised (as is the Bobcaygeon Lock); whereas in a boat lift lock, it is the chamber itself that rises and falls (such as the Kirkfield Lift Lock).

Navigation Aids and Tour Our Houseboat

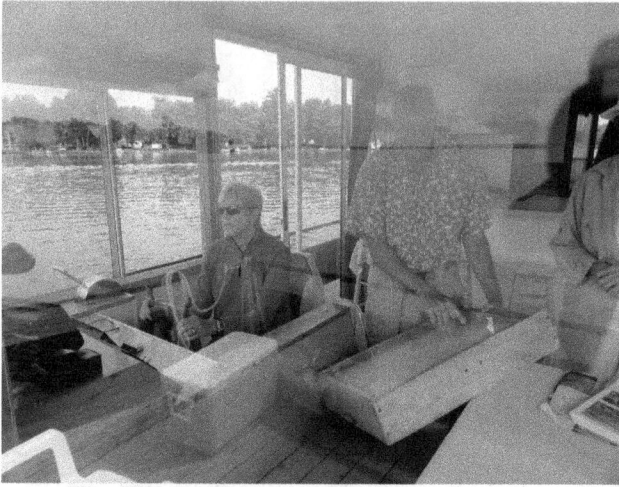

The Pilot and Navigator Work Together

We used navigational charts and a GPS to follow the Trent-Severn channel.

The houseboats are advertised for novice boaters, and the houseboat companies provide you (and require) an orientation course to include:

- Demonstrations on handling the boat (including docking it, starting/stopping) followed by each customer steering the boat thereby validating their hands-on abilities.

- Navigational skills to safely get you from here to there

- Location of all safety gear, onboard fire prevention, man-overboard procedures

- Channel markers, and river etiquette when overtaking and passing others (horn signals, etc.)

- A Final sign-off checklist of all things covered – and items located on the boat.

The entire training course is geared (before you cast off) to making your excursion a safe and rewarding adventure.

Personally, I would not recommend this trip for a complete boating novice without being sure at least one driver feels comfortable in big boats.

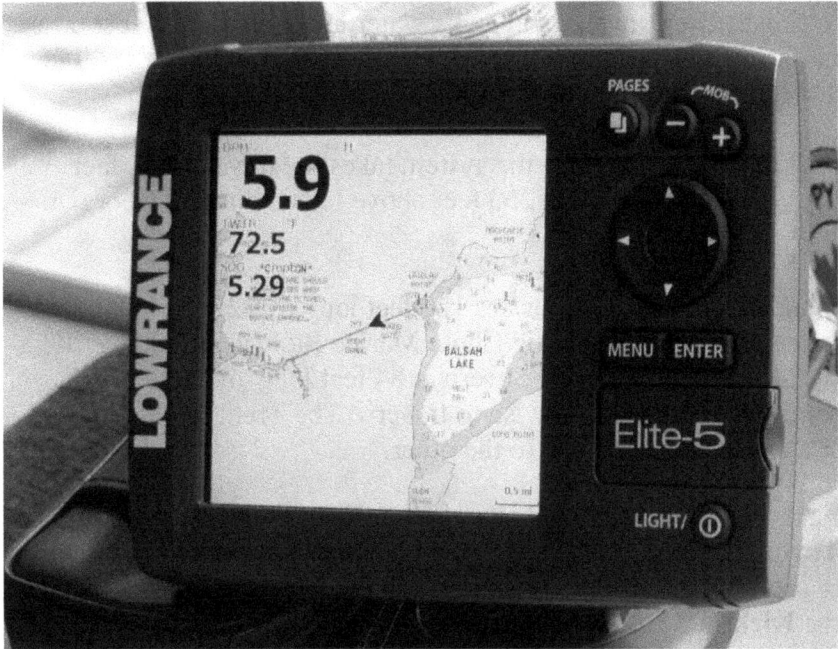

Our GPS - Where are we and how fast are we going?

My friend Dundee is a qualified boater on a variety of large boats. He is very comfortable with steering and navigating our 40 foot houseboat. Myself, I have a 19 foot deck boat, but admittedly it took me a while to calm my nerves on this "slow moving barge".

This was a large, slow to-turn boat. Initially, I was a bit nervous driving and navigating our 40 feet long and 14 feet wide houseboat into and out of the lock areas. Dundee's guidance and calming instructions certainly was a major plus for me when I was "Captain" of the boat.

History and Specs of The Trent-Severn Waterway
Construction began in the Kawartha Lakes region in 1833 with the lock at Bobcaygeon marking its beginning. It took over 87 years to finish the entire Waterway and only until after 1920 could a boat travel the whole route between Lake Ontario and Lake Huron.

The navigation channel runs an average depth of six feet from start to finish. The conventional locks water level vary by 20 feet or less in raising and lowering boats, whereas the Kirkfield Lift is 49 feet and the Peterborough Lift is 65 feet.

Peaking at Balsam Lake the system takes the traveler 600 feet above Lake Ontario and 250 feet above Lake Huron's, Georgian Bay.

Standard lock dimensions are 120 feet long by 32 feet wide. The two exceptions are the Big Chute Marine Railway at 100 feet long by 24 feet wide and Port Severn at 84 feet long and 23 feet wide setting the limits if you wish to traverse The Trent-Severn Waterway from one end to the other.

First, be sure to read the below **Seven Easy Steps for Locking Through**. Then, click on the two videos in the Videos Box below to see what it feels like to go through the **Bobcaygeon Lock** and the **Kirkfield Lift**.

"What Does It Feel Like Going Through a Lock?"

Seven
Easy Steps for
Locking Through

(1) Tie up at blue line. Wait for lockmaster to direct you to enter lock.

(2) Approach cautiously watching for wind and current. Follow directions of lock staff.

(3) Ready crew to loop (not tie!) lines at bow and stern around black drop cables on lock walls

(4) Once safely positioned in lock, turn off engine. Do not smoke or operate open-flame appliances. Keep bilge or engine compartment blower on while locking through.

(5) Be prepared to show lockage permit to lock staff, or be ready to purchase one.

(6) Tend lines carefully as the lock fills or empties.

(7) When lockage is complete, lock staff will direct you to re-start your engine and exit the lock slowly.

Seven Easy Steps Sign Posted at All Locks

"Did you spend all your time on the houseboat?"

There are many places to enjoy on the Trent-Severn and I cannot possibly discuss them all here. I will, however, refer to three that are special to me.

- The first is the *Buckhorn Canoe Company*. Dundee and I discovered this unique canoe building company owned and operated by Dick Persson.

  Dick's company builds, restores and outfits traditional all-wood, wood-canvas canoes, and small boats. We were immediately impressed with Dick's extensive historical knowledge of restoration of old watercraft, old canoe companies, and their boat and canoe models. His shop and showroom were museums unto themselves.

  Go to Dick's Blog (http://www.buckhorncanoes.com/) and read his passion and unique perspective for the history, research, building, repair, restoration, outfitting and use of wooden canoes.

  With Dick's permission I did a brief video of his comments on the differences between the Otter Tail and Beaver Tail paddles. Indeed, see the **Winter** section on using an otter tail to see if I improve my J-stroke by keeping my return stroke in the water.

- My next "must share" is my swimming in Burleigh Falls. I wanted so much to swim at least once on our trip, and this was my opportunity. The below Special Memories of Trent-Severn Waterway video has my brave five foot ledge jump into Burleigh Falls.

- Last, but not least, I strongly recommend a visit to the magnificent Canadian Canoe Museum (http://www.canoemuseum.ca/ in Peterborough, Ontario. This huge museum has exhibits and live hands-on demonstrations of canoe and kayak building. Found throughout the museum is the history of the native peoples of Canada and the historical importance that canoes and kayaks have played in the development of Canada's more remote wilderness areas.

See a below brief video of special moments at the Buckhorn Canoe Company, swimming Burleigh Falls, and the Canadian Canoe Museum at the blog post.

Never Say, "I wish I had locked the Trent-Severn Waterway"

The Tent-Severn Waterway was a wonderful and memorable experience, and now Cathy, Linda, Dundee and I will never have to say, "We wish we had house-boated the Trent-Severn Waterway in Ontario Canada.

References to the Trent-Severn Waterway

- Trent-Severn Tool Kit
  http://www.trentsevern.com/newsite/

- http://en.wikipedia.org/wiki/Trent%E2%80%93Severn_Waterway

- http://www.thetrentsevernwaterway.com/#top

- http://www.ontariowaterwaycruises.com/kawartha.html

- http://www.trentsevern.com/newsite/index.php?option=com_content&view=article&id=219&Itemid=328

- http://www.happydayshouseboats.com

- http://www.buckhorncanoes.com

- The Waterway (Kawartha Region Lock Dimensions)
  http://www.thewaterway.ca/kawartha_locks.html

- FAQ
  http://www.trentsevern.com/newsite/index.php?option=com_content&view=article&id=98&Itemid=165

Videos Available for Trent-Severn Waterway
- **Outdoor Adventures Blog: The Trent-Severn Waterway**
  http://outdooradventurers.blogspot.com/2012/09/the-locks-of-trent-severn-waterway.html
- **Special Memories of Trent-Severn Waterway**
  http://www.youtube.com/watch?v=C6whLjZi_yw&feature=player_embedded
- **Bob Caygeon Lock**
  http://www.youtube.com/watch?feature=player_embedded&v=63tgMKffMp0
- Kirkfield Lock
  http://www.youtube.com/watch?v=SOAE3a-R0-w&feature=player_embedded

---

Meeting a New Hampshire Good Samaritan

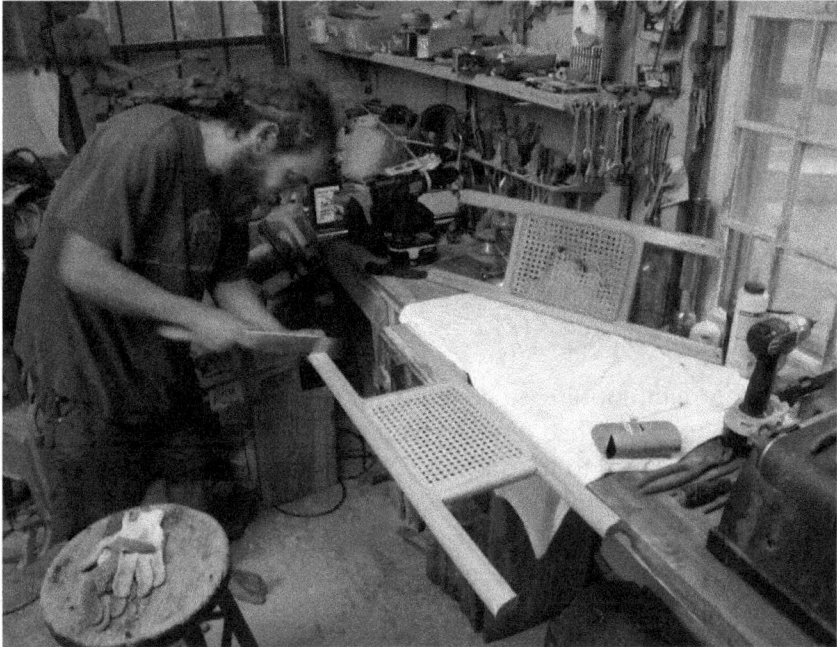

Our Good Samaritan

When you need help, a Good Samaritan appears.

My wife, Cathy, and I went to the Contoocook River to locate the kayak put-in and take-out for my Sunday triathlon, **The Contoocook Carry** (2-mile run, 5-mile kayak, and 14-mile bike). To scout together, we decided to use our Kevlar 25 pound 12 foot Lincoln canoe.

We came to a dead end road, and could not see the river or the put-in, yet the web site directions showed we were in the right spot. We spotted a man walking near a farmhouse, and yelled if he knew where Sunday's paddle race put-in was. He said, we could park there and he pointed to a path toward the river.

"Thank you."

We paddled to the Contoocook Dam - three miles - and then turned around and paddled back upstream - the current was no problem and with both paddling hard, we returned to the put-in in one hour.

And now our genuine memory of this trek started.

Cathy had a large hole in the middle of her cane seat. The first hour paddle was comfortable, rump wise, but as time progressed she had to continually reposition herself in the canoe to get the blood flowing.

We returned to the put-in, carried the canoe to the car and prepared to lift the canoe on to the car roof rack. It was then our Good Samaritan re-appeared.

The young man, looking to be in his mid-twenties and with dreadlock hair, who had kindly given us directions to park and get to the water, waved to us, and we yelled back our thanks for a great paddle. Carrying his 1 ½ year old blonde daughter, he walked over and he introduced himself as Mike. He admired our canoe, and then pointed to the torn cane seat. We certainly had noticed the seat, and it had given us "pain".

Mike commented, "I have a brand new caned seat in the barn, and you can have it." I responded, "Certainly, thank you." "Let's measure the seat to see if it is the same, and if yes, I will cut and install it," he said. He walked over to the barn, and returned with an identical seat!

Within ten minutes, he had the seat installed.

Who knew, here we were in a far-region of middle New Hampshire - near an old farm - and who should appear but Mike, our Good Samaritan, with an identical caned seat and the knowledge and tools to install it.

People helping people in New Hampshire. Thank you Mike for a personal experience of kindness we could never have foreseen.

Now I never have to say, "I wish I had accepted the kindness of a total stranger"

Video Reference A NH Good Samaritan
- Blog: A New Hampshire Good Samaritan
  http://outdooradventurers.blogspot.com/2009
  /09/meeting-new-hampshire-good-
  samaritan.html

National Senior Games Association (NSGA) Triathlon

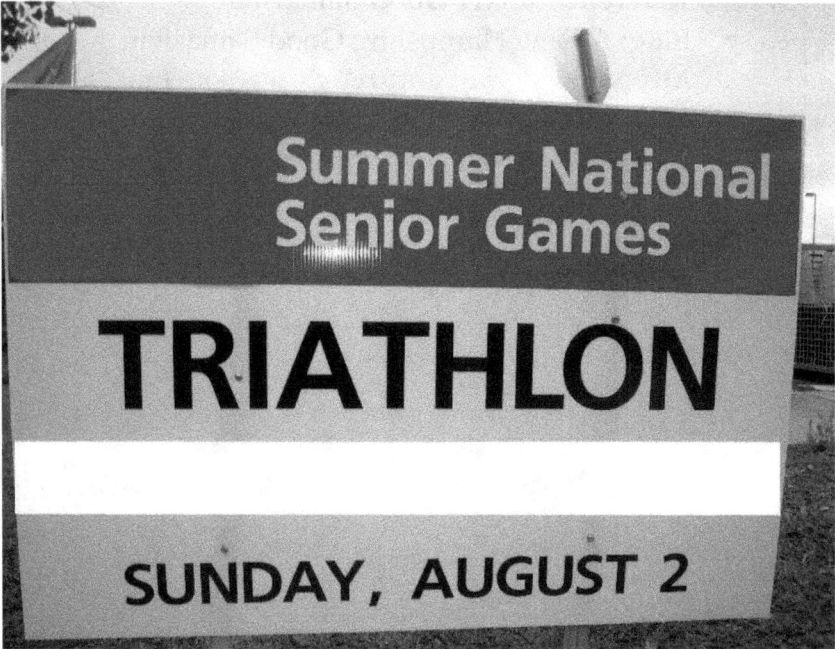

Wow! A year of training and anxiousness for the National Senior Games triathlon is now no more. On Sunday August 2 in San Francisco, I was the sole male representative for New Hampshire to do the Senior Games triathlon (1/4 mile ocean swim, 12-mile bike, and 3.1-mile run). I believe I did New Hampshire proud with a strong race in my age group.

To qualify to compete in the National Senior Games triathlon an athlete has to be over age fifty, and do two certified triathlons, or finish a State Senior Games triathlon in the prior year. I finished second in my age group at the prior year's Maine Senior Games Kennebunk Fireman Triathlon.

Here are my San Francisco Senior Games triathlon race highlights

• My wife Cathy was my support team and ardent fan.

• Coincidently, the Senior Games race director was Terri Davis, the same race director for the Escape from Alcatraz Triathlon, mentioned in my July 21 post. I introduced myself to Terri at the triathlon orientation session and encouraged him to visit this Outdoor Enthusiast blog.

• Elizabeth Bunce was the sole female triathlete from New Hampshire.

The Swim

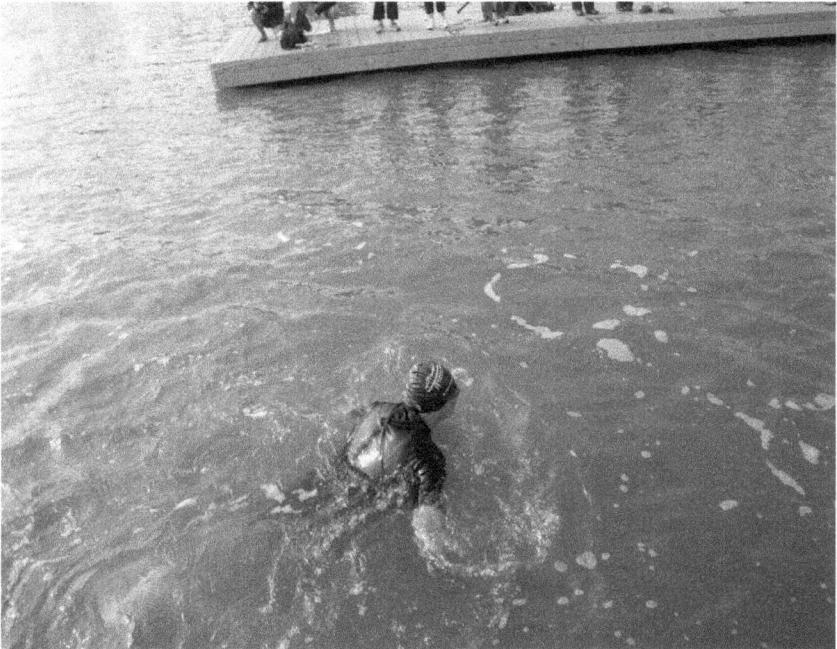

The First Leg Almost Finished!

The swim was in very salty 60 degree bay water of Port of Redwood City. I wore my short arm wet suit and was very comfortable.

We did a deep-water swim start - meaning we jumped from a dock, and swam to a channel where a start rope waited for our wave. All my previous triathlons had started ankle deep in water, or from shore.

- My swim was comfortable with low waves and tasted very salty. Ugh. However, I had no effects of the few times I inadvertently swallowed the water.

- I lost about 30 seconds in the swim to bike transition as I had mistakenly locked my suit's pull string. I did a Houdini type move to remove my wet suit.

The Bike

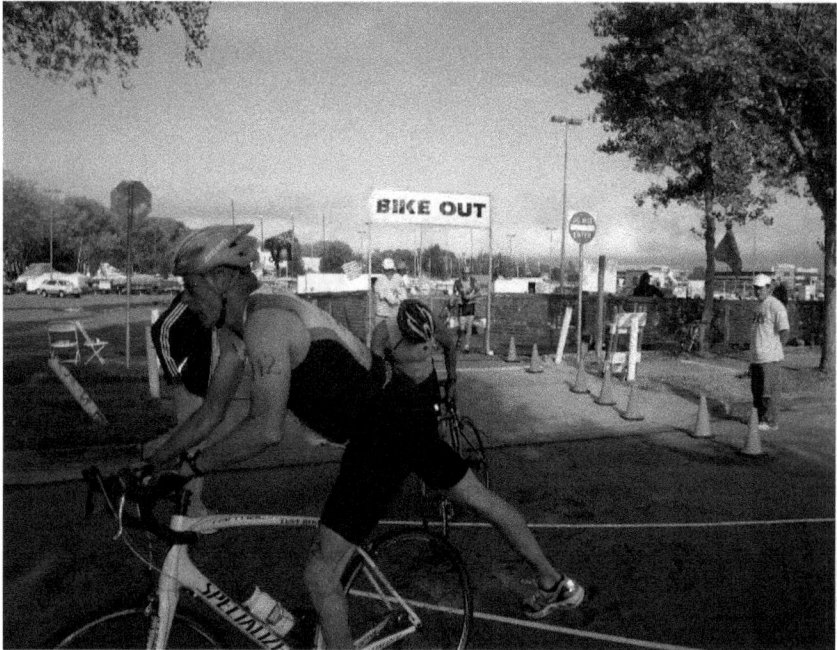

Transition from Swim to Bike

Rather than pay $125 to fly my own triathlon bike to San Francisco, I decided to rent one in Menlo, CA for $50. Overall, this was a very good financial move. When I called to rent the bike two months earlier, I was assured by the sales clerk the shop could match my bike shoes - so I did not bother to bring my own pedals.

My assumption the shop would match my bike shoes clip-ins was a mistake – I learned upon entering the bike shop that they could not match my bike shoe clips-ins. With not being able to pedal in my own bike shoes, I used the bike shop's toe straps and my running sneakers. I had not used toe straps for years, and I did not feel comfortable pedaling.

In addition to the pedal issues, the bike's seat and handlebars were not perfectly aligned for me, and I felt I was not pedaling efficiently.

No excuses here, as my closest competitor was way ahead of my time, and even with proper shoes and bike fitting, I could not have made up this time difference.

The bike route was three circular laps around an industrial park plus a straight roadway. The whole route was flat and for the first two laps no wind. In the final lap there were strong head winds. Of course, the wind was the same for all competitors.

During the bike component I saw three fellow cyclists on the roadside with an ambulance by their side. One cyclist had hit a road divider, whereas the others I could not determine how they spilled.

I did get frustrated a few times, as cyclists passed me on the left without saying "On your left". "On your left" is a warning that you are being passed. Once I was ready to pull out to pass a competitor, and nearly hit a cyclist passing me. I reminded them with a yell, "Remember to say "On your left!!" when you pass.

The Run

- The 3.1-mile run was four laps around a flat quadrangle. Before the race, I thought this method might have been too confusing and I might lose track of how many laps I'd completed, possibly affecting the pacing of my run. But as I made my laps, I found myself looking forward to seeing my support team, Cathy – and lap counting was no issue.

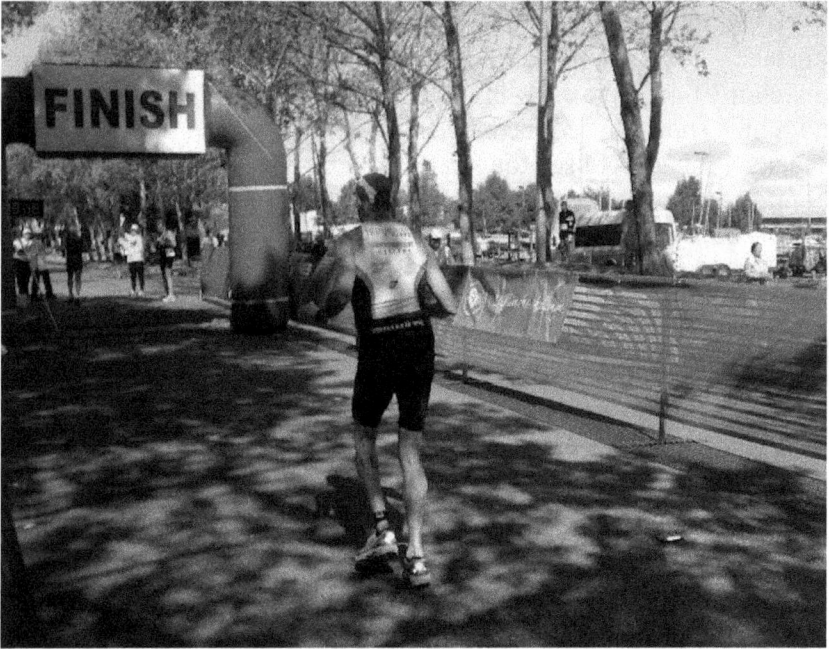

The Finish!

- The age of each runner was on the left calf of each runner, so knowing the age of my fellow athletes got my competitive juices up whenever I passed or approached a runner in my age category. But, I dared not ask which lap they were completing.

- As I neared my final lap my thoughts turned to concentrating on each stride to be sure I did not fall. I wanted to make sure the lone New Hampshire male triathlete finished the race!

Unorthodox Training Schedule

Two months before a triathlon I usually begin a mixture of a .8-mile weekly swim in Perkins Pond in Sunapee; two days per week of twenty mile bike rides immediately followed by one to two mile runs; and three or four five-mile weekly runs.

My regular training regimen was not followed for this Senior Games triathlon. Due to other commitments, my training consisted mainly of hikes, white water canoeing, and distance paddling. These certainly are cardio-vascular workouts, but my unease was did I train the muscles needed for a triathlon event.

Below is detail on my pre-race training for this event and my abnormal pre-race training standards

- I spent the third week in June in northern New Hampshire with three friends hiking the 4th Connecticut Lake, camping, and paddling five lakes in the Connecticut Lakes region. A week of zero running, biking and swimming.

- The 4th week in June in Standish, ME at Saint Joseph's College of Maine teaching two classes six hours each day. I managed one five-mile run, and zero cycling and swimming miles.

- During the July 4th week I managed one swim on Perkins Pond and ran five miles twice. Zero biking.

- The 2nd week in July I spent eight days paddling lakes and white water in the Allagash Wilderness Waterway (see July 31st post). A week of zero running, biking and swimming.

- 3rd week in July my grandkids joined us and we spent lots of time in canoes and kayaks. I did manage a one mile swim on Perkins Pond and two five-mile runs. Zero bike miles.

- 4th week in July my two sons, grandson, nephew, brother-in-law, and two friends climbed Mount Washington (an exhaustive cardio workout!), and then spent two days canoeing Lake Umbagog and the Magalloway River. A week of zero running, biking and swimming.

- Four days before I left for California, I did a five-mile run, rode my bike ten miles with my nephew, and mowed my lawn!

- Yes, I was concerned with my conditioning.

My Outcome in the National Senior Games Triathlon

I felt strong the whole race and thoroughly enjoyed it. However, I certainly would not recommend my atypical training schedule for an event like this to anyone.

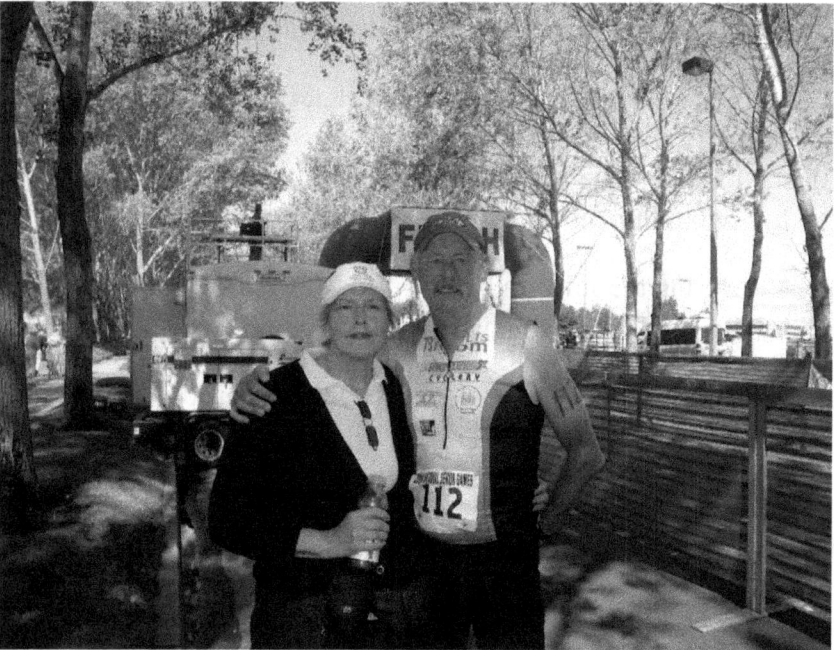

The Team

- I never have to say, *"I wish I had competed in the National Senior Games Triathlon!"*

Blog of Triathlon at National Senior Games
- http://outdooradventurers.blogspot.com/2009/08/2009-national-senior-games-association.html

Paddling the Allagash Wilderness Waterway

A Father-Son Paddling Trek

Ten of us just returned from paddling the Allagash Wilderness Waterway (AWW) in northern Maine. The ninety-eight mile AWW is composed of streams, rivers, and lakes, and shines as the brightest among the jewels of Maine's wilderness state parks and historic sites.

This was a father-son trip with four dads and five sons. Linwood "Loon" Parsons (http://www.loonsnest.biz/) was our guide. Loon's knowledge of the history and special sites around the Allagash meant many side trips and informative lectures on the unique history and lore of the Allagash Wilderness Waterway.

We entered the AWW at Indian Pond Stream on Saturday July 11th and exited Saturday July 18th at Allagash Village where the Allagash River and the St John River meet.

Wildlife

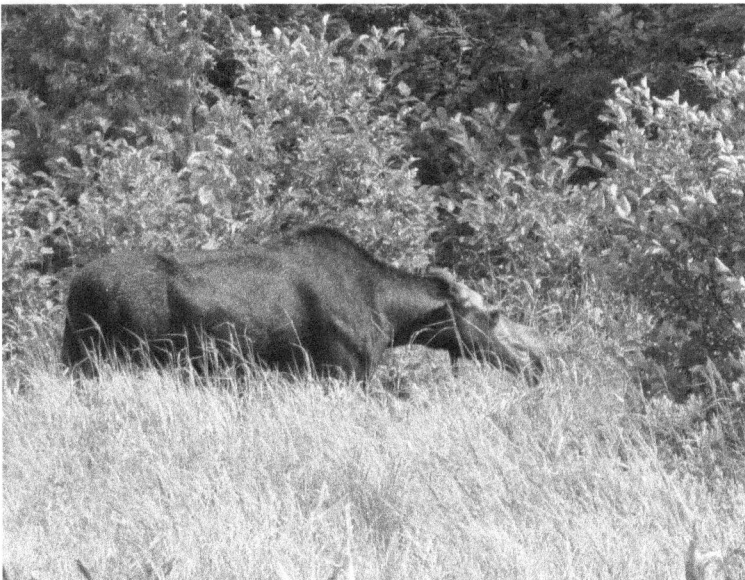

Shush…a Moose

A special treat for me was hearing the "snort" sounds of a moose. One evening a cow moose and her calf spent nearly an hour across the river from our camp, and we heard her many snort calls to her calf.

Each day we saw moose and we stopped counting moose at twenty-five.

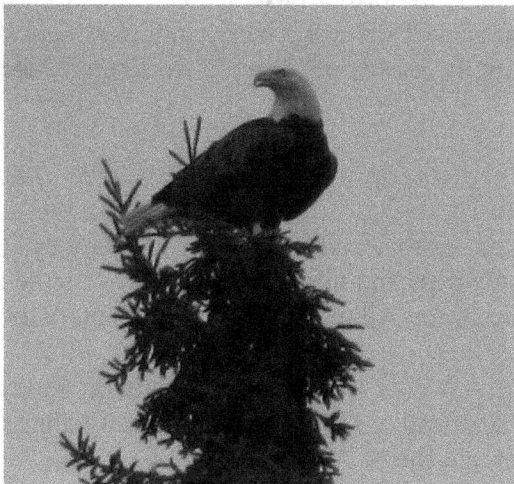

Look...There's an Eagle!

We saw many Bald Eagles, the national emblem of the United States and a spiritual symbol for native people. At one campsite a pair of eagles perched in trees across the river from our camp and made frequent screams as if warning us to stay away. We stopped counting eagles at ten pair.

A Loon Landing

A very unusual sight was seeing a loon land within a foot of our moving canoe. We spotted the loon coming toward us from afar, and we expected it to land. I have seen loons land hundreds of time, but what

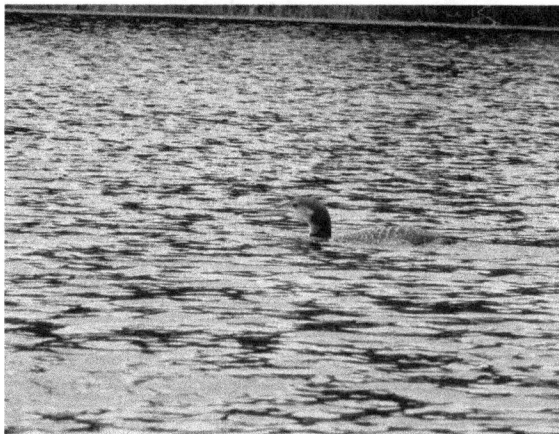

was unique this time was the loon did not land, but kept approaching us head on. It kept coming and coming, as if it was going to collide with us.

The loon reminded me of seeing a seaplane coming in low and long with its proud chest up and no legs showing.

Finally, after much anxiety on our part thinking the loon did not see us, the loon smoothly settled within a foot of our canoe and became one with the water – all this without making a ripple. Wow! What a sight to see.

Chase Rapids

This was my son Tim's and my third trip into the AWW in six years, and the water level was the highest and fastest we had seen. My earlier trips required us to frequently to get out of our canoe due to the low water conditions. This time we fought headwinds on Eagle and Long Lakes. Chase Rapids are five miles of Class 1 and Class 2 rapids with many thrills. We did short stretches of class 2 rapids over Long Lake Dam and below Allagash Falls.

My biggest thrill was paddling with my son, Tim. We did the first three days with me in the stern, including Chase Rapids. On day four, we switched ends of the canoe for the remainder of the trek. Tim's ability to read fast moving water, along with his paddling strength, resulted in an adventurous, fun, and safe trip though the rapids. Our last day, the eighth, it poured rain, but since we were on our way out, the rain getting any of our gear wet was of no consequence.

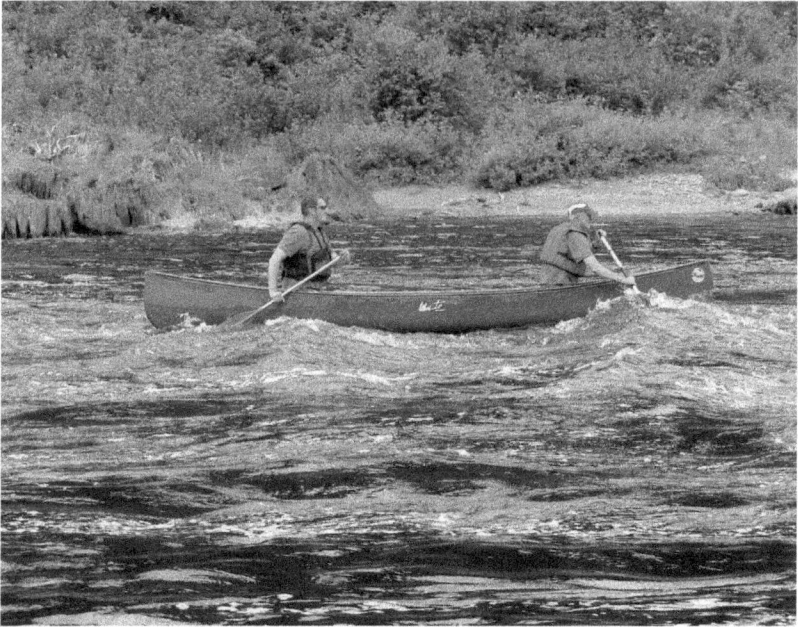

Eyes Focused Ahead in Chase Rapids

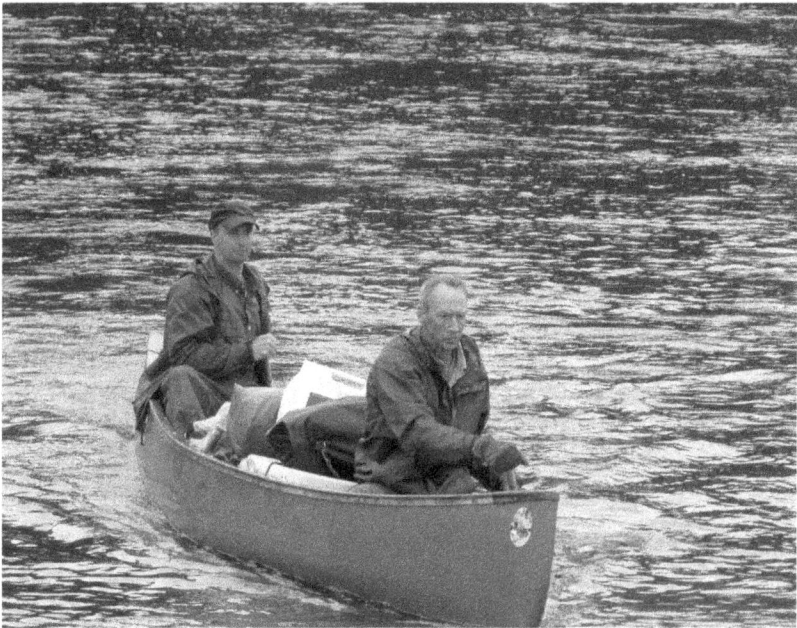

Notice the Loaded Canoe with Camp Gear

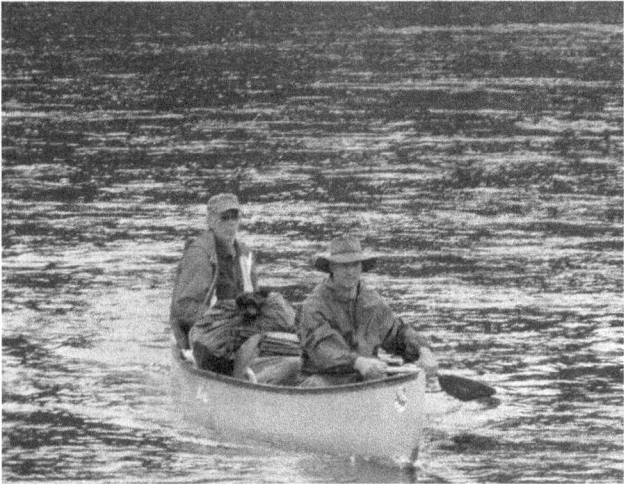

Time to Camp for the Night

Gourmet Meals

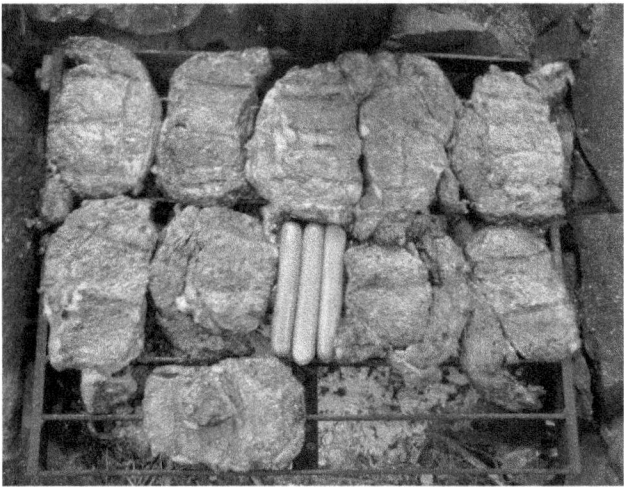

Our meals were simply delicious, well planned, and cooked by "The Loon". Rib-eye steaks and potatoes cooked over our open fire pit are just a sample of our eight days of gourmet dining. And since one of the paddlers was a "hotdog eater", our chef accommodated him for his own "special tastes".

Allagash History and Our Itinerary
Without a doubt, the Allagash Wilderness Waterway rates as one

of the grandest wilderness areas east of the Mississippi. Its mystique draws canoeists from all over America and the world. First roamed by native Abenaki Indians in search of food and furs, then in the 1800's by lumbermen in search of virgin timber for logs and pulpwood, it is today visited by the adventurist paddler seeking a deep wilderness experience.

The Allagash Wilderness Waterway is rich in historical points of interest from those by-gone eras. It abounds in wildlife of every description, from the majestic Moose to the ubiquitous White-throated Sparrow. Extending some 98 miles end-to-end, the Waterway offers the canoer both lake and river paddling environments.

Our trip began at Indian Pond Stream, flowed into Eagle Lake, and then proceeded northward for eight days ending at Allagash Village on the Canadian border. "Pongokwahemook", an Indian name meaning "woodpecker place" and today called Eagle Lake, is a most interesting spot on the Allagash. We pitched out tents at Thoreau campsite on Pillsbury Island, the northernmost point reached by Henry David Thoreau in his expedition of 1853. It is from this base encampment that we launched our exploration of the "Tramway" that connects Eagle Lake with Chamberlain Lake and of the old locomotives that ran between Eagle and Umbazooksus lakes in the early 1900's lumbering era. A strange sight indeed to see these 90 and 100-ton locomotives sitting alone in this vast wilderness.

By now, everyone's paddling skills have become finely tuned and in two days or so, we will be running the canoes down famous Chase Rapids, a beautiful and exciting run of nearly 5 miles ending at Umsaskis Lake. As the river enters Umsaskis Lake it meanders through an attractive marsh where we see moose feeding on the plant life. Canada geese often stop over here on their great migrations up and down the Atlantic flyway.

We next cross Round Pond, the last pond on the Waterway and spend the next few days being carried along by the current through easy rapids as the Allagash River descends toward the Saint John.

Trout fishing at the mouths of the many brooks and streams offered Eric and Garrett the opportunity to wet a fly. That evening Garrett shared his 14" brook trout cooked over our campfire.

We portage the most awesome spectacle on the river; 40-foot high Allagash Falls, a thundering, boiling cauldron of power and beauty.

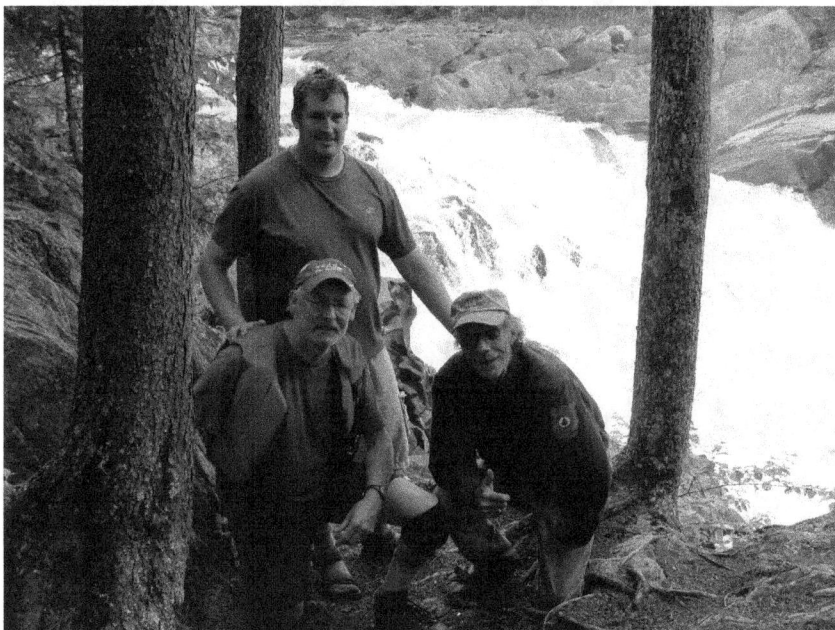

Overlooking Allagash Falls

Fourteen river miles below Allagash Falls through class 1 rapids, the Allagash River delivers us back into civilization and our wilderness river adventure becomes a treasured memory.

A special notation on this trip. We had planned this trek two years ago, but one of the Dads was diagnosed with throat cancer. We had made all the arrangements, and two weeks before the trek, we had to cancel the trip as he began aggressive treatment. Two years later, cancer free, he and his two sons, made his Allagash Wilderness Waterway dream come true.

Never say, "I wish I had …"

We now never have to say, "I wish I had paddled the Allagash Wilderness Waterway".

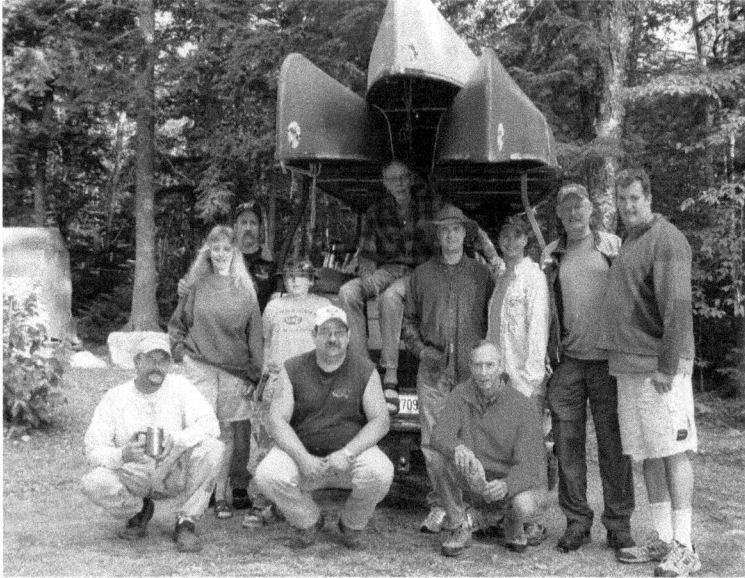

For more information go to Allagash Wilderness Waterway http://www.maine.gov/cgi-bin/online/doc/parksearch/index.pl) and Maine Bureau of Parks http://tiny.cc/58l6sw

> **Video References for Allagash Wilderness Waterway**
> - Blog: Paddling the Allagash Wilderness http://outdooradventurers.blogspot.com/2009/07/paddling-allagash-wilderness-waterway.html
> - Video of Pictures from Allagash Wilderness Waterway http://www.youtube.com/watch?v=5vND6qIj7UY&feature=youtu.be
> - Videos of Paddling over Long Lake Dam, Exiting Allagash Falls, and Canoe Poling the Allagash http://youtu.be/7OANcEldsUA

Hike Grand Canyon Bright Angel Trail Down to Indian Garden and Back to the South Rim

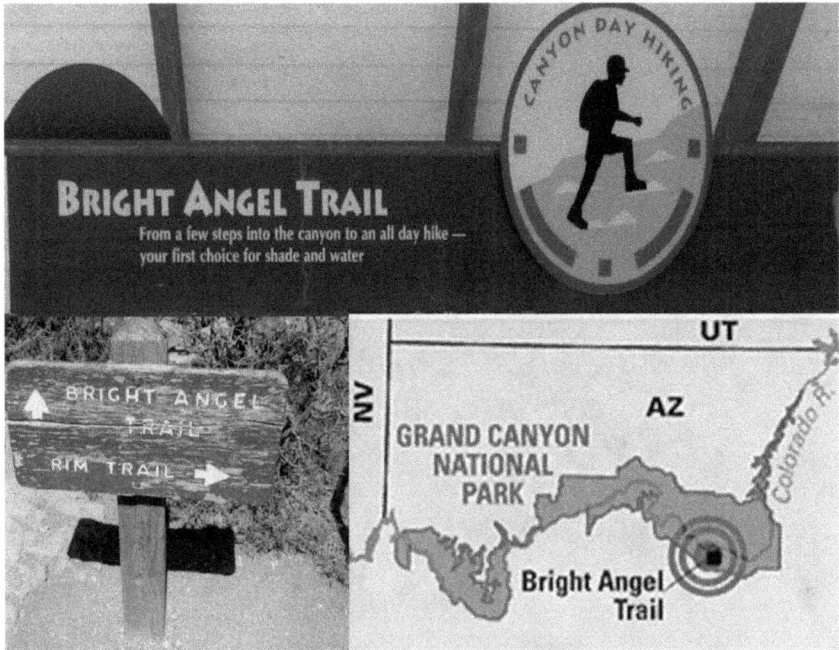

Bright Angel Trail

Last summer I had the privilege of being in Grand Canyon National Park in northern Arizona. Certainly as an outdoor enthusiast, I had to walk more than the Canyon's Rim Trail. My friend JK recommended a hike into the Canyon to Indian Garden via the Bright Angel Trail. The estimated hiking time was 6 to 9 hours for this 9.2 mile hike down and back to the south rim.

My enthusiasm for hiking into the Canyon was cautioned by my fears of:

1. My fear of height. The south rim of the Grand Canyon is nearly 7,000 feet above sea level. The thought of looking over a drop-off of thousands of feet was admittedly something I was not sure I could face.

2. Meeting Mules on the Bright Angel Trail. There are
   frequent mule trips passing hikers on Bright Angel Trail.
   Could I squeeze close enough to the mountain side to let
   mule riders pass me on the Trail?

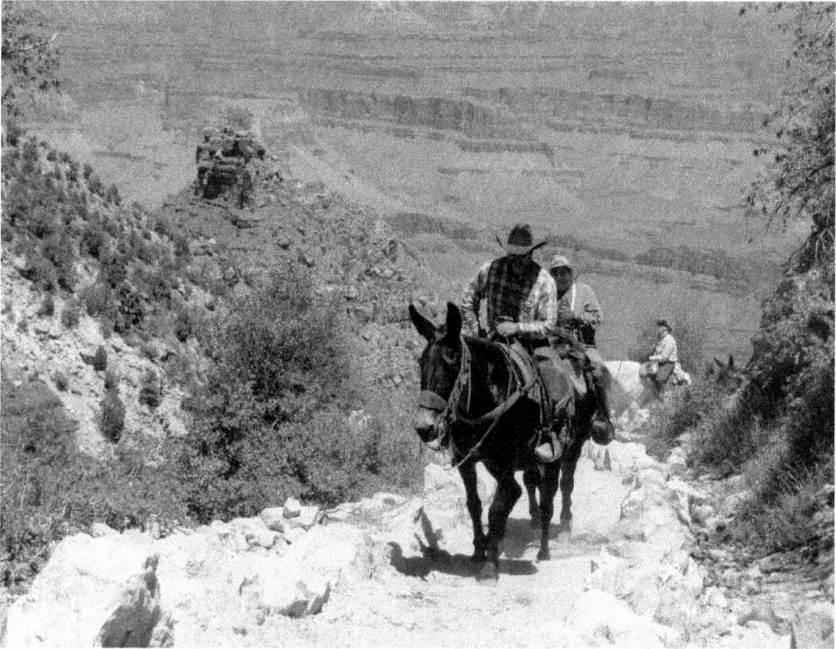

"Mules ahead" is Common on Bright Angel Trail

3. Width of the Bright Angel Trail. Would the Trail down into
   the Canyon be so narrow as to force me to hug the
   mountain?

4. On Thursday morning at 6:40 am I began my hike on the
   south rim at the Bright Angel Trailhead. Two and a half
   hours and 4.6 miles later I reached Indian Garden. The hike
   down was fabulous, and I stopped frequently in awe of this
   incredible landscape and to take pictures and "smell the
   roses" of my America's beautiful country.

   The four ½ hour return trip from Indian Garden to the rim
   was quite the challenge. The only thing that kept me going
   was I knew I had a six-pack sitting on ice in my cooler!

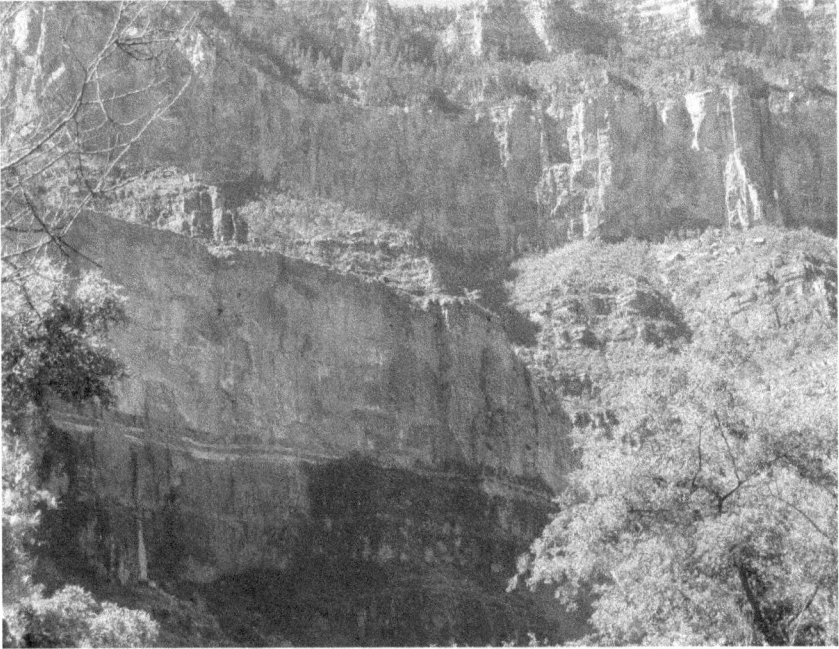
Looking Up from Indian Garden

I believe the main reason for my exhaustion on the return trip from Indian Garden to the south rim was because I had not trained at 7,000 feet above sea level. My daily Bedford, New Hampshire training runs were at an elevation of 275 feet.

Lessons learned from my six plus hour hike from the south rim on Bright Angel trail to Indian Garden were:

• Height. My fears were for naught. The width of the trail was four to six feet, and most often the cliffside of the trail had trees and rocks that eliminated any fear of falling hundreds or thousands of feet

• The width of the trail was more than enough to accommodate mules passing. I had three groups of mule riders pass me on the way up. As they passed I simply sat on the mountain side with plenty of room to relax, drink water, and take pictures, as you will see in the video.

• The three rest areas (Mile-and-a-Half Resthouse, Three-Mile

Resthouse, and Indian Garden) all had water sources for refills of my water bottles.

• The dust from the limestone was choking and blinding. Following another hiker up the trail put me in a dust cloud and I had to wait until the hiker was way ahead before I continued my trek. The mules passing generated even more dust. Certainly a person with breathing issues needs to be very aware of this situation.

• Shade was plentiful in my morning trek down. However, my journey back to the rim started around 10 am and shade was less prominent and the bright sun was hot resulting in sweat mixed with suntan lotion (a mandatory item) burning in my eyes.

• There were four-foot timbers every three to four feet on the trail to prevent trail wash away. This meant on the return to the rim I had to constantly lift my feet six to twelve inches with every step. My thighs began aching before I reached the Three-Mile Resthouse.

• My approach to the hike back was to divide my trek into three phases: (1) Hike from Indian Garden to the Three-Mile Resthouse, (2) Hike from the Three-Mile Resthouse to the One-and-a-Half-Mile Resthouse, and (3) Hike from the One-and-a-Half-Mile Resthouse to the Canyon's rim.

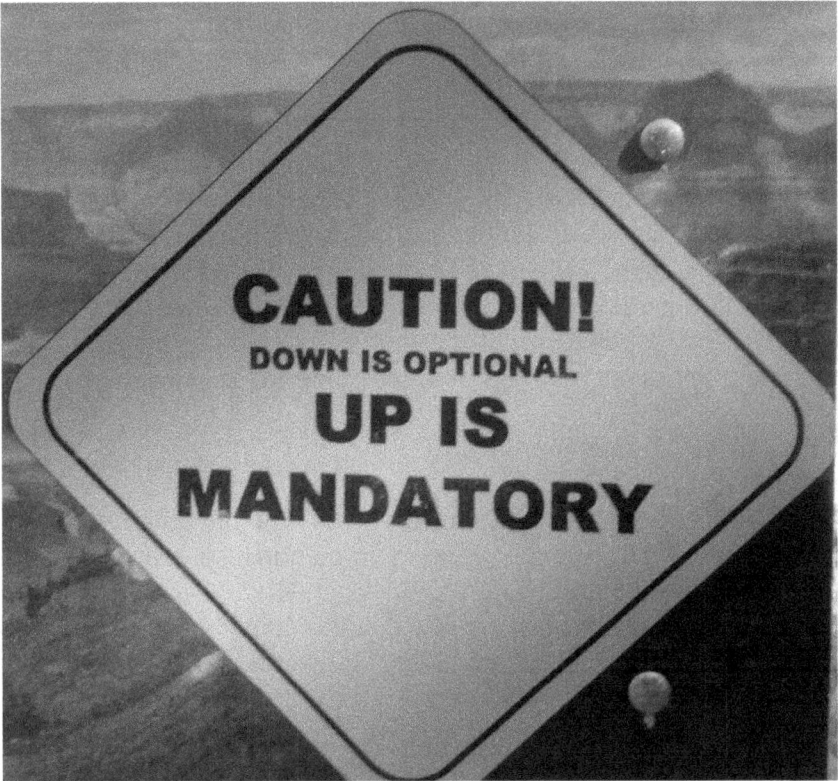

Sign at Three-Mile Resthouse: Down is Optional – Up is Mandatory

Hmm, I trust the picture of **Down is Optional, Up is Mandatory**, caused you to ask yourself, "What does **Down is Optional – Up is Mandatory** mean?" Well, as noted, hiking down the Canyon is essentially an easy stroll. Your main concern is to lift your feet so as not to trip over the log sections and rocks. Thus "Down is Optional" means go down the canyon knowing you must be able to climb back up – thus "Up is Mandatory" means you are responsible for getting yourself back up to the canyon rim. There are over 200 heat-related rescues in Grand Canyon National Park each year, and most of them on the Bright Angel Trail. So, a word to the wise.

The need to replenish water is a lifesaving concern in a desert environment. Water replacement in May is no issue as my 4.6 mile descent of the Bright Angel Fault to Indian Garden had three springs. Only Indian Garden has water year-round.

The steep decent is made easy through switchbacks curling down the mountain. You will also be returning up the same trail – and that is where the rub lies. The climb back to the upper rim of 7,000 foot above sea level, and the dust from the path, the constant lifting of your legs, the hurt of your thighs, minimal shade, and your level of cardio fitness, the return trip can be a life-threatening decision. So, **"Up is Mandatory"** means overcoming all these barriers that can prevent you from returning to the rim.

Memorable Moments

• As I hiked I began thinking this trail would be runnable, similar to my winter wild experience described here in an earlier blog post. Then, just before the One-and-a-Half-Mile Resthouse, I was passed by a person running. A few minutes later I met him at the Resthouse. We introduced ourselves, and he said he was 63 years old and "out for an early morning run". He turned around at this point and ran upward toward the rim.

• As I neared Indian Garden the trail leveled off, and I would run a bit – both to reduce the time to Indian Garden as well as to change my gait and vary the use of different leg muscles.

• On my return to the rim, I could see a woman walking very slowly in front of me. She was stumbling and stopped frequently to grasp the wall. She appeared to me to be in trouble. I caught up with her, and we spoke as we rested against the wall. I asked her if she needed any assistance, and she replied "No". We both were near finishing, and I waited for her near the Bright Angel Trailhead. We did a high-five. Certainly she was close to not understanding, **"Down is Optional – Up is Mandatory"**

• Because of my early morning start, almost my entire down hike was in the shade. However, my return hike was mostly in the sun - and it was very hot.

• Going down I did not touch the wall. On my trek back, I

frequently would use the wall to help support my upward progress - and the wall was cool. I kept thinking a hiking stick would be nice about now.

Enjoy my video and hike into the Grand Canyon to Indian Garden and my return to the south rim.

I never have to say, "I wish I had hiked Bright Angel Trail into the Grand Canyon"

See all my below **Video References** for pictures and videos of the Bright Angel Trail hike.

References to the Bright Angel Trail

• http://en.wikipedia.org/wiki/Bright_Angel_Trail

• http://www.bobspixels.com/kaibab.org/bc/gc_tr_ba.htm

• America's 10 Most Dangerous Hikes - Bright Angel Trail, Grand Canyon, AZ

Video Reference Grand Canyon Bright Angel Trail Hike
  • **Blog: Hike Bright Angel Trail**
    http://outdooradventurers.blogspot.com/2011/05/
    hike-from-grand-canyons-bright-angel.html

  • **Hike on Bright Angel Trail**
    http://www.youtube.com/watch?feature=player_
    embedded&v=IoCJWOdOjCc

Escape from Alcatraz Triathlon

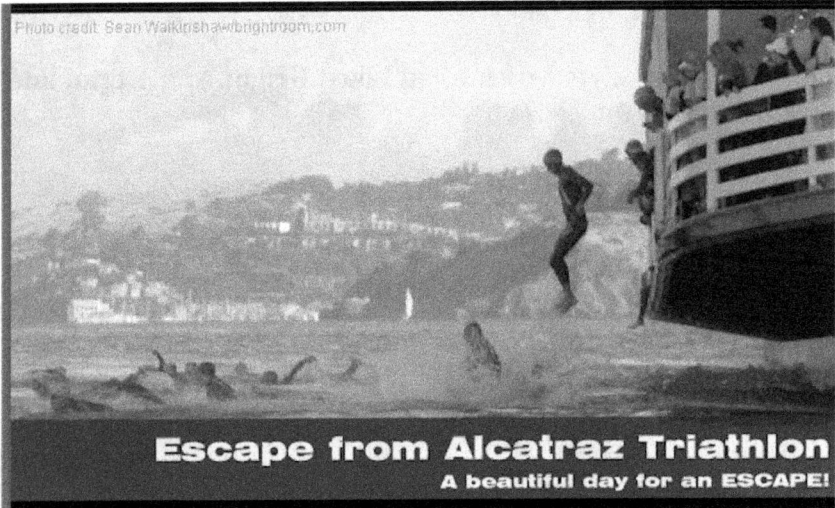

Photo credit: Sean Walkinshaw/brightroom.com

Escape from Alcatraz Triathlon
A beautiful day for an ESCAPE!

The Start of the Alcatraz Triathlon Begins with a Jump

I have always been intrigued with the Escape from Alcatraz (EFA) triathlon. The strong currents passing Alcatraz Island make a swim to the mainland unthinkable. I heard many years ago about this extreme event, and envisioned attempting it only in my dreams. Last week I listened, enthralled and full of questions, as Jim Graham, a fellow member of the Blue Steel Triathlete Club (http://www.bluesteeltri.com/), excitedly shared with me his recent "up front and personal" conquest of the EFA race.

The Escape from Alcatraz Triathlon includes a 1.5-mile swim from Alcatraz Island in San Francisco Bay. The race continues with an eighteen-mile bike ride out the Great Highway, through the Golden Gate Park, and concludes with an eight mile run through the Golden Gate National Recreation Area.

In addition to Jim, other Blue Steel club members. Tim, Jeff, and Carlo participated in the Escape from Alcatraz (EFA) Triathlon (http://www.escapefromalcatraztriathlon.com/).

Jim Graham gave permission for me to publish his narrative of the race. Jim's account of the race is also found at the Athletic Alliance web site (http://athleticalliance.com/), which Jim, Tim and I am members.

As described by Jim Graham

Tim Wolf, Carlo Carluccio, Jeff Litchfield and I traveled to San Francisco to do the "Escape from Alcatraz" Triathlon on Sunday June 14th. Carlo, Tim and I got into the race via the lottery, having put our names in online in December. Jeff qualified by having raced in New York last fall.

I was impressed with the EFA race on so many different levels: venue, organization, and difficulty, and I felt compelled to do a detailed write up. I have this great urge to go back and do it again next year, so I figure I will plant the seed now for people to think about joining me.

Jeff and I arrived in San Francisco on Thursday June 11th - a few days early to do a little reconnaissance. Our 1st stop after we left the airport at noontime was China Town, for a nice lunch.

After lunch, we drove the bike course in the car to check it out. It was a bit difficult to follow the course with the map we had as it lacked a bit of detail, but we managed. Our first impression was, "wow, this course is hilly!" We were staying at a house in Mill Valley on the other side of the Golden Gate Bridge. Each day we had a beautiful ride back and forth over the bridge.

On Friday, the plan was to pick up Tim at the airport, then swim in the bay and run part of the run course. We also found out we could pick up our bikes as well. We had shipped our bikes using "Tri Bike Transport". The out and back service cost about $250 round trip and was definitely worth it aside from the fact that you are without your bike for 10+ days on either end of the trip.

When we arrived at Aquatic Park for our swim, which is a couple of miles east of the transition area, there were a few dozen EFA participants already there doing practice swims. We put on our wetsuits and dove right in. Much to my surprise the water temperature was not that bad and there was only a little bit of rolling chop. This was a sheltered cove, but it gave us a taste of what we were up against.

Jon recommended we get a feel for the terrain and run the middle 4 miles of the run course, the "sand ladder". We dried off, changed into our running gear, and headed over to the "Warming Hut", which is right under the Golden Gate Bridge. We were starting our run about 2 miles away from transition, all of which is flat and straight. From underneath the bridge, you begin to climb, first on steps, which then changes to a narrow walkway, which then changes to a dirt single track trail. I estimated there to be about 250' of elevation gain over a mile. Once at the top you make a fast trail decent down onto Baker Beach where you run on the loose sand for about 3/4 of a mile before climbing the Sand Ladder back up to the top to reverse course back the way you came. We were running the course alone, except for a few people hiking and some people fishing along the beach. Most of this section of the course was tight, with little possibility for passing people.

We picked up our bikes at the "Sports Basement", a gigantic outlet selling all types of sporting goods that included an entire Triathlon section! Jeff could not control himself, purchased a new short sleeve wet suit, while I for the first time in a while was able to exhibit a sliver of self-control, and kept my wallet in my pocket.

Saturday we went to the Muir Woods to check out the giant Redwood trees and had lunch at Joes Tacos (Great pre-race meal). In the afternoon, we went for packet pickup and a mandatory athlete meeting where they went over how to sight the course on the swim leg and several other details about race morning. Tim had the foresight to get a hotel room four blocks from the transition area for Saturday night. This way we would not have to drive into the city early Sunday morning and could get some extra time staring at the ceiling waiting for the alarm to ring!

Sunday – EFA Race Day!

The alarm went off at 4:30am. Pre-race jitters, along with fire trucks, late night party goers etc., kept me awake for most of the night. Since we could not get a late AM checkout, we had to put all of our bags in the rental car to store them because we were heading back to Jon's house after the race. We rode our bikes down to the transition area with our transition bags. We had to drop off our T1-A bag that includes shoes and water bottle needed after exiting the water. It is about 3/4 of a mile run from the water to the bike transition.

You then rack your bike and set up your bike transition area. There were coach buses waiting to take you from transition down to Pier 3 where you boarded the boat that takes you to Alcatraz Island. You get body marked and wait in the usual "porta-potty" lines before getting on the boat that was set to depart at 7am sharp. I was wondering how the boat would look with 2000 Triathletes lying around, and it was impressive.

There are three decks on the boat, and the second deck we were on was a large ballroom that was empty of all tables and chairs and triathletes were sprawled and napping all over the floor.

Somehow, despite the crowd, Tim, Jeff, Carlo Rich Eichorn from Hopkinton, and I managed to come together and hang out for the 60 minutes it took to get out to Alcatraz Island and get positioned onto the swim exit deck.

As the boat slowly made its way out I was surprised at how calm the water looked, which as it turns out did not reflect what we were about to jump into. People were supposed to depart the boat based on their swim wave. I started heading for the door as soon as they were finished with the National Anthem, and I was surprised to see all different color caps on the way down the stairs. It occurred to me that nobody really cared about their wave time and was heading for the door. Chip timing and going over a timing mat before you jumped in took care of timing issues. I approached the doorway where everyone was leaping off the boat in chaos, and before I knew what hit me, I was leaping off the boat and hitting the water. I remembered to hold my goggles and scissor kick as I entered the water so I did not go very deep. My next thought was to get out of the way so nobody landed on my head.

The first few minutes of the swim seemed to be smooth water and I felt good, although I had a tough time seeing the radio tower we were supposed to be sighting. All of a sudden, the water became very choppy with very large swells. The water temperature was the least of my problems, as I was concerned with gulping seawater, sighting my line, and staying calm. I kept being caught in the wave's rhythm and getting hit in the face every fifth breath making it difficult to get a fix on my line. At one point I swam over the top of a large "something" that my hand hit that really scared the crap out of me. It was tough to swim a straight line at the radio tower because you were being knocked around by the swells and having to dodge other swimmers.

I ended up overshooting the perfect line by about 50 yards and forced me to swim the final 50 yards parallel to the beach against the tide.

As I exited the water, I was psyched that I had made it through the swim. A glance at my watch had my time at 44 minutes, which under the circumstances I was happy. I quickly found my transition bag in T1A, stripped off my wetsuit, put my shoes on, grabbed my bottle of Heed and started the 3/4 mile run to T1. I was VERY glad I had that bottle of HEED in my bag. I really needed to wash the ocean water out of my mouth and dilute the pint of salt water I had swallowed.

I managed to find my bike and made my way out of transition and onto the course.

The first couple of miles on the bike are straight and flat, and there was hardly a headwind. It was about this time that you hit the first of what are many climbs. We had ridden the bike course in the car a couple of times, so I knew what to expect. However, riding it on the bike was a rude awakening! I tried to temper the climbs and not blow up while trying to be aggressive on the descents to try to make up a bit of time.

Between the number of people on the course, the nasty pavement and tight turns, you were always braking or adjusting and not able to get in a good rhythm. The course did have some great views if you dared or were able to pick your head up to look at them. As I descended the final hill and got onto the final flat 2 mile return to run transition, helped by a significant tailwind, I finally felt like I was getting into a rhythm, too little too late!

I entered transition knowing all I had left was an 8 mile run and I would be finished with this beast. On the first 2 miles of the run, which are flat and along the ocean, I saw all of the pros running by. Andy Potts had a big grin on his face as if he was out for a leisurely jog, while some of the other pros who were four or five minutes back looked like they were turning themselves "inside/out" to get to the finish. It is humbling knowing they are beating you by more than 60 minutes!

As I approached the 2-mile mark, the course changes from flat dirt path to stair climbs and uphill single track. The stair climb was 4 feet wide with 2-way traffic, and it was difficult to pass. As you crested the hill, you were directed from the single track out onto a paved road, which also had race bikers on their return trip. The paved road section was about 1/2 mile downhill before you were directed onto a trail that led down to "Baker Beach". You entered Baker Beach and took a left heading towards the half waypoint of the run. Everyone had made their way down onto the hard packed sand at the water's edge rather than run in the loose sand, which made it very difficult.

After the turn around, you made your way back along the beach 1/2 mile towards the dreaded "Sand Ladder". The Sand Ladder consists of about 350 ladder type steps in the sand that ascend up the side of a large hill that brings you back up to the road you descended from. As you approached the ladder, it looked like a "death march" as two single file lines of racers made their way up, one line on the left and the other on the right.

You could hear loud music at the top where they had a DJ blasting tunes. They had timing mats at the bottom and top of the ladder so you could get your ladder split. My ladder split was 3:56, OUCH! There was a 1/2 mile of single track climbing as you were repeating the route of this out and back run. As you crested the hill, you began a wild downhill trail run that retraced all of the trails, paths and steps you climbed during the accent. It was tough running downhill on tired legs while trying to pass people and avoid any uphill runners making passes. Once down at the bottom, all that was left was 2 miles of straight and flat. Good news - you're almost done. Bad news- it's still 2 miles!

Down the finish chute, I gave it every last bit I had. I crossed the finish line and I wobbled over to the fence and leaned on it to hold myself up because I was ready to black out. I laid on the ground rather than pass out. I was completely wrecked and lifeless. Tim came over and gave me a bottle of water, and then Jeff came over to tell me to get my lazy ass off the ground! What great buddies!

It took 36 ounces of liquid to quench my thirst over the next 15minutes, so I guess I was a bit dehydrated.

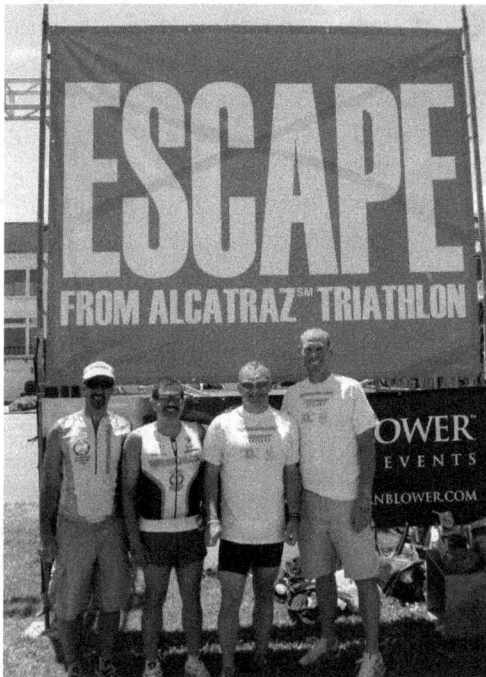

L-R: Carlo, Tim, Jim, Jeff

After the boys got their massages, we all grabbed our bikes from transition and brought them over to the Tri-Bike Transport tent to drop them off for their shipment home.

At that point, we decide to find some place to eat in this beautiful Marina Green area. We all agreed with Tim that a HUGE burger was a perfect post-race meal, so we set off in search of a burger joint and stumbled upon "Bistro Burger" that served huge gourmet burgers.

We managed to be seated at a beautiful outside sidewalk table under sunny blue skies! Menu: Huge char broiled burgers topped with bacon and avocado with a huge basket of sweet potato fries and an ice coffee.

Carlo headed home Monday morning, and Jeff, Tim & I rode the Trolley Cars around San Francisco taking in the sights.

After getting my ass kicked by a racecourse, it usually takes me awhile to want to go back and do it again. I am ready to sign up for next year's EFA right now! As this is an expensive race/trip, I will begin digging the change out of my seat cushions saving up for next year's race. Who is coming with me?

For a complete race recap, go to Escape from Alcatraz Triathlon http://www.escapefromalcatraztriathlon.com/

Video References Escape from Alcatraz Triathlon
- Blog: Escape from Alcatraz Triathlon http://outdooradventurers.blogspot.com/2009/07/escape-from-alcatraz-triathlon-i-have.html

---

FAQ from the July Escape from Alcatraz Triathlon

As a result of my **July 5, Escape from Alcatraz Triathlon blog posting**, I received many emails with additional questions for Jim Graham and Tim Wolf. Their responses to these inquiries are posted below.

Jim and Tim, we learn all the time from fellow outdoor enthusiasts. In fact, this sharing is a major reason for this blog. As such, I have follow-up questions for you to expand upon a bit on the details of your EFA.

Q. You said it was ¾ miles from where you exited the water to the bike transition area. Did you wear your bike shoes in this run from water to bike – or did you wear running shoes?
• Jim: I used an old pair of running shoes. The EFA organizers suggest using a different pair than what you are going to run the race in as they get soaked and full of sand. No socks either.
• Tim: There is a transition area just out of the water where you have a bag of stuff. In mine, I had water to wash out the salt, a towel and a pair of old running shoes that I put on for the run to the bike. You could not run that far in bike shoes, nor would it have been smart to try to run it barefoot as a large section of the course was on concrete with lots of little rocks, glass etc.

Q. The current/tide factor obviously makes it an entirely different length than an ordinary 1.5 mile swim. Any idea what the current was and how far you might have swam? In other words, how would you describe swimming one direction against the current in order to reach another direction? Does this course mean you can never relax in the swim, because if you do, you might never recover to get back?
• Tim: A lot depends on the weather conditions on the day of the swim. I have seen times that indicate the swim to be more like a mile (in terms of time in the water), and up to 2 miles. In this EFA,

I was out of the water in 35 minutes. In a normal flat 1.5-mile swim, I would expect to be out of the water in 31 to 33 minutes, so it was not far off.

While it is true that the current is pushing you towards the Golden Gate Bridge, many other factors slow you down, so in this case it worked out that time in the water was about equal to a 1.5-mile swim.

The things that made the swim tough were:

- You had to sight at the top of the wave; otherwise you could not see the point that you were aiming at.

- You had to swim for a point way to the left of where you were planning to exit the water. This was tough mentally because you really "wanted" to swim to the exit. We were warned repeatedly that if we did not swim to the left we would miss the exit point and would not be able to swim against the current to get back.

- When the sun came out it was in your eyes if you took a breath to the left, so sighting your swim marker was often very difficult, if not impossible.

- The wind was from the right and caused you to be hit in the face with water when you breathed to the right. I was forced to drink a little seawater when this happened.

- There were a lot of people that jumped off the boat in front of me and therefore a lot of people that I had to get around

- No Sharks but I saw jelly fish the size of basketballs that would scare the hell out of you if you ran into one.

- The cold was not really an issue as you were too worried about the above to be worried about the cold.

- I saw a number of people pulled out of the water by rescue staff.

- Q. Tim, how difficult was the EFA compared to other triathlons you have done?

    o I was pleased with my effort. Jim's description is accurate, and from my standpoint, it is the toughest race I have ever done both mentally and physically. There was never a point in the race where you could mentally relax and regroup; you had to stay focused the entire time. It was definitely NOT just a "run-of-the-mill" triathlon.

- Q. Steve, do you intend to do the Escape from Alcatraz Triathlon?

    o Absolutely not! The EFA is way beyond my skill and endurance level. I posted Jim and Tim's EFA experience on my blog because as a triathlete I knew this extreme event took an exceptional triathlete. Knowing these two men, and hearing their account of the EFA, was a chronicle I wanted to share with other outdoor enthusiasts. To me, hearing their tale was like sitting with Neil Armstrong and hearing him talk to me about what it was like to go to the moon.

Video References FAQ for Escape from Alcatraz Triathlon
- Blog: FAQ Escape from Alcatraz Triathlon http://outdooradventurers.blogspot.com/2009/07/faq-from-july-5-2009-escape-from.html

---

Sea Kayaking and Camping on the Maine Island Trail

My cousin Linwood suggested I join the Maine Island Trail Association (MITA). (http://www.mita.org/) The Maine Island Trail (MIT) is a 375-mile chain of over 180 wild islands along the coast of Maine. The MIT is a must do for any outdoor enthusiast.

The Planning Phase

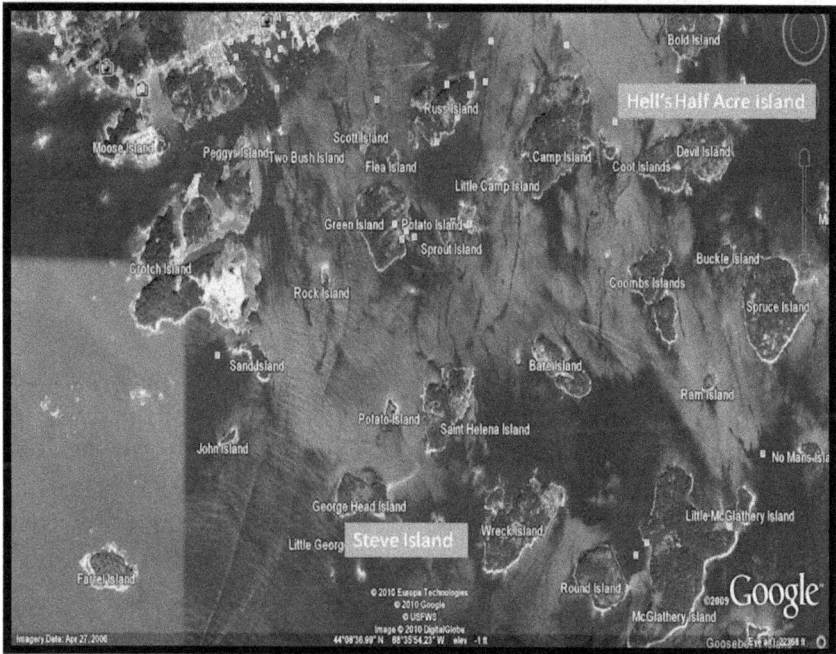

Maine Island Trail Map of Our Trip

Kayaking and camping on islands in the Atlantic Ocean is not something one does on a whim. Who would like to go with me? When do we go? Where do we put-in? Where do we park the car for three days? Which islands do we camp on? Do we need fire permits? Do we need camp site reservations?

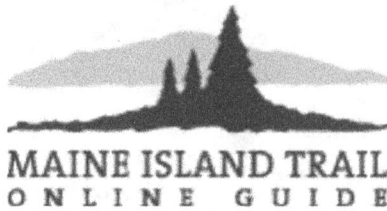

I invited my regular camping and paddling buddies, and Dundee was the sole positive responder. Dundee and I selected Stonington on Deer Isle as our put-in because it offered a plethora of islands close to shore for our maiden trip.

I emailed the office of MITA, and Eliza quickly responded answering my questions about island fire permits (there is a telephone number at the MITA website (http://www.guide.mita.org/) and also in the hard copy guidebook); camp site reservations (There is no need for campsite reservations on any of the islands - a MITA member has access to all sites on the trail, at any time, unless the guide descriptions indicates otherwise); The Deer Isle overview page of the guide has a list of put-ins available, and we selected **Old Quarry Ocean Adventures** with parking and launch facilities at a discount for MITA members.

Linwood sent emails on maps (http://www.charts.noaa.gov/OnLineViewer/13313.shtml) for nautical navigation charts. He cautioned us to plan transits from the islands and mainland using a favorable following tide flow. Tides can be 2 to 4 knots in some of those channel passages, and if we end up bucking the tidal flow, we won't make much headway toward our destination and may run out of energy and/or daylight.

He sent us tide charts (e.g. http://www.maineboats.com/tide-charts/tides?t=augstn10) as tide knowledge is critical for camp sites and campfires, since the fires must be below the high tide line. The velocity of flow is maximum at mid-tide and slackens toward either end, reaching null at the direction of change. In the Stonington areas the tide will run about 12 feet (give or take the phase of the moon effects). We needed to remember to drag our kayaks a boat length or two above the high tide mark. When the tide rises 12 plus feet, we do not want to find our transportation has gone out to sea.

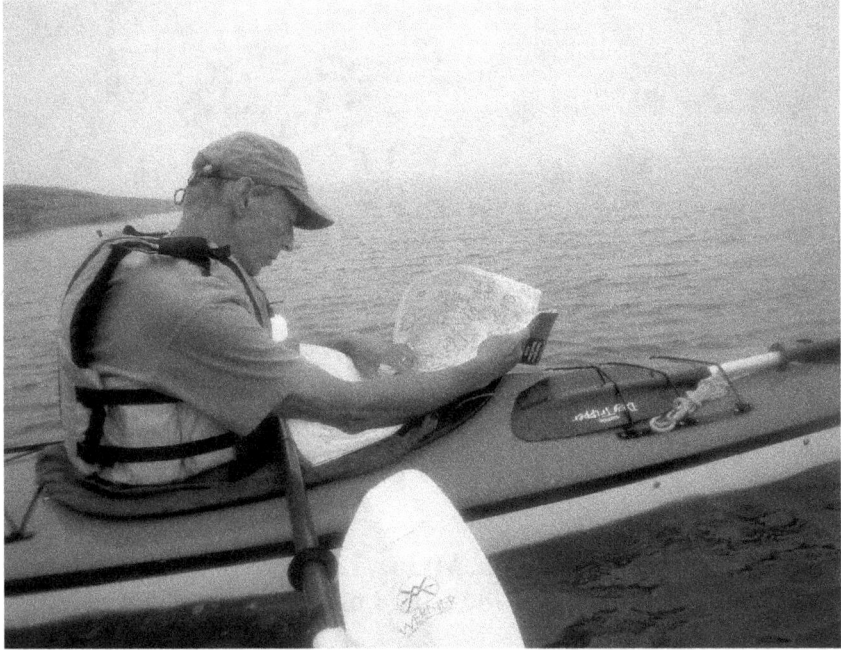

A Good Navigator with a Map and Compass

Our gear included compasses, relevant guides and charts, the MITA guidebook, and a plastic water resistant nautical chart.

Packing our kayaks for our three day paddle meant tough decisions on what to bring and what to leave. My wife Cathy thought we would never pack the gear we had readied, but indeed we managed without sinking our kayaks.

Our Itinerary

Hells Half Acre Island on Wed Night and Steves Island on Thurs Night with a 4 pm Fri Return to Old Quarry.

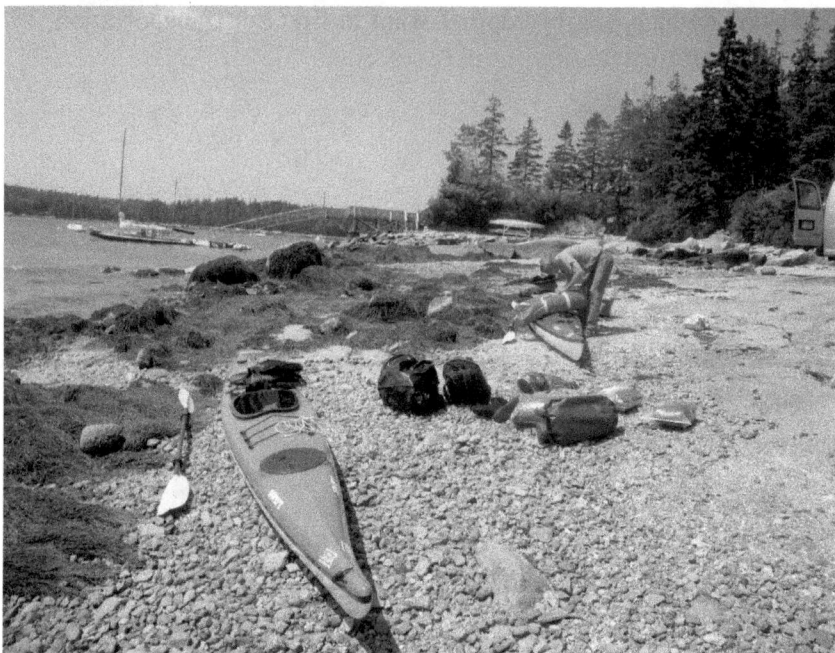

Our Put-In at Stonington, Maine, Located on the Southern Portion of the Island of Deer Isle.

I sent emails to friends to follow our progress on their email with Google Maps (the app is called **Where's My Droid** (http://sites.google.com/site/alienmanfc6/wheresmyandroid). I also downloaded an app called **My Tracks** (http://mytracks.appspot.com/) to follow our island trail paddle.

Day 1 – Wednesday

We registered our itinerary with Old Quarry. The Old Quarry staff were extremely accommodating with information on selecting alternative islands to camp on (e.g. "too buggy", "be careful of lobster boats when crossing channels and between islands", etc.)

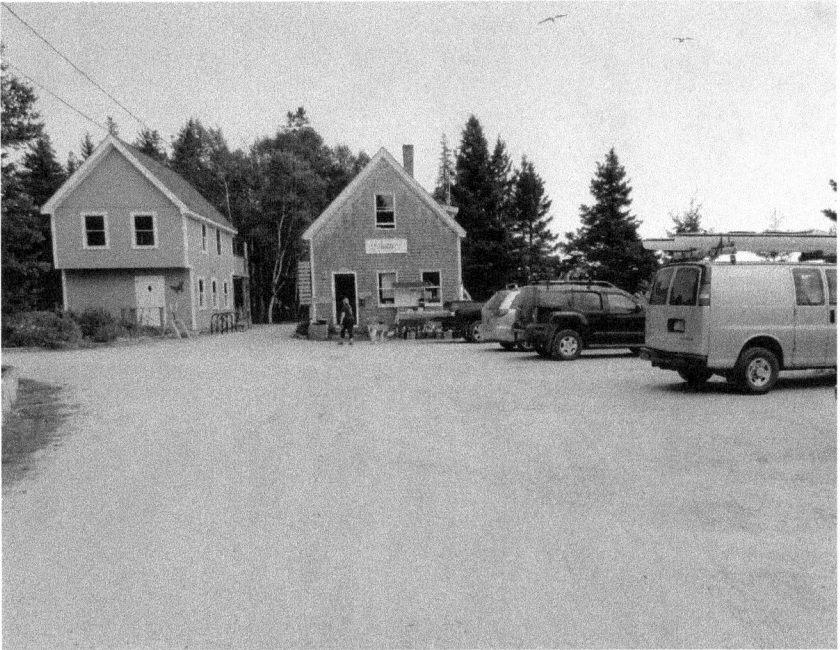

Old Quarry Ocean Adventures

We had a smooth put-in at Old Quarry, and with a smooth paddle we were at Hells Half Acre island in just over thirty minutes. We were in awe of the island and the view of the bay. We took a walk about this two acre island, and located a nice spot on the east end of the island and pitched our tents on two wooded platforms.

Our initial plan was to save a camping spot by pitching our tent, and then doing some paddling to other islands. However, we were in awe of this paradise, and after some adult beverages, we decided to cool it for the night right where we were. This proved to be the right decision as shortly after we landed a three mast schooner, the "Victory Chimes", with five sails full, tacked into our harbor. It was a magnificent sight.

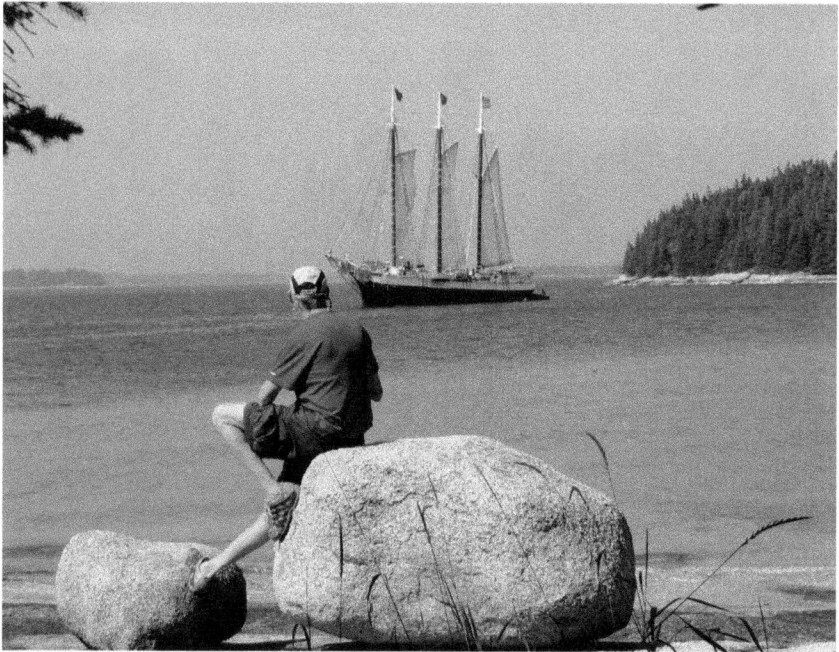

Watching "Victory Chimes" from Hell's Half Acre Island

Dundee was chief chef for this evening's dinner. We made a campfire below the high water line, and he proceeded to prepare beans and franks. Fabulous meal.

The sunset was dreamlike on this beautiful summer evening with a gentle breeze.

On Wednesday night we went to sleep surrounded by beautiful islands with clear skies and overhead stars.

Day 2 – Thursday

We awoke Thursday morning on an island in the middle of the ocean! We were completely engulfed in pea soup fog!

We had a lazy breakfast hoping the fog would clear. It did not.

At 10 am we decided to use our map and compass skills, and find our way to Steves Island. Dundee's experience at reading a nautical chart and steering by compass were impressive.

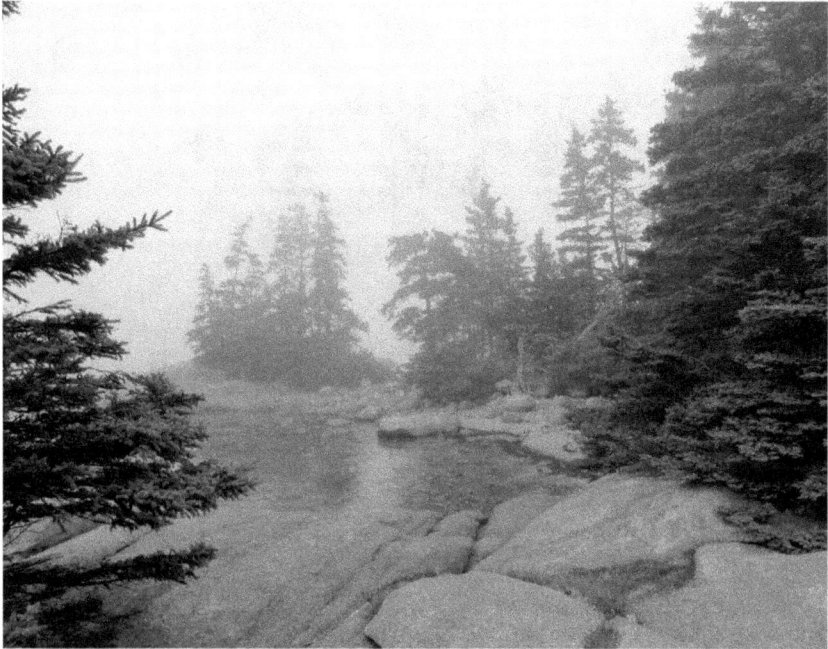

The Fog

I felt comfortable with Dundee leading the way, but I must admit it was a weird feeling paddling into pea soup fog and hoping to find our next marker to know we were on course to Steves Island.

It took us about an hour to paddle to Steves from Hells Half Acre, as we meandered between a few islands enjoying this surreal experience of fog paddling. We could see about thirty feet ahead, so when we located an island, we paddled around it so as to take in the scenic pleasures of the spruce and granite topography along its shoreline, and if truth were to be told, to be sure we could recognize the island on our navigational map so we knew where we were.

Paddling Away from Hell's Half Acre Island

When we found Steves Island, we were met by a couple, Taylor and Catherine, who had spent the prior night there, and because of being fog bound today, they intended to spend another day on Steves trusting that Friday's sun would burn away the fog.

We found a delightful campsite to pitch our tents. We toured this rock bound island, with balsam trees in the middle. Of course with the fog, our views off the island were essentially nil. We could hear lobster boats, but did not see them.

During the day four kayakers in beautiful hand-made sea kayaks found the island for lunch. Interestingly, I knew one of the kayakers, so it was fun talking old times. They had all the appropriate navigation equipment for foggy weather, and after lunch left to make their way back to their campsite at another MITA Island.

A Fresh Muscle Feast

Given we were now friends with Taylor and Catherine, we invited them to join us for Steves Island fresh muscles and pre-dinner Hors D'Oeuvres. The **Video References** box below offers a link to our ocean muscle feast.

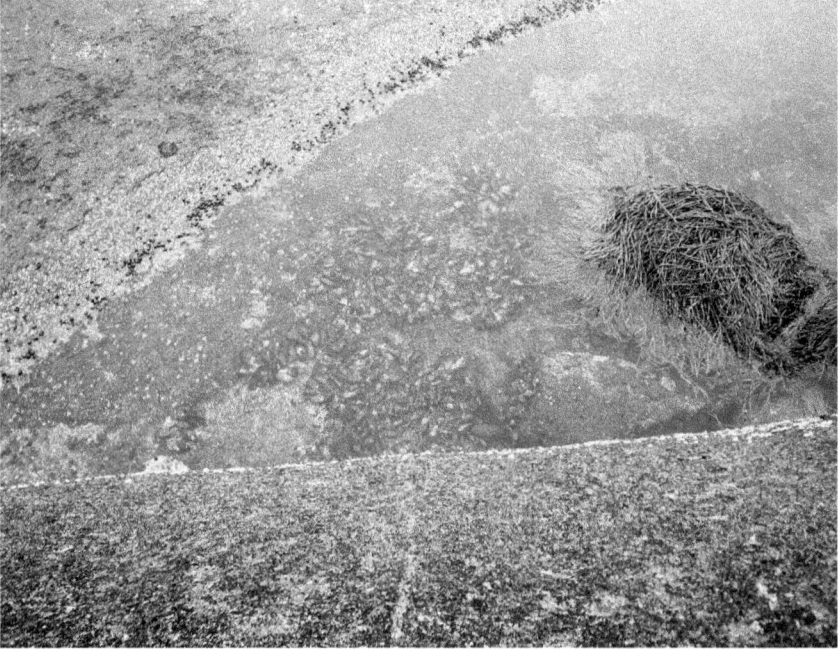

Muscle Bed at Low Tide at Steves Island

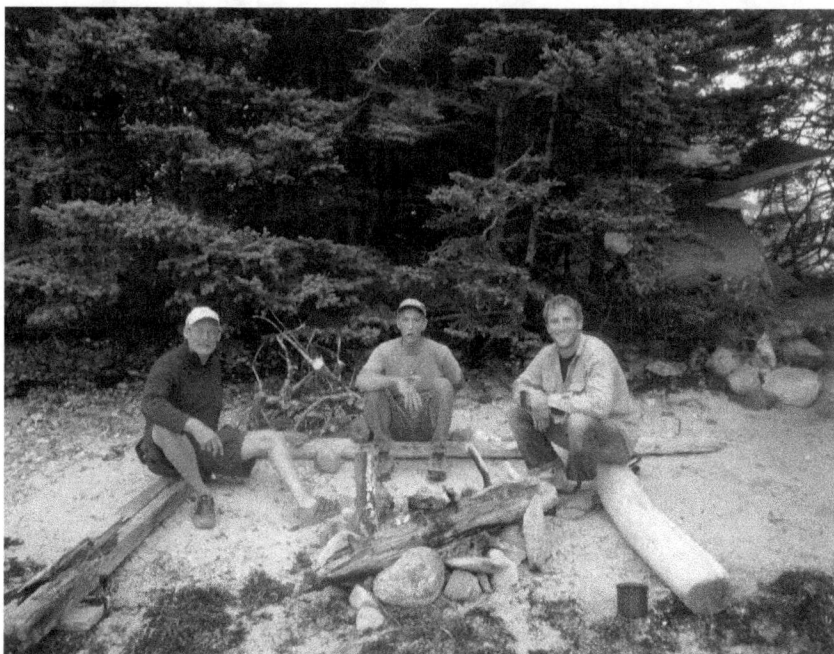
Steves Island and Steamed Muscles

Day 3 Friday

We awoke at 5:30 am Friday hearing the working lobster boats
getting an early morning start. The fog was lifting and we knew the
day would be clear. Around 9 am we began to be surrounded by
views of the islands, as indeed they had been depicted on our map.

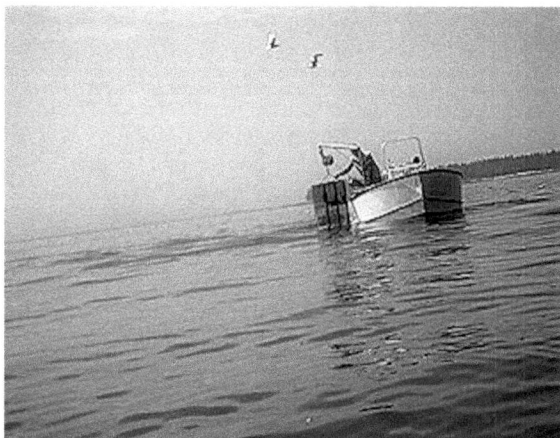
An Early Morning Working Lobster Boat

At 10 am we started a gentle paddle back to our Old Quarry take-out via Crotch Island and Stonington. We left Steves Island with wonderful memories of ocean muscles and new and old friends. Crotch Island used to be a stone quarry, and was loaded with monstrous granite cut stones. A lot of the granite blocks used in the construction of many government buildings and monuments in our nation's capital were mined off this island.

We paddled along the shorefront of Stonington harbor, and around 1 pm we pulled into our take-out.

We reported our return at the **Old Quarry Ocean Adventures** office, and after buying three freshly caught Maine lobsters, we headed home to New Hampshire.

Shared Learning

• My Droid Incredible ran out of power in less than 7 hours after its full charge, so my expectations for **Where is my DROID**, and **My Tracks** was a big negative (although some friends used GPS My DROID on day one and it worked great.

• Always bring a water resistant nautical map and compass – and certainly know how to use it BEFORE you go

• Join the Maine Island Trail Association (MITA)

• Most assuredly I will return many times to enjoy and explore the 200 plus islands cared for by the Maine Island Trail Association (MITA) membership.

• Enjoy the below **Video References** taken on MIT

• Never say, "I wish I had paddled the Maine Island Trail"

Video References Paddling the Maine Island Trail

- Blog: Sea Kayaking on the MIT
  http://outdooradventurers.blogspot.com/20
  10/08/sea-kayaking-and-camping-on-
  maine.html

- Hells Half Acre's Island Pea Soup Fog
  http://www.youtube.com/watch?v=k4G4K
  mqLIp8&feature=player_embedded
- Eating Ocean Muscles on Steves Island
  http://www.youtube.com/watch?v=NhfMK
  al5DWo&feature=player_embedded
- Old Quarry Ocean Adventures
  http://www.oldquarry.com/
- Maine Island Trail Association
  http://www.mita.org

Paddling, Hiking & Camping at Connecticut Lakes & Lake Francis

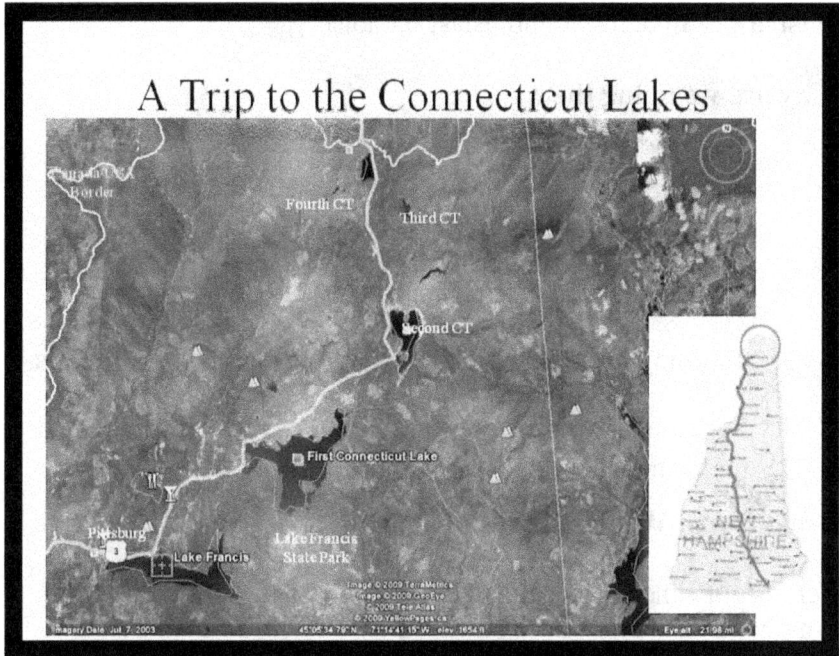

A Trip to the Connecticut Lakes

Route 3 Goes the Length of NH as Shown on the Side Map. The Great North Woods is Circled.

Pittsburg, New Hampshire – The Great North Woods

When you say or hear, "Connecticut Lakes and Lake Francis", or "Pittsburg", you are talking about the most northern area of New Hampshire near the Canadian border.

On a Monday in mid-June, John, Dundee, Dick and I drove to the Lake Francis State Park in Pittsburg, NH. Pittsburg has an estimated population of 900 and is the northernmost town in NH and the largest town by area in the state. U.S. Route 3 is the only major highway in the town ending at the Canadian border. Contained within the boundaries of Pittsburg are the Connecticut

(CT) Lakes and Lake Francis. These lakes are the headwaters of the 410 mile Connecticut River.

Pittsburg is known for snowmobiling and ATV trails, fishing and hunting, canoeing and kayaking, and its moose. Some of the folks jest, "There are more moose than people."

Pittsburg is an outdoor enthusiast paradise.

Why are we doing this?

1. To visit Moose Alley and almost assure ourselves of seeing moose.

2. We want to straddle the Connecticut River at its 4th Connecticut Lake headwaters outlet.

3. To enjoy my fellow trekkers and The Great North Woods.

4. Because we never want to say, "We wish we had paddled the Connecticut Lakes and Lake Francis."

Great North Woods Itinerary

Here is our schedule for this four-day paddling, hiking and camping trip:

- Monday: Drive to Lake Francis State Park, set up camp, and paddle the lake as daylight permits. The Park will be our camp site for three nights

- Tuesday: Hike to the 4th Connecticut Lake, paddle the 3rd Connecticut Lake, and continue our Lake Francis paddle.

- Wednesday: Paddle 2nd Connecticut Lake, East Inlet and Scott's Bog.

- Thursday: Take down our campsite, paddle 1st Connecticut Lake in the morning, and return home in the afternoon.

The Fourth, Third, Second, First Connecticut Lakes, and Lake

Francis flow into each other starting with the tiny Fourth CT Lake on the Canadian border. The water connections are small streams with intermittent sections of white water. Paddling these connections is not really feasible due to the narrowness of the stream, its shallow depth, obstructing rock formations. For each lake we portage our canoes/kayaks on our car carrier racks.

I used **Google Earth** for maps to orient ourselves and determine distances. **Google** search found the website **Paddling.Net** which had a wonderful article titled, **Connecticut Lakes - Kayak Trip / Canoe Trip.** This article contained a detailed narrative of an earlier trip.

Young's Store was our primary hub for information, food, and adult beverages. "If they do not have it, you do not need it." Next to Young's Store was a wonderful breakfast and lunch café.

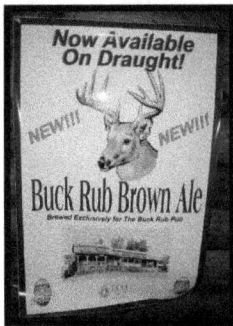

The **Buck Rub Pub** was a great place to quench your thirst and have dinner.

They even have their own specially made **Buck Rub Brown Ale**!

Statistics of Connecticut (CT) Lakes
- 4th CT 78 acres (on the Canadian Border)
- 3rd CT 231 acres (fed by the 4th CT)
- 2nd CT 1,102-acres (fed by the 3rd CT)
- lst CT 3,071 acres (fed by the 2nd CT)
- Lake Francis 1,933 acres (fed by lst CT)

For detail statistics on the Connecticut Lakes go to
http://en.wikipedia.org/wiki/Connecticut_Lakes

Pictures are Worth a Thousand Words

Rather than give a narrative of this beautiful area, I will simply show pictures of the areas we visited. At the end of this section I have listed references for more detailed information on The Great North Woods for those outdoor enthusiasts that may want to visit this most beautiful area.

Lake Francis

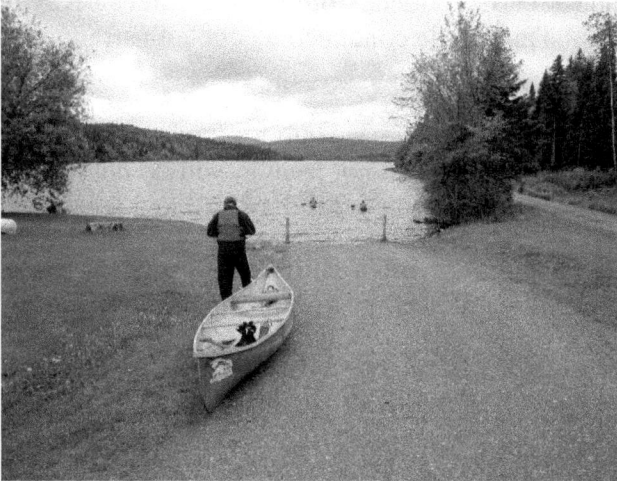

Put-in at Lake Francis State Park

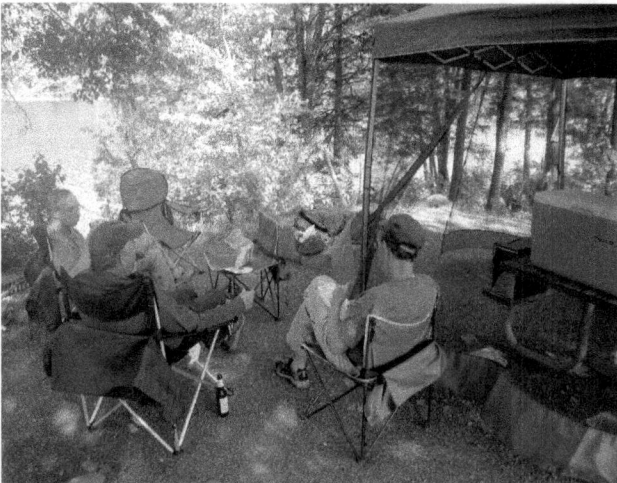

Relaxing at the Campsite

Republic of Indian Stream

Did you know that there once was a country between New Hampshire and Canada? Read on.

- For a few years in the 1830s, an area of today's Pittsburg, NH was an independent republic, not part of New Hampshire and not part of the United States.
- The US attempted to tax the 360 inhabitants, and Canada tried to make them serve in its military, so the people decided to establish their own sovereign nation – **The Republic of Indian Stream.**
- The existence of the republic was ended by New Hampshire in 1835.
- The Webster -Ashburton Treaty of 1842 established the border between Canada and the United States.
- Pittsburg is the largest township in the United States, covering over 300,000 acres.

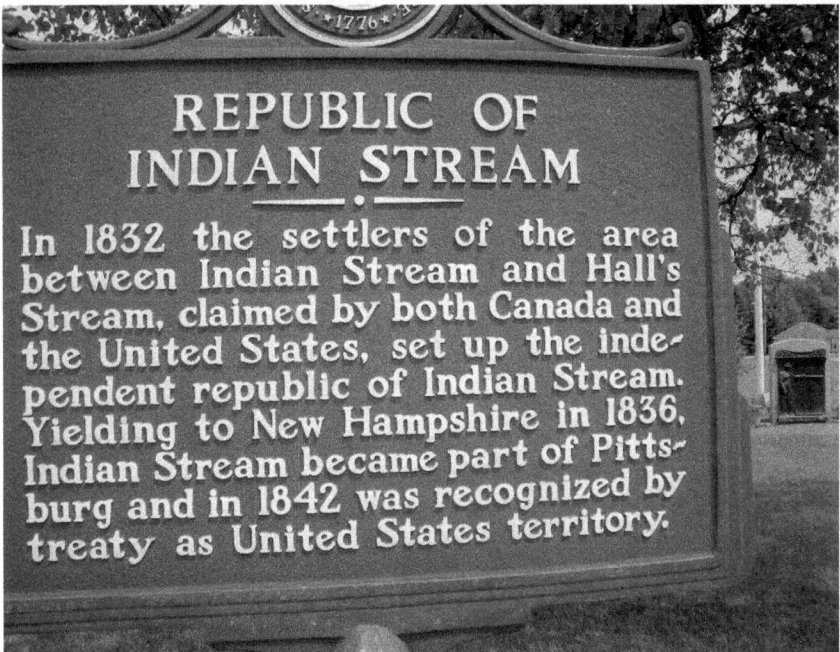

REPUBLIC OF INDIAN STREAM

In 1832 the settlers of the area between Indian Stream and Hall's Stream, claimed by both Canada and the United States, set up the independent republic of Indian Stream. Yielding to New Hampshire in 1836, Indian Stream became part of Pittsburg and in 1842 was recognized by treaty as United States territory.

A Country Between the United States and Canada

Fourth Connecticut Lake - Headwaters of the Connecticut River

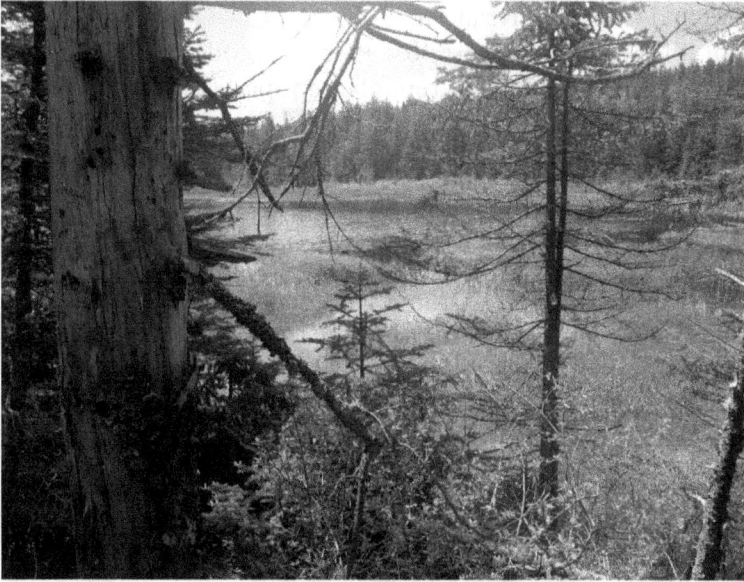

A View of the4th CT Lake

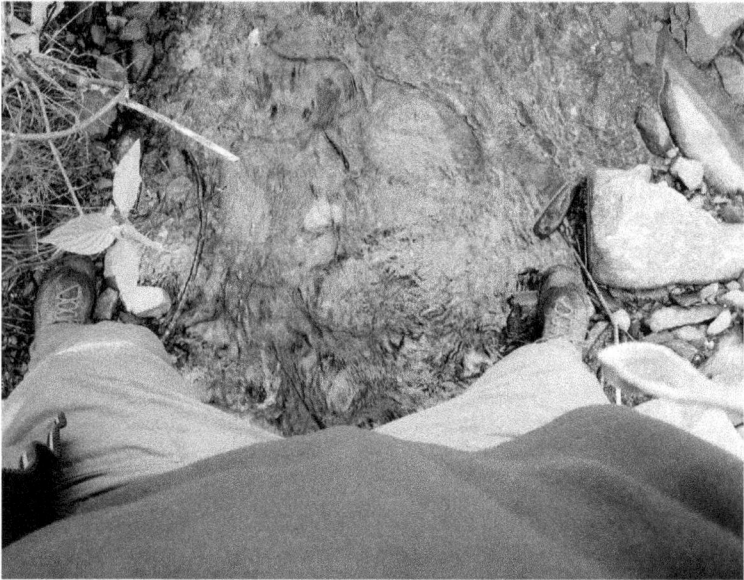

Outdoor Steve Standing with one foot on each side of the Connecticut River

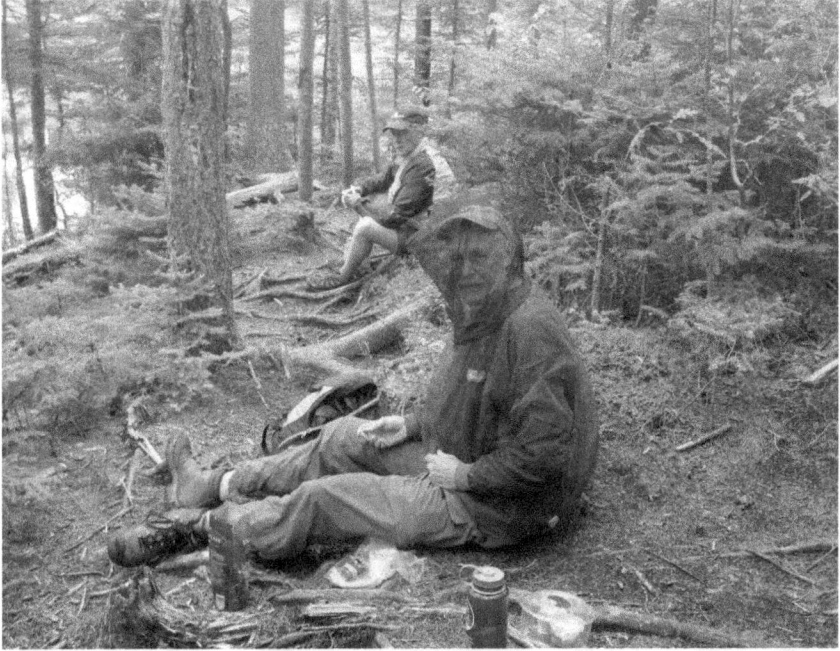

Using the Bug Baffler!

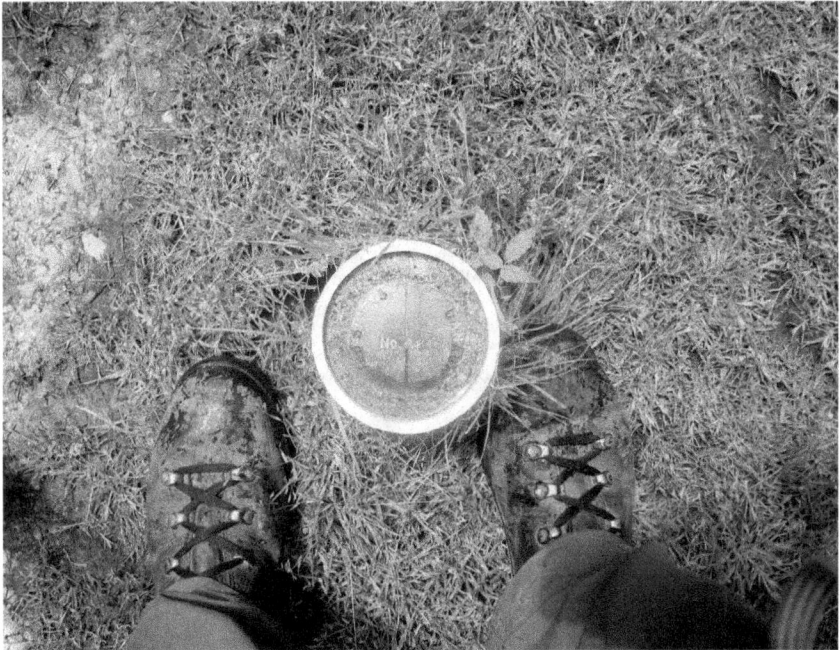

Straddling the USA and Canada Boundary

Third Connecticut Lake

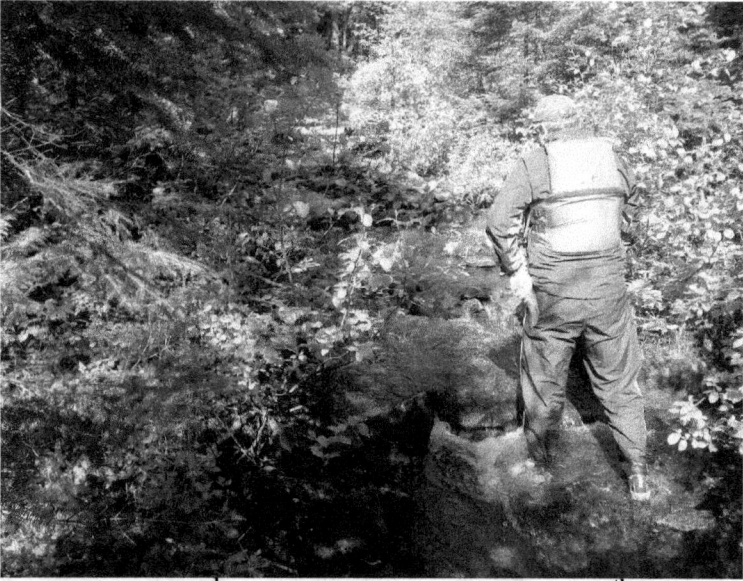

Is this the 3rd CT Inlet of Water from the 4th CT?

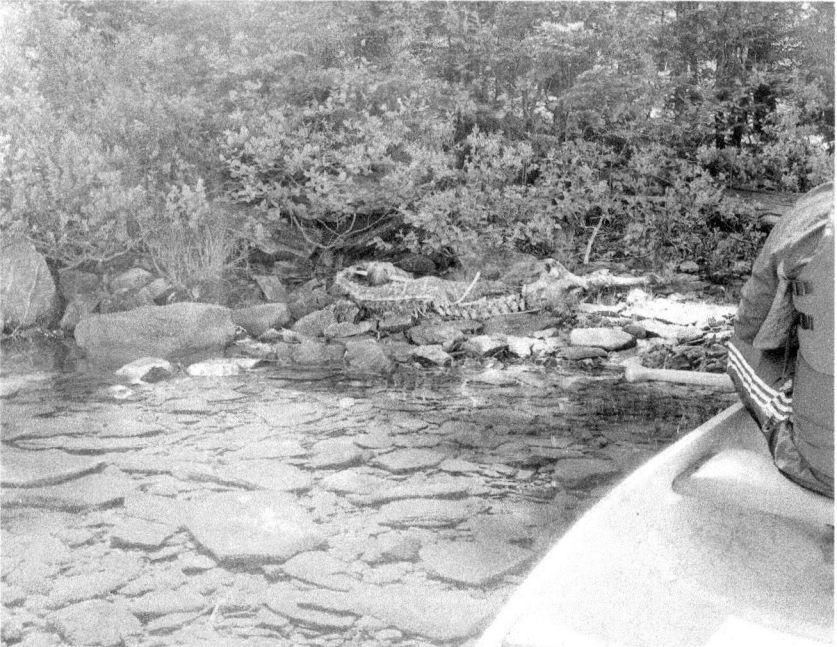

We Spot a Moose Skelton on the 3rd CT

First Connecticut Lake

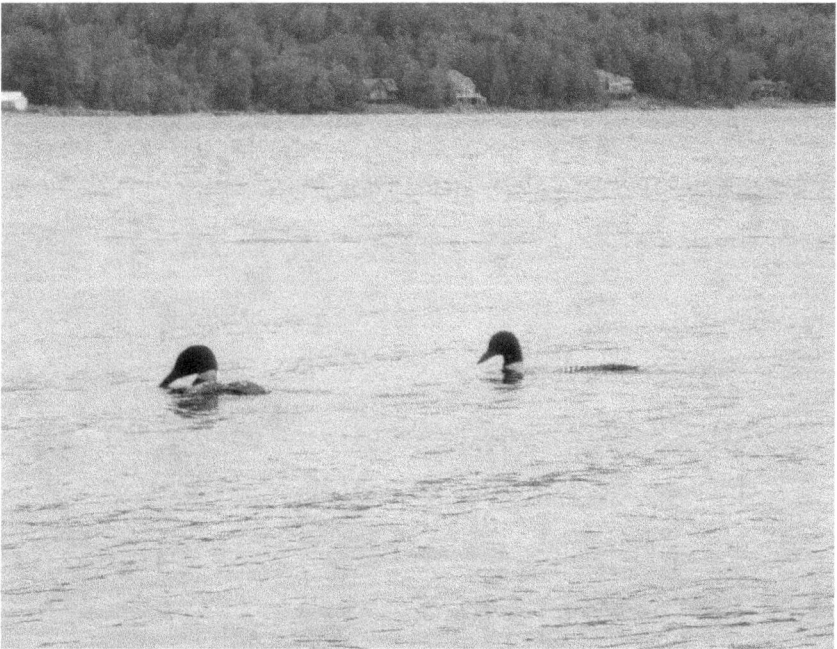

A Mating Pair of Loons

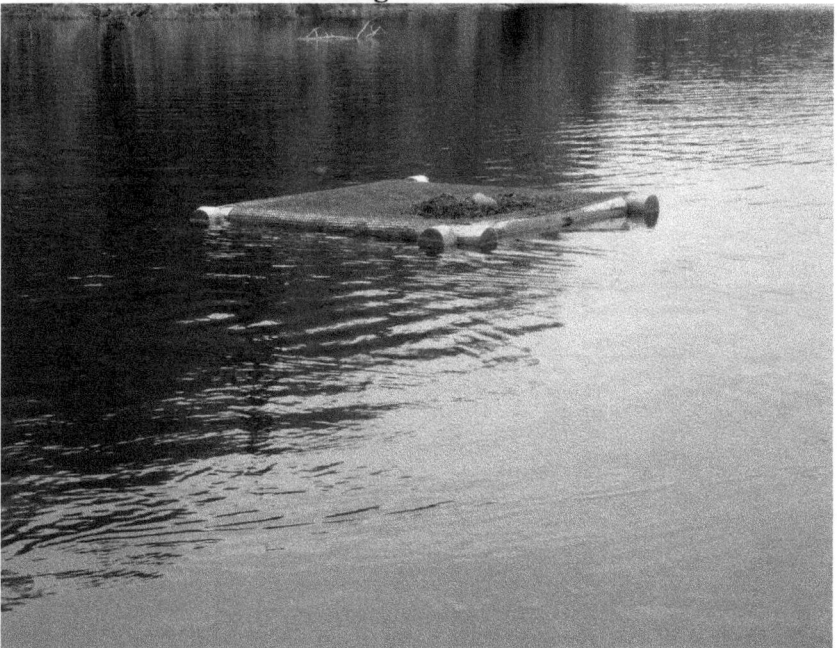

See the Loon Egg on the Man-made Loon Nesting Platform

East Inlet

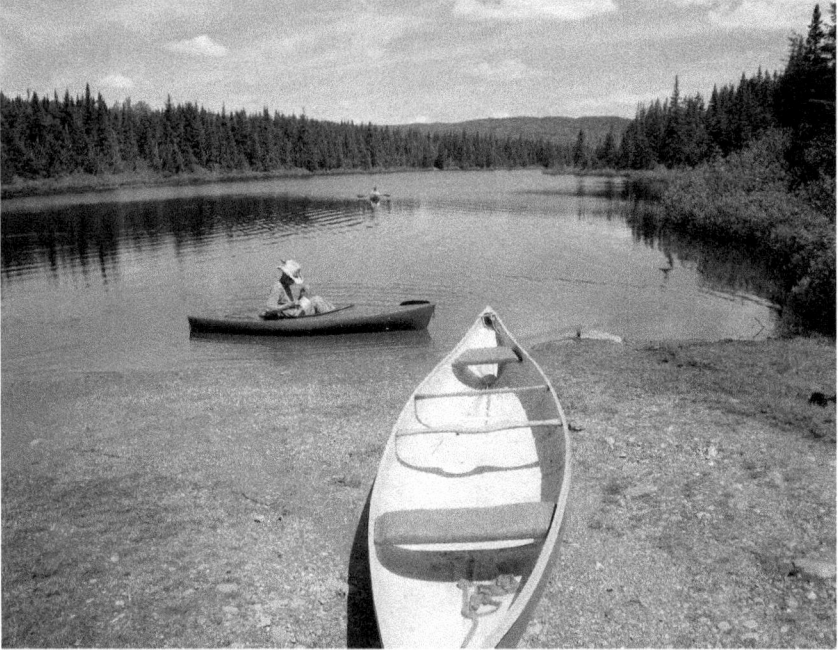

Put-in and Take-Out at East Inlet

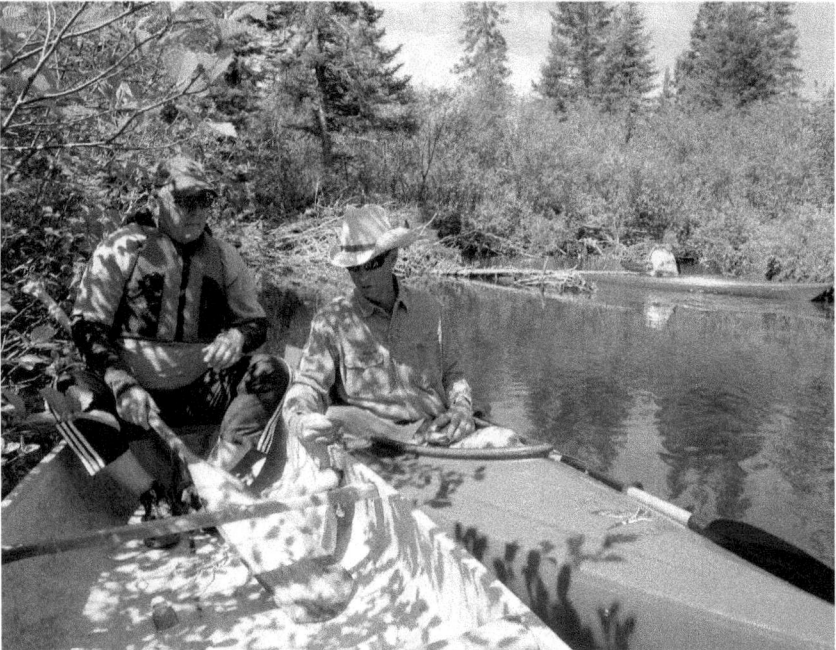

Beaver Lodge in East Inlet

18 Mile Moose Alley

I get asked, "What is the best way to see moose in the Great North Woods?" My response is to drive Route 3 (the last 18 miles in NH is nick-named "Moose Alley") and when you spot a stopped car, pull up behind it, as they most likely have spotted moose.

It is safe to say, you will see moose everywhere – including in the middle of the highway – so be careful when driving anywhere in Pittsburg.

"Once you see one, you see them all" is not a valid expression with moose. Each time I see a moose it is a thrill – however, do not get close as these are huge animals. An adult moose can stand close to seven feet high at the shoulder, and males (or "bulls") can weigh as much as 1,500 lbs. Females with a calf are especially dangerous, and during rutting season, a male moose may charge anything. A word to the wise.

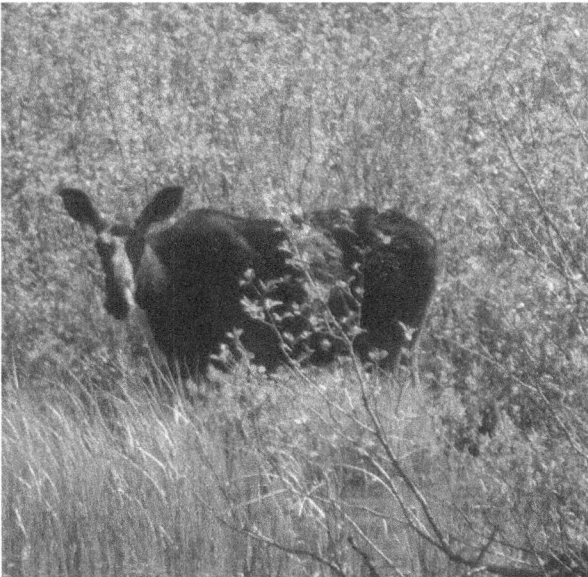

Moose - Scotts Bog from My Canoe

Never say, "I wish I had been to the Great North Woods of New Hampshire"

Video Reference Planning a Paddle to Connecticut Lakes and Lake Francis

- Blog: Paddling the Great North Woods of New Hampshire
  http://outdooradventurers.blogspot.com/2009/04/paddling-and-hiking-connecticut-lakes.html
- Lake Francis State Park
  http://www.nhstateparks.org/explore/state-parks/lake-francis-state-park.aspx
- Buck Rub Pub
  http://www.buckrubpub.com/
- Youngs Store
  http://www.yelp.com/biz/youngs-store-pittsburg
- Connecticut Lakes – Canoe and Kayaks
  http://www.paddling.net/places/showReport.html?450
- Moose
  http://en.wikipedia.org/wiki/Moose#Size_and_weight
- Connecticut Lakes
  http://en.wikipedia.org/wiki/Connecticut_Lakes

Never say, "I wish I had swum across Perkins Pond"

Enjoy a description of seven friends doing a group endurance swim of nearly one mile at Perkins Pond, Sunapee, NH.

The swimmers, accompanied by a safety boat, go across the pond, around a raft, and then return back to the start. The swim takes approximately 40 minutes. The video describes the requirements the athletes must meet before they can swim with the group.

The maps, pictures, and video show snippets of the swim and will give you an "up front and personal" perspective.

The history of this swim started when my 7 and 8 year old boys, Shaun and Tim, asked to drive our 6 horsepower motorboat by themselves. Cathy and I knew the boys could swim, but if an emergency should occur in the boat, we were unconvinced about their ability to swim a long distance to shore.

We told the boys they could only take the boat alone if they could swim across Perkins pond, and then swim back, all without a life vest. Of course we would accompany them by boat to insure their safety.

Our challenge proved to be an incentive for these young boys to improve and practice their swimming skills. Later that summer they fulfilled their swim agreement, and they were allowed to use the boat, wearing a life vest, by themselves.

Now, with close friends and family, we annually gather to repeat this original challenge – and this time with our grandchildren.

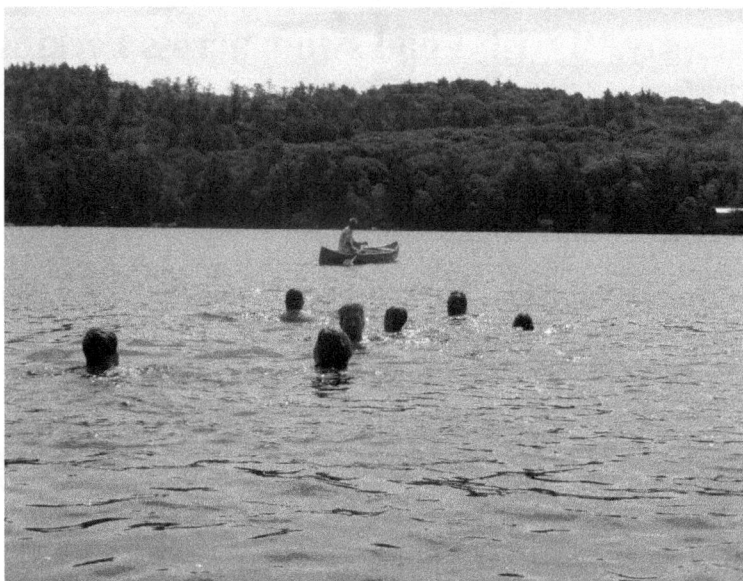

**The Swimmers Watched by a
Canoe Lifeguard Carrying Life Jackets**

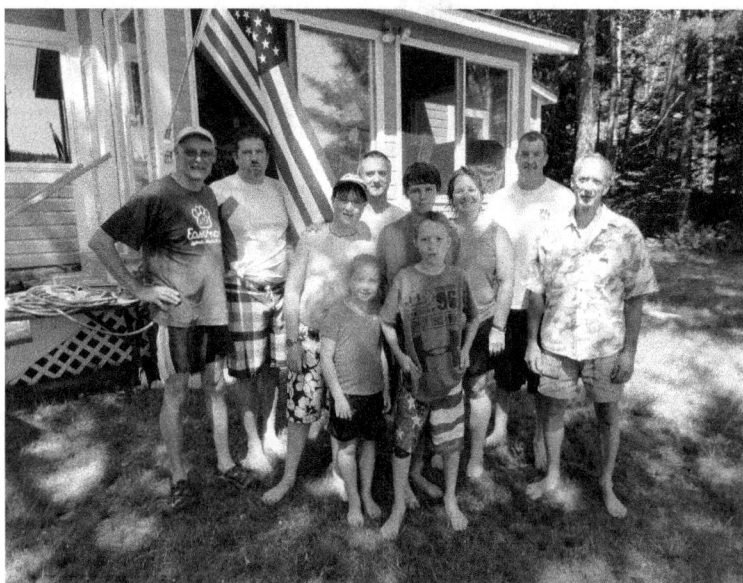

The Swimmers & Lifeguards After Their Annual 1 Mile Swim

Whether as a swimmer or supporter, enjoying the outdoors with friends and family is something you do to never have to say, **"I wish I had swum across Perkins Pond."**

Video Reference Swimming Across Perkins Pond
- **Blog: A Family Swim**
  http://outdooradventurers.blogspot.com/2010/07/never-say-i-wish-i-had-swum-across.html
- **Video The Swim**
  http://www.youtube.com/watch?v=6NGRfADxPVU&feature=player_embedded

---

A Hike to Table Rock, Dixville, New Hampshire

Please join me in a hike to Table Rock in Dixville Notch, NH.

My wife Cathy and I spent an enjoyable three days at the magnificent Balsams Grand Hotel Resort, located in the great north woods of New Hampshire. Looking out the window from our room, I was enticed to hike to Table Rock.

Table Rock is without question the scariest, most spectacular overlook of my New Hampshire hiking experiences. Table Rock is the tip of a chiseled natural elevation that towers over the Dixville Notch highway. Table Rock jets out at the highest point of the Notch, seemingly a sentry guarding the Balsams property hundreds of feet below it. On a clear day, the view from Table Rock can include the mountains of Canada, Vermont, and Maine.

Reaching Table Rock requires a one plus hour uphill climb on a narrow tree-canopied forest trail with 30 – 50 degree grades with rocks, roots, streams, and mud.

A Mount Monadnock in Vermont and in New Hampshire

Our guide mentions in the blog post that on a clear day you can see Mt Monadnock. Huh? Can you really see Mount Monadnock from Table Rock? To some this may be an odd question, but yes, there is a Monadnock in northeastern Vermont and a Mount Monadnock in southern New Hampshire.

Vermont's Mount Monadnock (3,148 foot elevation) is located near the Canadian border in northeastern Vermont. To get to the trailhead for Vermont's Mt Monadnock - Follow Rte. 3 north to Colebrook NH - go past the intersection with Rte. 26 and take your next left onto Bridge Street. Cross the river into Vermont and take a left onto Rte. 102. Take your first left into the gravel pit. Follow the road to the left and park just before the sign Vehicles are not allowed beyond this point. Head up the road on foot and turn left at the trailhead sign. Follow the trail and then head to the right corner where you will see a blue surveyor mark at the start of the trail. http://en.wikipedia.org/wiki/Monadnock_Mountain_(Vermont) and http://www.rbhayes.net/monadnock.html.

New Hampshire's Mount Monadnock (3,165 feet elevation) is located near the central Massachusetts border just east of Keene, New Hampshire. There are trails to the Mt Monadnock summit from virtually any of the roads surrounding the mountain.

To reach the New Hampshire Mt Monadnock area see information and directions at http://www.qcc.mass.edu/brink/trav-rec/mt_monad/directions_to_mt.htm) and http://en.wikipedia.org/wiki/Mount_Monadnock

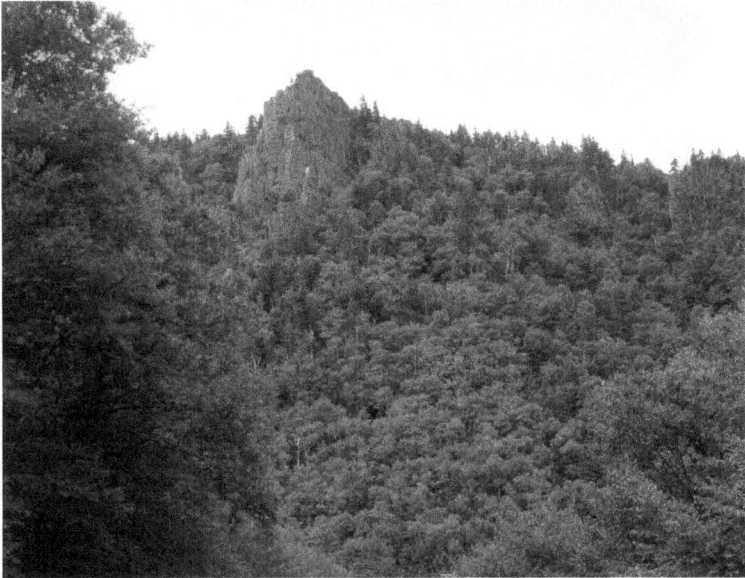

Outcrop of Table Rock from Dixville Notch Road

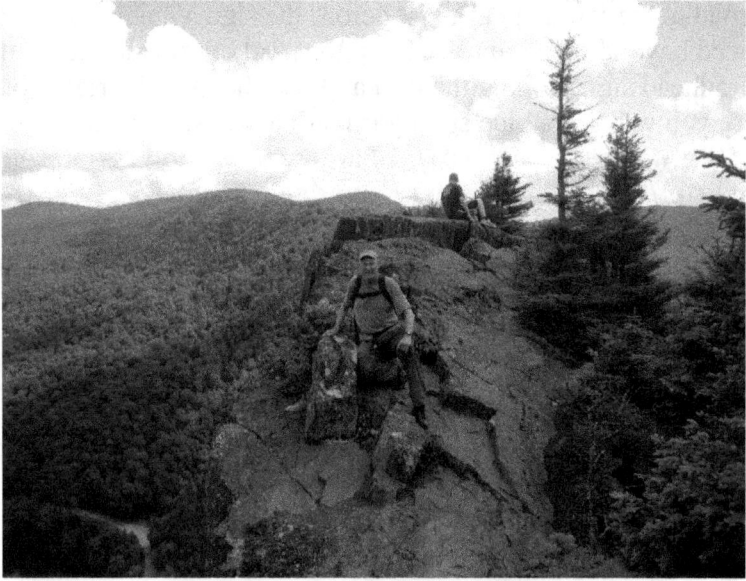

Sitting on Table Rock Outcrop

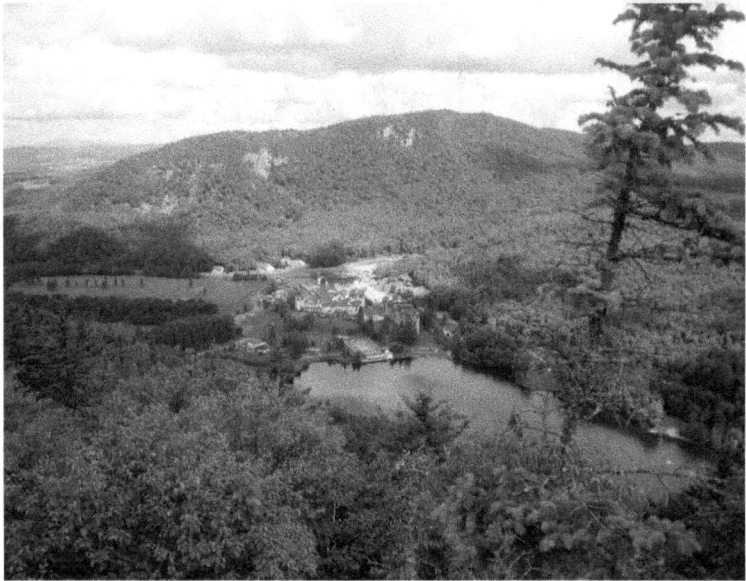

Looking Northwest at Balsams Grand Resort

Cohos Trail

Table Rock is located at a junction of the Cohos Trail (http://www.cohostrail.org/). The Cohos Trail is a rugged isolated wildness trail, similar in concept to the Appalachian Trail and Vermont's Long trail.

The Cohos Trail is a hiking trail running 162 miles through northern New Hampshire to the Canadian border at the Connecticut lakes area of Pittsburgh, NH. Certainly the Cohos Trail is something an avid hiker needs to "bag".

Never say, "I wish I had hiked to Table Rock.

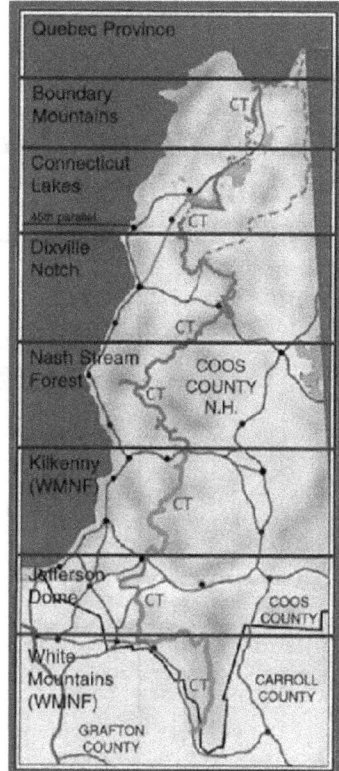

Video Reference Hike to Table Rock Dixville, NH
- **Blog: TableRock**
  http://outdooradventurers.blogspot.com/2010/07/hike-to-table-rock-dixville-new.html

- **Video Table Rock**
  http://www.youtube.com/watch?feature=player_embedded&v=S87AKkLEFeU
- **Cohos Trail**
  http://www.cohostrail.org/

Hiking Mount Chocorua - White Mountain National Forest

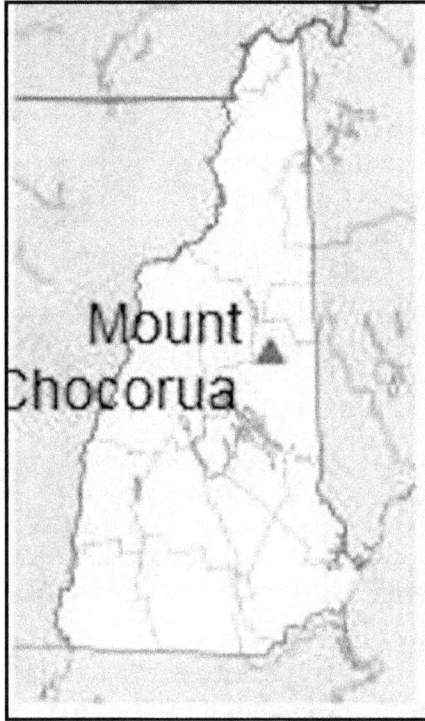

We do 360 degree turns in the middle of Champney Falls with arms lifted knowing if this were springtime we would be engulfed within a roaring waterfall dropping hundreds of feet! We see majestic Mt Washington with its Presidential brethren - over twenty-five miles away! Breathtakingly, Lake Chocorua is thousands of feet below from where we had stopped hours before for pictures of where we now stand on Mt Chocorua.

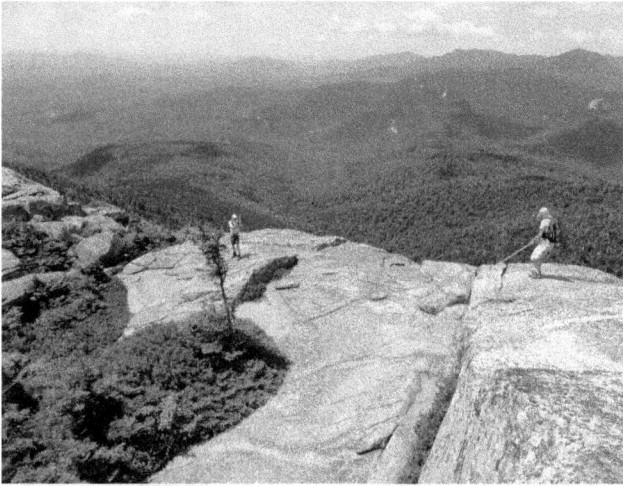

A View of White Mountains from Mt Chocorua

For years I have viewed Mt Chocorua as I motored along the Kancamagus highway, drove south from Conway on Route 16, or viewed this magic mountain while watching dogsledding on Lake Chocorua. I asked, "What mountain is that?", and in response to "Mt Chocorua," I say, "If opportunity presents I want to hike it".

Well, opportunity presents only when you make it happen. I asked my friend George if he wanted to hike Chocorua, he said "yes", followed by Dundee's immediate response of "Absolutely".

Mt Chocorua Statistics and Trail Choice

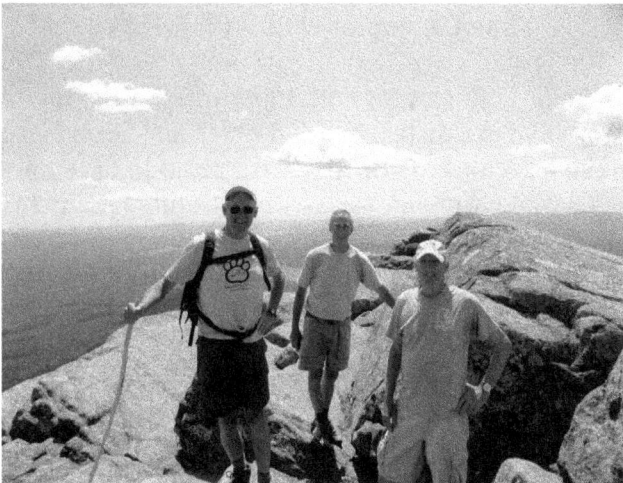

While Mt Chocorua at 3,480 feet is not one of the prized 4,000-foot peak-bagger mountains in New Hampshire, its rocky summit is readily visible from all directions. Viewed from the South at Chocorua Lake it appears as a rock pyramid, from the East it is more like a camel's hump, and from the North a shark's fin. (http://en.wikipedia.org/wiki/Mount_Chocorua).

Six major trails lead to the top of the mountain. We chose Champney Falls Trail.

Champney Falls Trail

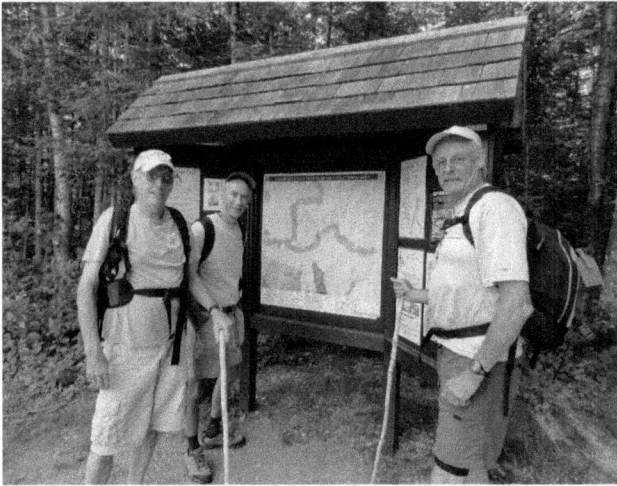
The Champney Falls Trailhead

Champney Falls Trail merges with Piper trail for the final ascent. The one-way hike is a distance of 3.8 miles and 2300 feet elevation gain from the Kancamagus Highway trailhead to the summit of Mt Chocorua. Our hike time for the ascent was three hours, whereas our descent was two and a half hours.

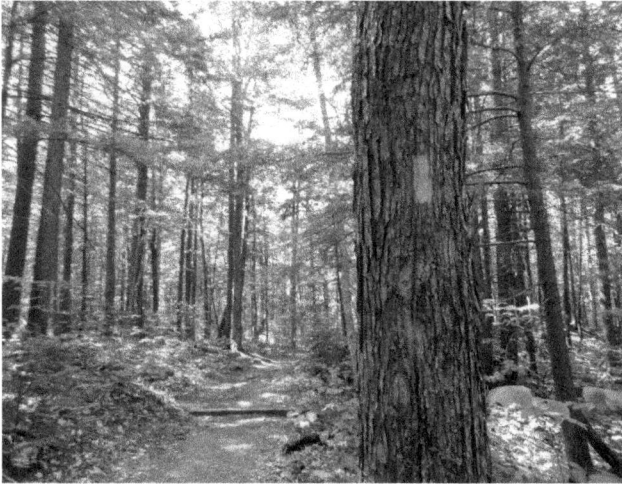
The Trail is this way! Follow the Painted Strips.

We follow a yellow paint stripe trail sign. Above tree line all trails join in a single jagged rock path requiring scrambling and extensive use of hands, planting of feet against boulders for more lift traction. Being hesitant about heights, I resist the urge to look down into the drop-off. Close to the top the yellow markers are faded and harder to see, and we often guess whether we are on the correct trail, and then once again we spot the bleached and nearly unrecognizable yellow stripe. Whew.

The last hundred yards finds you surrounded above and below by massive granite rock. You look up toward the seemingly far away Mt Chocorua summit, and second-guess yourself as to whether you can reach it.

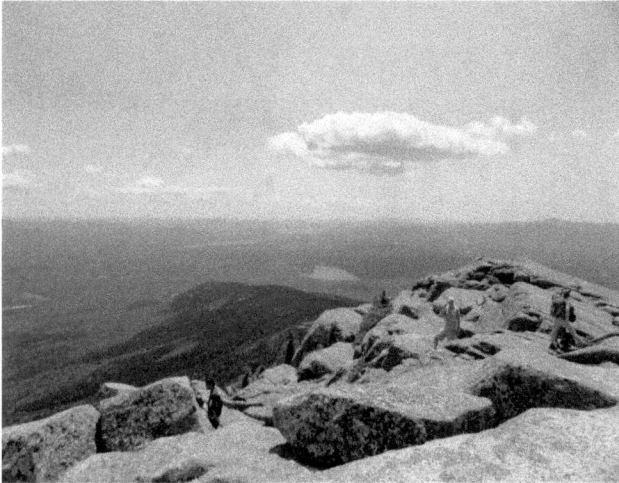
A Magnificent View from the Peak of Mt Chocorua

Mount Chocorua Name History

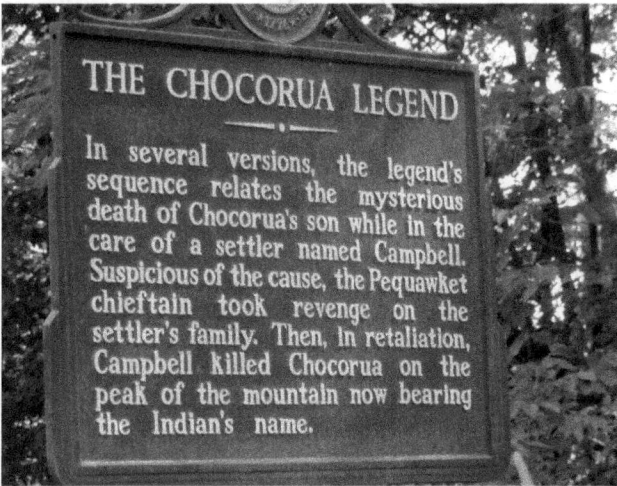

THE CHOCORUA LEGEND

In several versions, the legend's
sequence relates the mysterious
death of Chocorua's son while in the
care of a settler named Campbell.
Suspicious of the cause, the Pequawket
chieftain took revenge on the
settler's family. Then, in retaliation,
Campbell killed Chocorua on the
peak of the mountain now bearing
the Indian's name.

As noted on the Wikipedia web site, there are many versions of
the Chocorua legend, one of which is displayed on a historical
marker near Chocorua Lake.

Special Memories

- Standing in the middle of Champney Falls with its hundred
  plus foot drop.

- A Mother Black bear and her cub ran across our trail.

- The last few hundred foot climb of Chocorua is grabbing ledges, positioning my feet, and pushing myself up, then re-grabbing, positioning feet, and pushing again, etc.

- Standing on a cloudless seventy-degree day on the summit of Mt Chocorua with a 360-degree view that includes northern New Hampshire's presidential range, lakes and peak bagger mountains. (In northern New England peak bagger mountains are considered to be over 4,000 feet.)

- This hike in wet weather would be extremely slippery and not recommended for the beginning hiker.

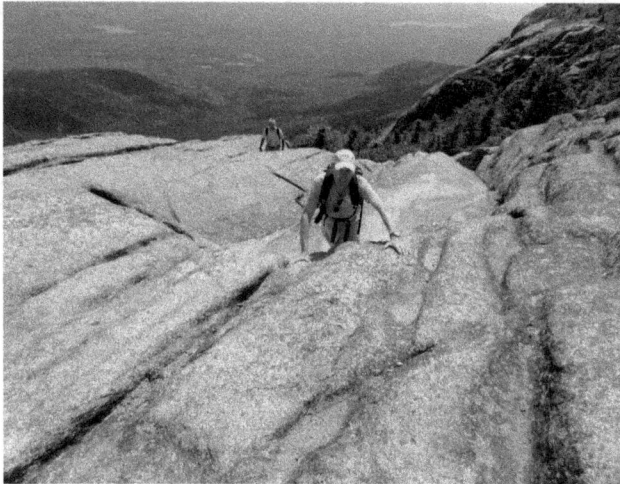

A few more feet to the top

Now, George, Dundee and I never have to say, **"We wish we had hiked Mt Chocorua!"**

Video References
- Blog: Climbing Mt Chocorua in White Mountain National Forest
  http://outdooradventurers.blogspot.com/201 1/08/hiking-mount-chocorua-white-mountain.html

---

Kayaking on Cape Cod at the Great Salt Marsh

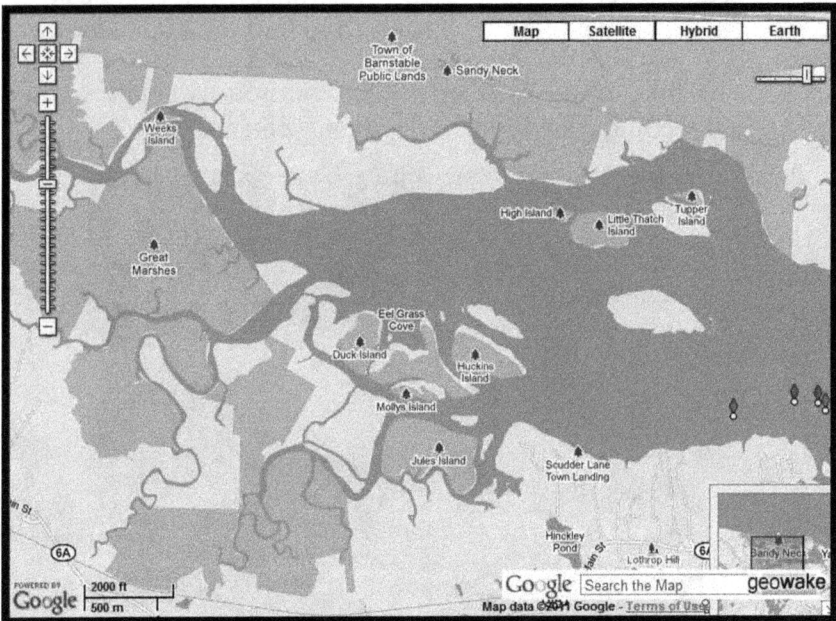

- Our friend John invited Dundee, my son Tim, and me for a day's kayak paddle near John's Cape Cod home. We expected an easy paddle in Barnstable Harbor's protected waters.

  The 11 AM put-in at Scudder Lane's paved ramp began an hour before low tide. Due to winds of 10 to 15 miles per hour, mixed with the change to incoming tide, we experienced choppy water and one to two-foot waves -- and a somewhat exciting paddle.

  We had light winds as we crossed the harbor to Sandy

Neck and paddled along its beautiful sand beach. We saw
the power of the ocean on the great salt marsh as you will
see in the below video of chunks of sand being pulled into
the bay.

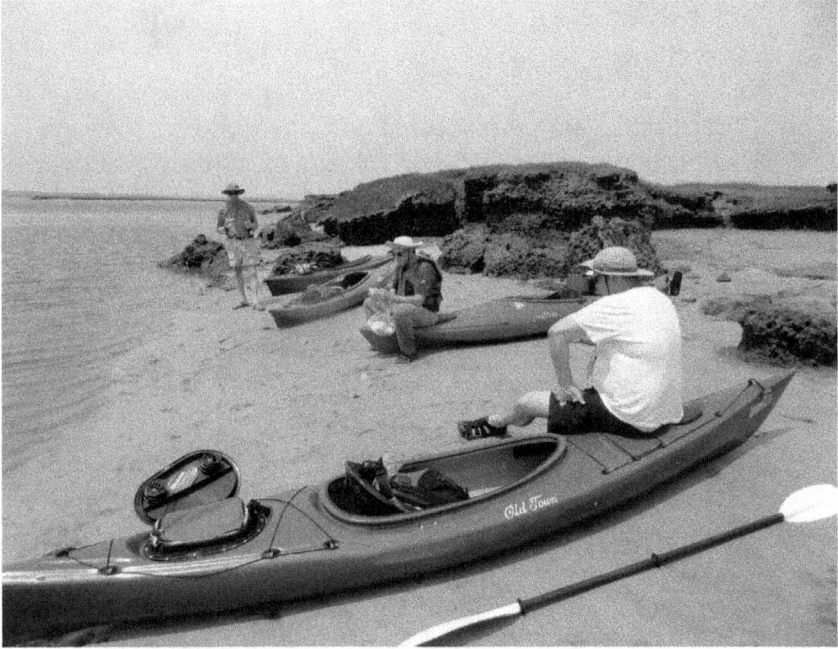

- We walked on Sandy Neck beach – and this required
  pulling our kayaks over low tide sand bars.

- We did not paddle the extreme marshes as low tide left
  only mud lanes like quick sand. Our brief venture into the
  marsh required stepping ashore and going through one to
  two foot-deep mud to get to the high water grass. My water
  sandals were nearly lost as the sucking mud would only
  release my feet after I removed my sandals.
- When the tide changed, we experienced tidal phenomena at
  spots where low water sand bars and deep water met. You
  will see in this brief video water frothing, similar to white
  water flowing over rocks – but rocks were not present.
  Indeed I was at first hesitant to cross this very real white
  line, but after passing through a few of these areas I
  realized the froth was only the outgoing and incoming

135

water meeting on the low tide turn.
- We paddled by oyster farmers "up close and personal" as they cultivated their oyster beds.
- Our water tour of Barnstable Harbor and its Great Salt Marsh lasted four and a half hours.

Directions:

"Barnstable Harbor is located on Cape Cod Bay between the barrier beach of Sandy Neck and an extensive saltmarsh estuary between Sandwich and the Cape Cod Canal to the northeast and Wellfleet to the southeast. It's roughly nine nautical miles from the entrance of the Cape Cod Canal to Barnstable Harbor.

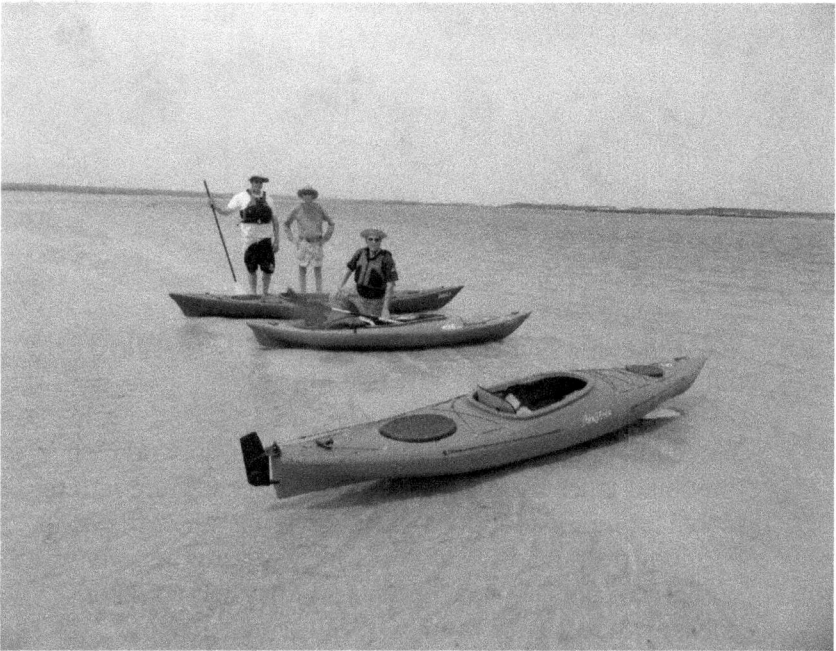

It's important to note the tide and weather conditions. If it's particularly nasty, you may not want to go because of the Barnstable Harbor entrance is shallow water and east-west tidal currents that shift north to south in the harbor channel. A tidal range of nearly 10 feet makes the harbor prone to shoaling and sandbars. It is best to enter the harbor on a rising tide. Once in the harbor channel, stay well within the markers, as the areas off Beach Point and Sandy Neck Light are very shallow and prone to strong currents.

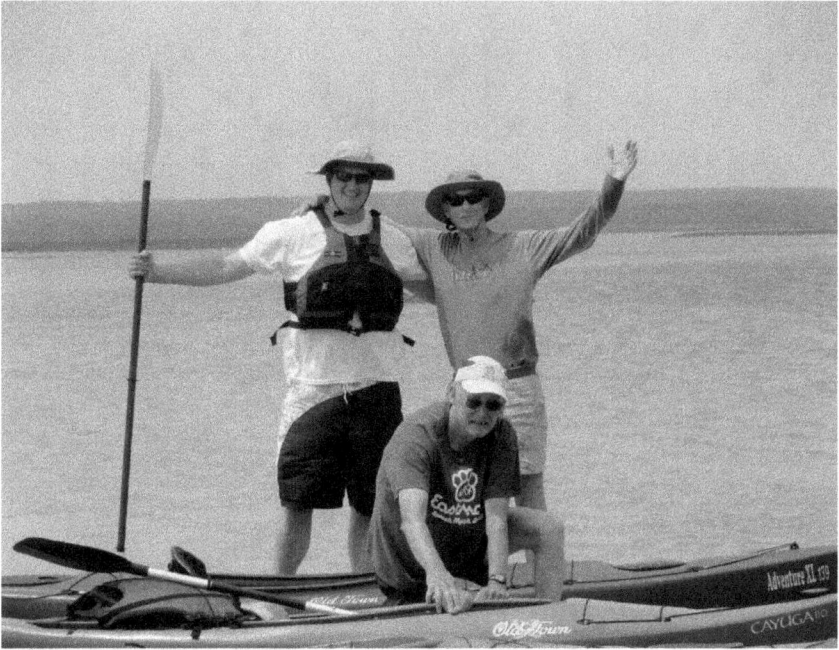

Nearby Scudder Lane has a paved ramp that launches into the harbor, but it has limited parking. Finally, while boaters would be wise to avoid Barnstable Harbor's tricky network of creeks and marshland, kayakers and paddlers will love it. However, if embarking on an unguided trek, be sure to take along a GPS and/or a cell phone, as it's easy to become stranded or lost in the Great Marshes' maze of creeks. Use NOAA chart 13251."

I never have to say, "I wish I had kayaked the Great Salt Marsh of Cape Cod"

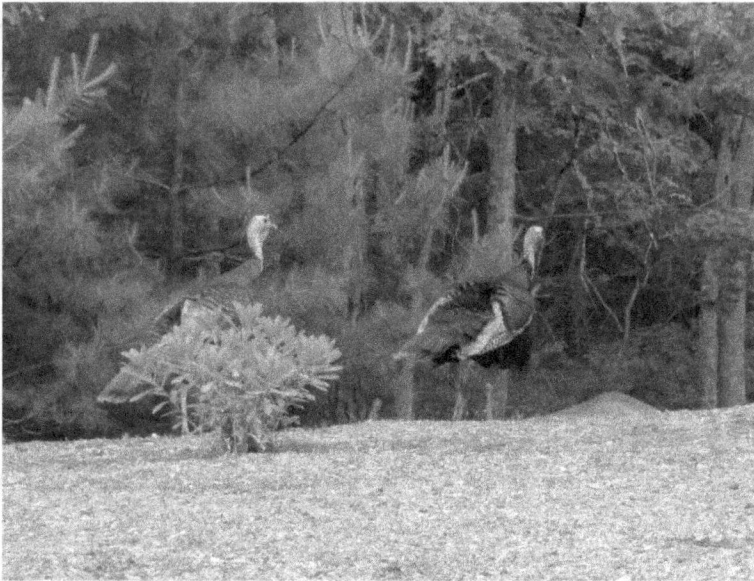

Yes, there are Turkeys on Cape Cod

Read more at:

- http://www.trails.com/tcatalog_trail.aspx?trailid=CGN029-026
- http://www.greatmarshkayaktours.com/naturalists_dream_tour.htm

---

Video References Kayaking on Cape Cod

- Blog: Kayaking on Cape Cod at the Great Salt Marsh
  http://outdooradventurers.blogspot.com/2011/06/kayaking-in-barnstable-harbor-and-great.html
- Kayaking at Cape Cod's Great Salt Marsh
  http://www.youtube.com/watch?v=4x8vx6J8Kzk&feature=player_embedded

---

Camp OutdoorSteve Training Youth in Canoe Rescue

An afternoon learning canoe rescue and self-confidence.

My teenager grandson was visiting our camp in Sunapee, NH. We were sitting around a campfire with his Sunapee friends. In the course of our campsite storytelling, I shared with them my experience participating in a canoe rescue on one of my paddling trips to the Allagash Wilderness Waterway of Maine.

The message I wanted to convey to these youths was, "practice makes perfect."

Briefly, on a canoe trip to the 34 mile Moose River Bow Trip, two of our group flipped their canoe in the middle of Holeb Pond. My friend John and I were nearby, and we quickly paddled over, tied a rope to the overturned canoe, and towed them to shore – an exhausting paddle that took nearly a half hour. My cousin Linwood, a Master Maine Guide, asked, "Why did you not rescue them?" My response was, "We did!"

Linwood then proceeded to tell us we should have righted the swamped canoe in the middle of the lake – and at our next campsite he would teach us how to do this.

The next day for nearly four hours, myself and six companions, under the tutelage of Linwood, learned and practiced two types of canoe rescue scenarios:

1) Two or more canoes are paddling together and one flips over. An upright canoe assists the capsized canoers by righting their boat, retrieving their gear, and standing by while they re-enter their boat (even in deep water)
2) Two paddlers, alone, flip their canoe and need to upright it without outside help.

Interestingly - and here was my message to the youths about "practice makes perfect" - the next year myself with the same group of friends were paddling across Eagle Lake on the Allagash Wilderness Waterway. Suddenly, one of our canoes capsized in the middle of the one-mile wide lake.

By the time we reached them, the two occupants were swimming holding onto the canoe with their tents, food, and other camping gear drifting nearby (all protected by dry bags). With hardly a word said, this group, who had practiced the canoe rescue the prior year, immediately began their learned "two or more canoers paddling together" rescue technique. Within minutes, both paddlers were back in their canoe with their gear intact, and we continued to our next campsite. Thus, the message is "practice makes perfect."

Camp OutdoorSteve Teaching "Practice Makes Perfect" Canoe Rescues

The next day after this heroic fireside chat, my grandson and his friends knocked on my door asking if they could learn the canoe rescue. The below sequence of pictures and the following video is a wonderful afternoon of fun and learning. Most importantly, it demonstrated the value of practice and the resulting self-confidence if one day they face what might be a real canoe rescue situation.

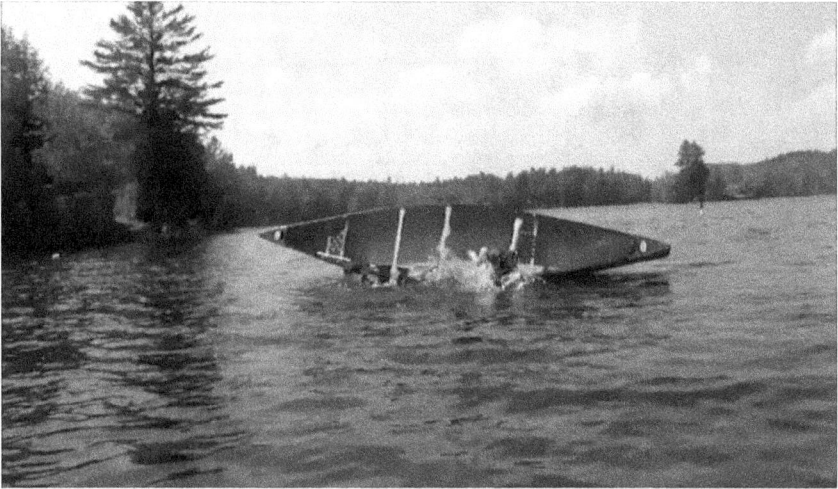
The Flip!

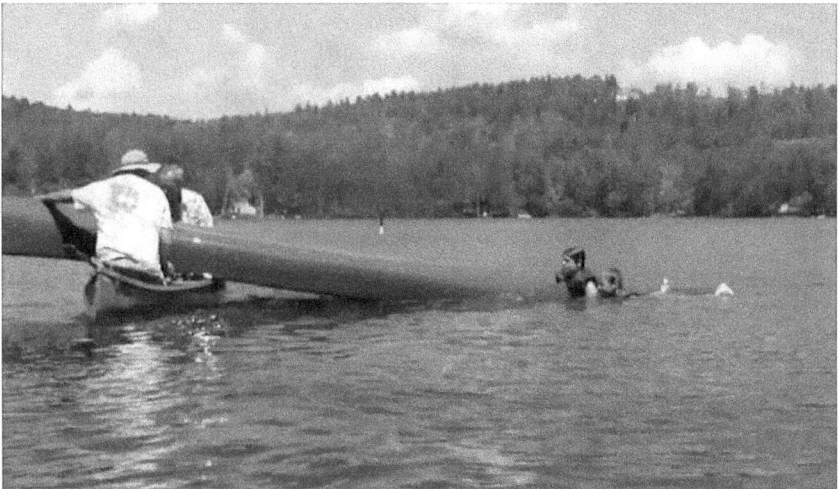
Emptying the Canoe of Water

The two paddlers in the water get on one end of the overturned canoe and push down until the other end of the canoe releases its vacuum and rises out of the water. The canoe is then pulled onto the rescue boat and slid perpendicular across to its midpoint (i.e. no water in the canoe).

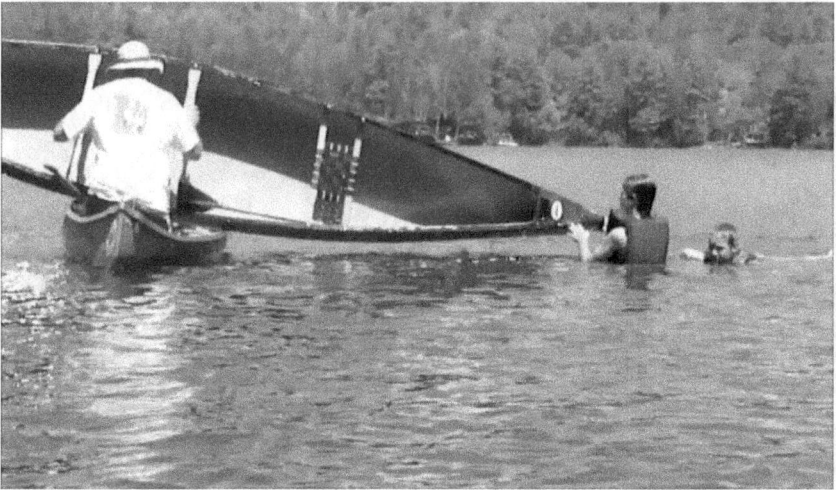

The Canoe is Rolled Right-Side up and Slid into the Water

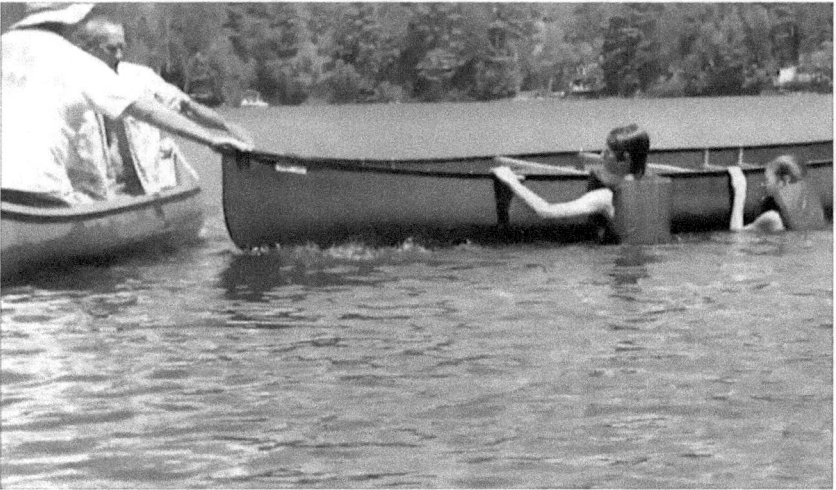

Dry Canoe is Brought Alongside the Rescue Boat (Parallel) and Braced by the Rescuers While the Swimmers Climb Back in from the Side.

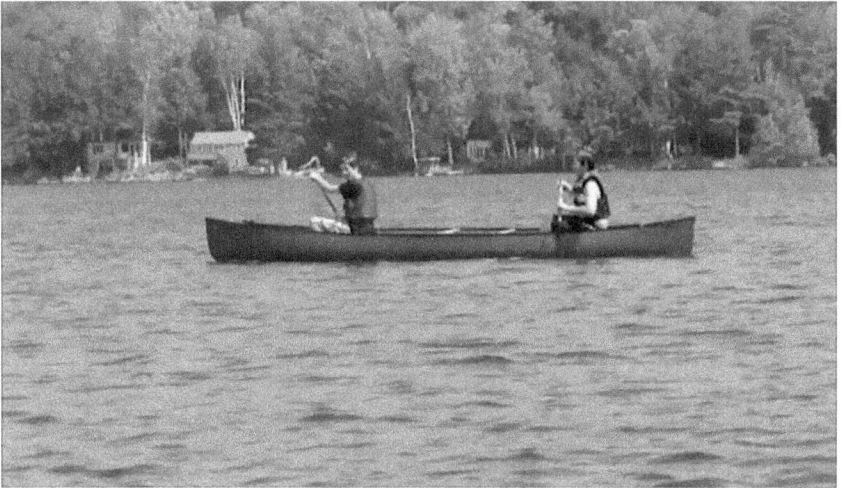

Away They Go!

Practice – Practice – Practice – Then the Actual Rescue is Easy.

> **Video Reference Practicing the Canoe Rescue at Perkins Pond**
> http://youtu.be/gRFsWovoQ3g

Fall

The roads are lovely dark and deep. But I have promises to keep, and miles to go before I sleep, and miles to go before I sleep. – Robert Frost

Touching a Paddle in the Boundary Waters of Minnesota

Cathy said, "I want to visit Minnesota". So off we went.

We flew to Minneapolis, rented a car, and spent seven days traveling in northeastern Minnesota. We saw beautiful country, visited unique places in the Lake Superior area, and most of all we met wonderful Minnesotans. We now have new friends and great memories of Minnesota and the Boundary Waters Canoe Area Wilderness (BWCAW).

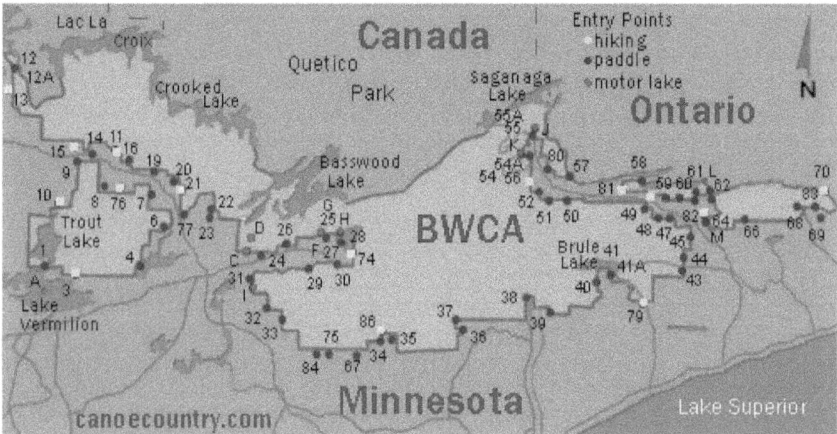

The BWCAW is a region of wilderness straddling the Canada–United States border between Ontario and Minnesota. It is composed of over 1 million acres of forests and thousands of miles of water routes. No motorized vehicles or boats are allowed within the perimeters of the wilderness area. Permits are required for all visitors to the BWCA. A limited number of permits grant access to each BWCAW entry point.

Cathy and I spent three days in Ely, Minnesota at the Blue Heron Bed and Breakfast, close to entrance 31 of the BWCAW. Being in Ely provided us opportunities for:

- A two hour kayak paddle to South Farm Lake in the BWCAW

- A three hour canoe paddle from North Farm Lake into the Kawishiwi River, another entrance into the BWCAW

- Visiting the **International Wolf Center** to see wolves in a two acre habitat. Attend a Wolf Howling seminar.

- Visiting the **North American Bear Center** and seeing black bears in their natural environment

- An evening at a lakeside campfire learning how to "howl" like a wolf to see if we could get a reciprocal howl from wild wolves that may be nearby.

Enjoy our **Video References** below as Cathy and I share a taste of the boundary waters and the Ely attractions. Two of our Minnesota friends will give you an upfront demonstration of wolf howling.

Next September friends and I will never have to say, "We wish we had paddled a week in the Boundary Waters Canoe Area Canoe Area Wilderness."

To get more information on the boundary waters visit:

- **BoundaryWatersCanoeArea.com**
  http://www.BoundaryWatersCanoeArea.com

- **Discover Ely, MN**
  http://www.wolf.org/wolves/visit/visitingely.asp

- **CanoeKayak.com**
  http://www.canoekayak.com

International Wolf Center
http://www.wolf.org/wolves/

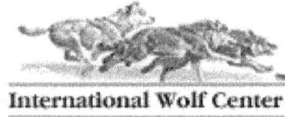
International Wolf Center

North American Bear Center
http://www.bear.org/website/

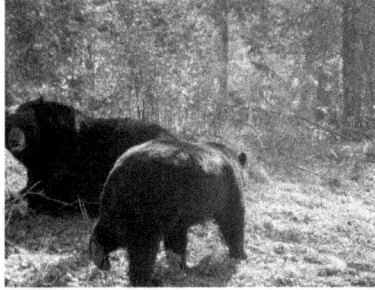

Video References: Researching a Trip to Minnesota's Boundary Waters

- **Blog: Touching a Paddle in the Boundary Waters**
  http://outdooradventurers.blogspot.com/2010/10/touching-paddle-in-boundary-waters-of.html
- **Wolf Howling, Ely, Black Bears and Boundary Water Research**
  http://www.youtube.com/watch?feature=player_embedded&v=PsWzoIYVwvA

Exploring Lake Umbagog – a Gem in the Great North Woods

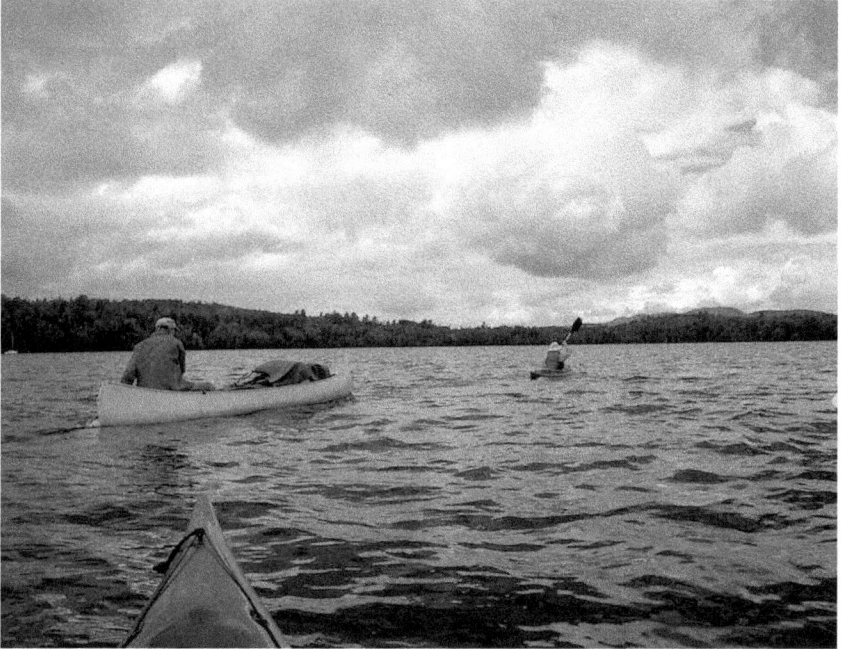

Ominous dark clouds were overhead. White caps on Lake Umbagog were building. The wind was gusting. Do John, Dundee and I continue paddling north three miles, or do we head back to our campsite?

We had left our Big Island remote camp two hours earlier paddling on the west shore of Lake Umbagog with the plan to reach the northern end of the eight mile long lake, and then return south to our campsite via the east shore. On the way we would explore the headwaters of the Androscoggin River and the terminus of the Magalloway River.

Fortunately, we heeded a fellow paddler's storm warning, and decided to do a one-mile paddle across the lake to Tyler Point before heading south. Or did we delay our turnabout too long?

Planning the Trip

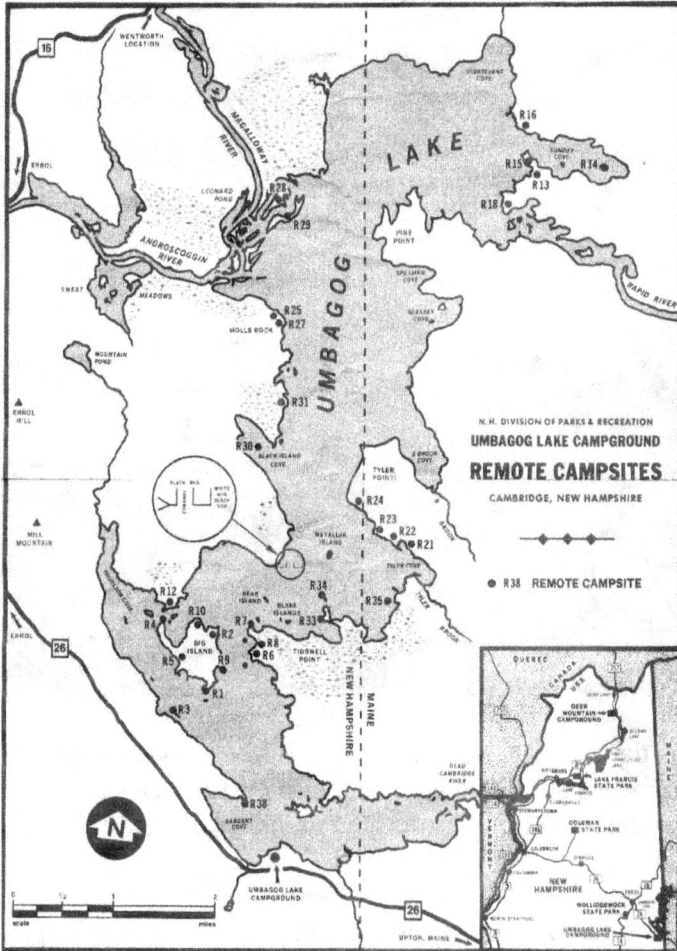

Weather is always a major consideration for us. Originally we planned to do a ten-hour hike in Baxter State Park, Maine to the terminus of the northern end of the Appalachian Trail. Two days of heavy weather were forecast, and we decided against this trek. Dundee suggested paddling Lake Umbagog. We went to www.weather.com/ and www.noaa.gov/ for satellite views, and our consensus was the weather would be light scattered showers in the Lake Umbagog area.

The weather in this region can change rapidly, and the literature notes the lake can become very challenging in moderate to high winds. Regardless, we decided it was a go!

Lake Umbagog

The Lake straddles the border between Maine and New Hampshire. Lake Umbagog is 7,850 acres with a north-south length close to eight miles. Using Google Earth (www.google.com/earth/index.html) we estimated at least 12 miles of paddling hugging the western shoreline to the northern terminus of the lake. Shoreline campsites are operated by the State of NH. The web site to make reservations is http://newhampshirestateparks.reserveamerica.com/

The Lake Umbagog State Park offers 34 remote campsites in isolated locations around the lake accessible only by boat. Wildlife viewing includes deer, moose, loons, eagles, osprey, and other varieties of birds.

For more information about canoeing and kayaking Lake Umbagog go to http://www.fws.gov/northeast/lakeumbagog/boating.html

To see a Lake Umbagog map with its 34 remote sites go to http://netrailhead.com/nh/sp/umbagog.html

The Trip - Day 1

We arrived at the Lake Umbagog State Park in early afternoon for three days of paddling and camping. Two park rangers welcomed us and were most accommodating. Upon our comment to them that we wanted to paddle the whole lake, and were seeking a remote site to help us accommodate our goal, they suggested campsite 4 on the north side of Big Island. Big Island is about three miles up the lake from our put-in at the southern tip of the lake.

Our paddling crafts: John (Old Town Cayuga 110 kayak), Dundee (Grumman 15' aluminum canoe) and I (Old Town Adventurer 139 kayak).

We paddled north near the western shore, and arrived at our campsite in about two hours. We set up our tents, including tarps over the camp table to protect us from rain. We started a fire in the fire ring, and relaxed to enjoy our earthly presence on this remote wilderness island.

Day 2

We awoke at 6 am. Chief Chef John made a delicious egg, bacon and cheese omelet wrapped in tortilla shells. These, along with Dundee's coffee, made a great start for the day. By 9 am we are paddling north along the western shore. The wind is calm and the water as smooth as glass.

Around 11 am we reach Black Island cove. The wind had begun to pick up and the lake became choppy with small waves forming. Fortunately, we heeded a camper's advice to abandon our trip north and to head back to camp as the wind was expected to increase and the already rough waters to build even higher. We still wanted to see as much of the southern half of the lake as we could, and we felt we could return safely on the eastern side of the lake. We paddled across the lake to Tyler Point with the easterly wind and with the waves at our backs. As Dundee said, "With the wind at our backs we were surfing fast across the tips of the wave crests. Yes, it was fantastic!"

We went ashore at Tyler Point, and there we introduced ourselves to Leonard and Camille, two brothers raised in the area. Leonard suggested on our return paddle we stop at Tyler Cove for a ¼ mile hike to a natural flowing spring.

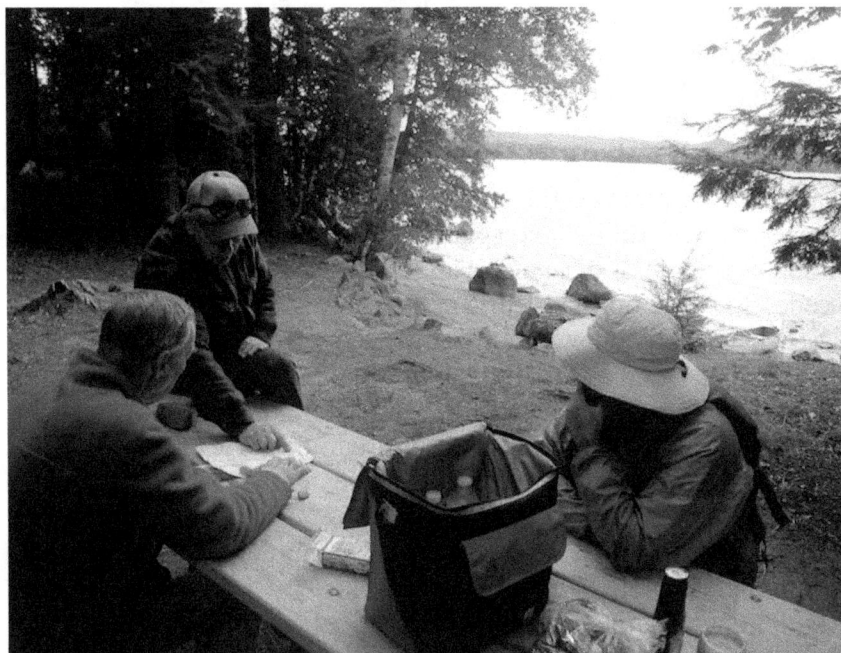

A Suggestion to Stop at Tyler Cove on Our Return Paddle

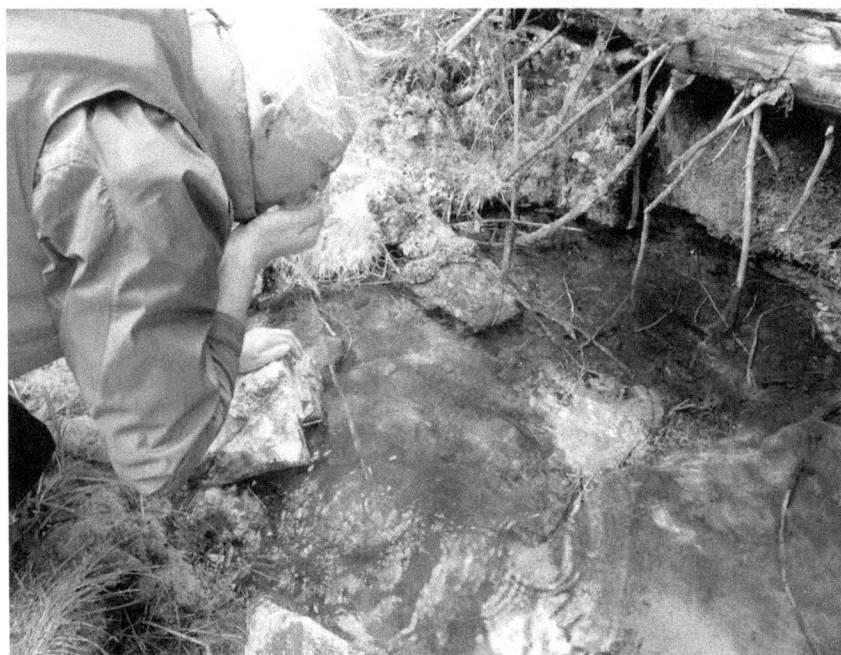

Sipping from the Fountain of Youth at Tyler Cove

The short hike to the spring at Tyler Cove was certainly worth our time, and as I scooped the delicious cold spring water into my mouth, I wondered if we had discovered the fountain of youth!

The wind was now gusting and causing us serious concerns, and the waves were rolling and splashing such that I had visions of an ocean launching of our kayaks and canoes at high tide. We now needed to prove our mettle to get back to our Big Island campsite. The wind was blowing directly at us, and we needed to go perpendicular to it in order to move south along the eastern shoreline. We used whatever protection from the shore and trees we could fine to minimize our exposure to the strong winds and heavy rain now blowing across the lake from the west.

Dundee had the toughest paddle, as his aluminum canoe was like a sail in the wind. He had to paddle with his bow into the wind, at a near 90 degree angle in order to go parallel with the shoreline and not get swamped by the pounding waves. His paddling expertise and confidence were apparent as he gently moved along the shoreline.

John and I pointed our kayaks at a 45 degree angle into the western wind in order move south. We both wore kayak skirts, but some water did manage to leak into our kayaks. Our hope was to not take on too much water in order to avoid the need to go ashore to bail the kayaks, or in the worst case end up being swamped. Bailing was nearly impossible in these winds and lake conditions, as constant paddling was needed to maintain both our direction and uprightness.

Indeed, after a three hour return paddle journey, we made it safely back to Big Island – a bit wet, but none-the-less without a "tip over". We had beaten the winds and white caps of Lake Umbagog.

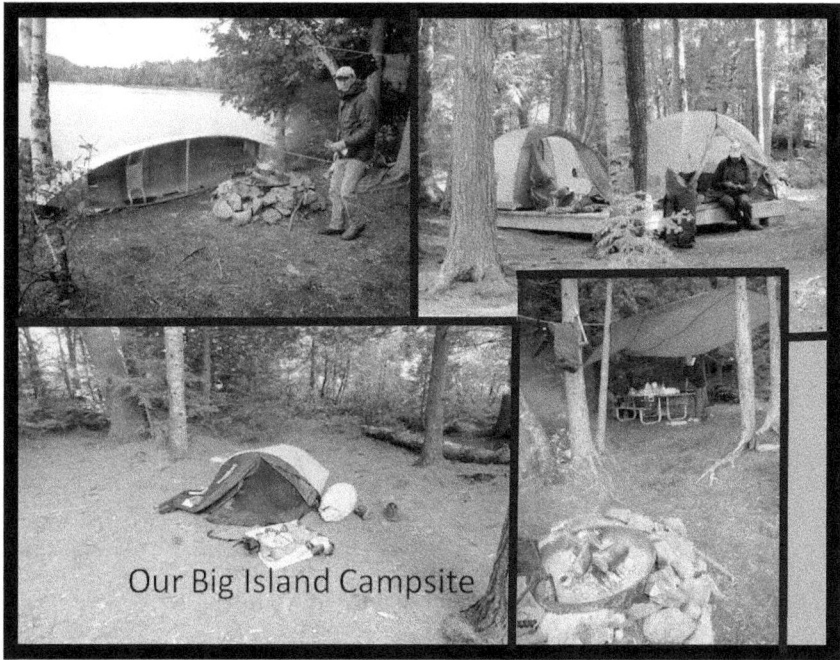
Our Big Island Campsite

We were drenched from the rain and water, and certainly cold, so once reaching our camp we immediately built a roaring campfire, changed into warm clothes, and boiled water for hot soup.

Never say, "I wish I had paddled Lake Umbagog".

We would certainly return to Lake Umbagog for another paddle to explore the northern half of the Lake, including the headwaters of the Androscoggin River to the Errol Dam, and the terminus of Lake Magalloway from the Lake Umbagog Wildlife Refuge on Route 16.

Certainly, we never have to say, *"I wish I had paddled Lake Umbagog."*

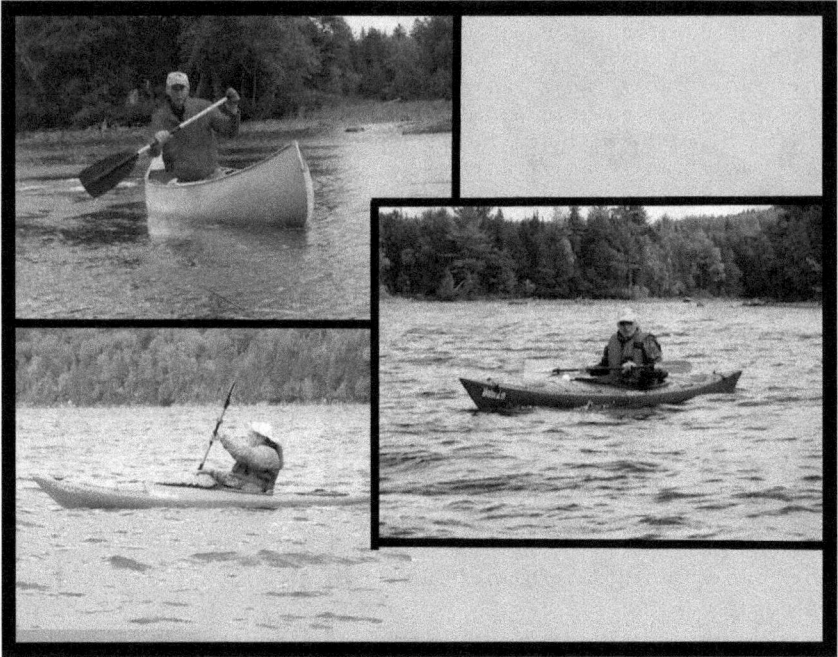
Paddling Lake Umbagog

Video Reference Lake Umbagog Paddle and Tenting
- Blog: Exploring Umbagog – a Gem in the Great North Woods
  http://outdooradventurers.blogspot.com/2010/09/exploring-lake-umbagog-gem-in-great.html

Paddling the Waters of Quetico Provincial Park in Ontario, Canada

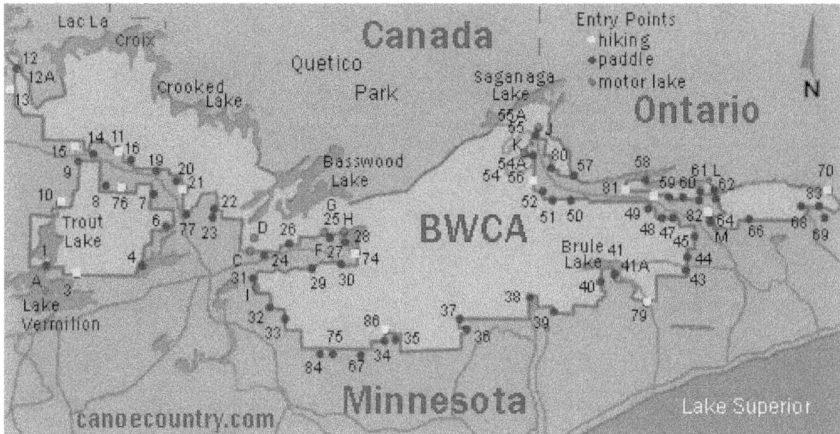

Quetico Provincial Park is a region of isolated Canadian wilderness straddling the Canada - United States border between southwestern Ontario and northern Minnesota. Quetico is composed of over 1 million acres of forests and thousands of miles of water routes. Permits are required for all visitors.

In mid-September three outdoor enthusiast friends and I paddled a six day 35 mile loop in the Quetico Provincial Park region of Ontario.

We all agreed we had the most physically and technically demanding portages we have ever attempted. We balanced these challenges against seeing some of the most beautiful wilderness, pristine water, and wildlife in the country. Indeed, the boundary waters provided us with a very memorable and impressive paddling experience.

The Portages

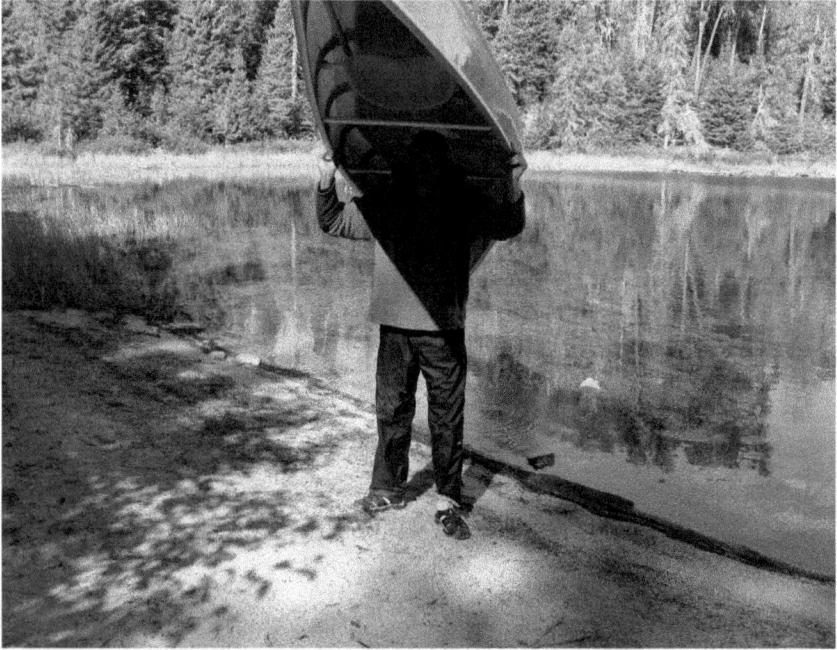

Notice the Shoulder Yoke for One Person to Carry a Canoe

We had seventeen portages for eight plus portage miles. (See the **Video References** below to see my spreadsheet for the lake sequences, their portages, and the portage distances).

My son Tim and I were in an 18' 6" 43 lbs kevlar ultra-light Wenona canoe, and Dundee and his son Paul in a similar model canoe. The portages were through dense woods with extremely narrow and rough granite rocks of all sizes and shapes, up and down hills, over fallen trees, mud, and water.

At each portage one person from each canoe carried the canoe on their shoulders using a leather padded neck yoke. I portaged the canoe 5 times, whereas Tim did the other 12 portages. Dundee and Paul likewise worked a similar type of division of labor to carry the canoe at each portage. Our backpacks (in each canoe - a food pack and two packs for each of our personal gear) averaged 50 plus lbs for the first few days until the food weight eased.

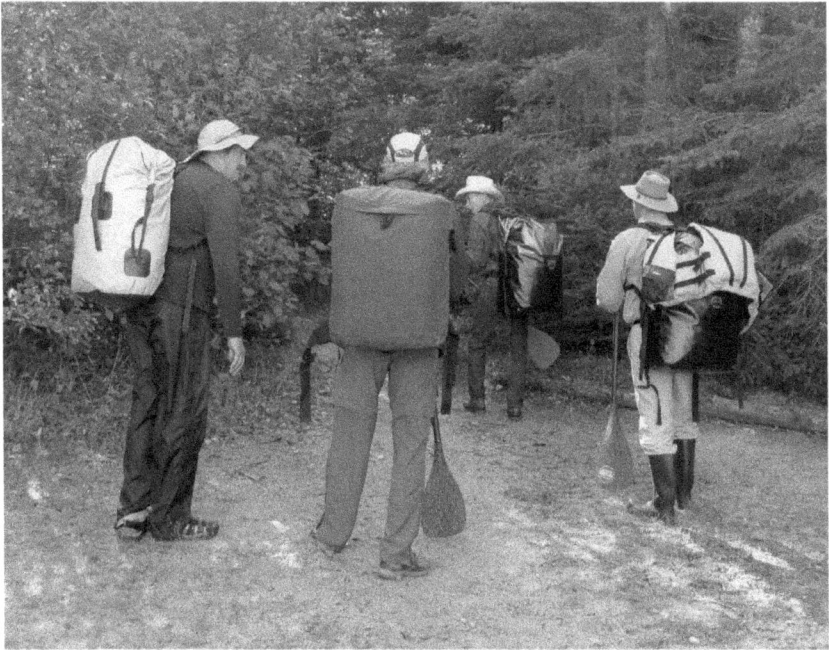
Beginning a Gear Portage

To get the full feel of our physical effort of the seventeen portages, you must realize the four of us had to make three trips each across the portage. Because of the narrow and rough terrain and its length, each canoe was carried by one person, while their canoe partner carried the food pack. We then returned over the portage for the remaining gear to carry our personal packs and other hand carried gear such as paddles, fishing poles, tent dry bag, and maps.

We had no injuries of hernia, sprained ankles or whatever. Amen!

As you see from the portage spreadsheet, our first day of paddling had the three longest portages, and since it was our first day, we had the heaviest weight of our entire trip. I must confess - after we selected a campsite on the Meadows Lake island, set up our tents, and went for a much needed refreshing swim - we all took a one hour nap. Exhaustion was upon us. Thereafter we began preparations for dinner.

Our Team

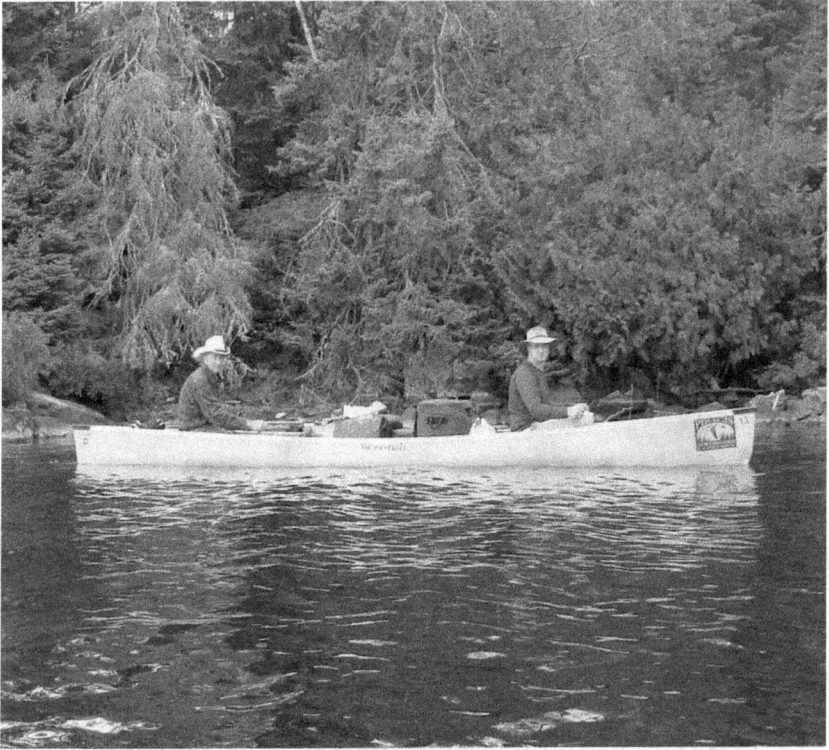

Dundee and Paul Paddling Lake Agnes

Paul, our Meal Planner and Chief Cook, did a fabulous job in providing wonderful meals. My son Tim shared with Paul the meal preparation, camp setups, cleanup, etc.

Dundee was the navigator with excellent map reading skills and keeping us on our water trail as we paddled through fifteen or so lakes. There were no trail signs or lake signs – our only guidance was the detail map and our compass showing the portages– and Dundee's innate sense of direction and recognition of where we were in reference to the map.

As the days passed, we realized we were following a waterway highway as we portaged from lake to lake in a very logical manner.

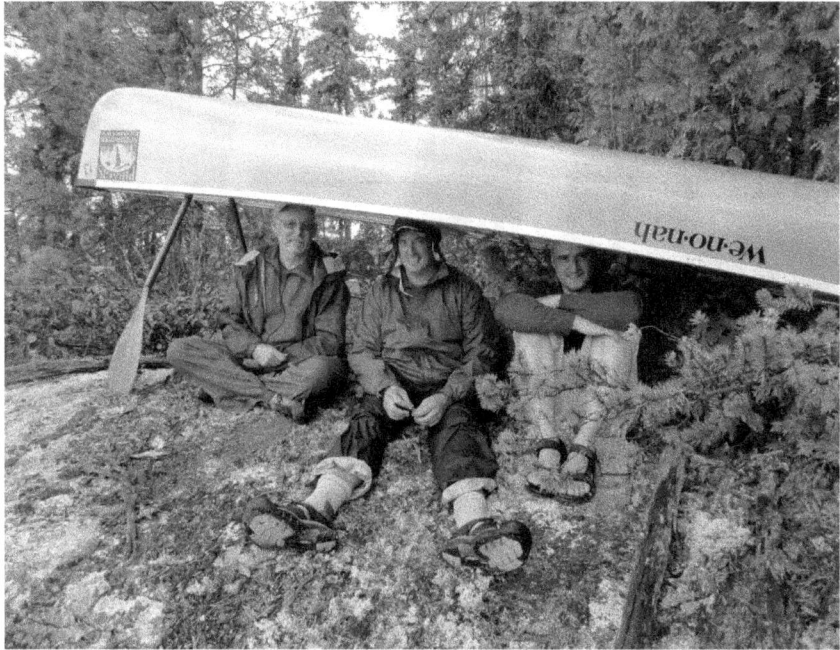

Just in Time to Get Out of the Rain/Snow Storm

On all five of our evenings we slept on islands - as we felt this would provide more security from bear and wolves.

Wildlife and Indian Pictographs
We saw a variety of wildlife, including eagles, loons, mink, beaver, otter, grouse, signs of moose, heard wolf calls, and had warnings of black bear from Quetico rangers, but no sightings.

We saw ancient Ojibwe Indian pictographs (paintings on the lakeside granite) and petroglyphs (images etched into the granite) along the lakeside cliffs. We had bought a book, **Magic on the Rocks** by Michael Furtman on the Pictographs of Quetico, and we read the book in camp to prepare ourselves with some education on these little understood Ojibwe artifacts (http://www.michaelfurtman.com/magic.htm).

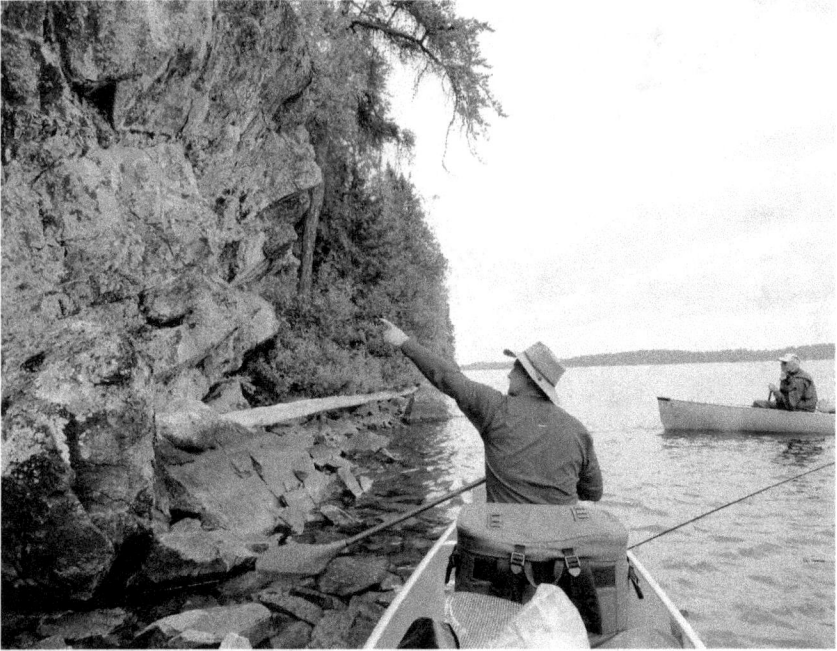
Paul Points to Ojibwe Pictographs

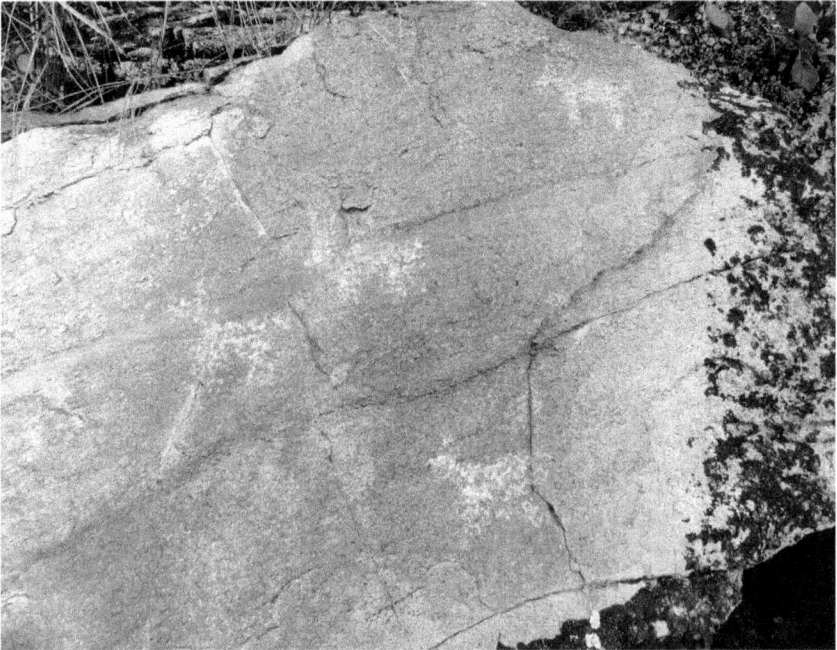
Can You See the Four Pictographs Paul Sees?

Louisa Falls
We swam the first two days – day one off our island campsite in Meadows Lake and the second day in the middle of Louisa Falls - a one-hundred foot waterfall flowing from Louisa Lake into Agnes Lake. Halfway down the falls is a neat natural bathtub including a stream of water for a great back massage from the rushing water into the tub.

The following day we had a brief flurry of snow and cold rain, and of course, swimming was over. We fished as we paddled, but caught nothing of a size we could eat.

Forest Fire
There was a massive forest fire in the area - we could see and smell distant smoke from our island campsite on Summer Lake, but we were not in any danger. The Quetico ranger at Prairie Portage told us they leave these most generally lightening started fires to burn out by themselves, as they are a natural process of the wilderness ecosystem.

Rough Water and Cold Weather

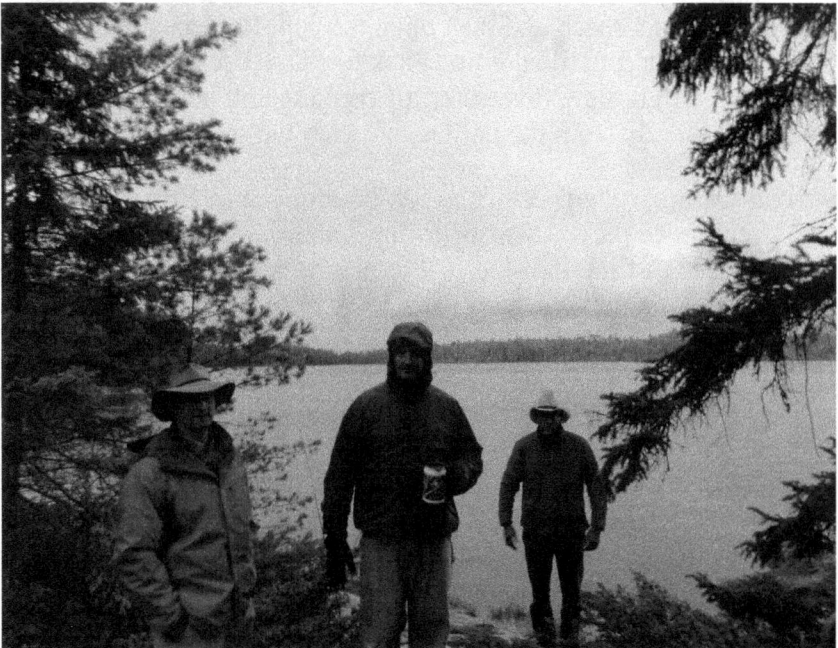

From Swimming Weather to Freezing Weather – Be Prepared!
We had three days of on and off heavy rain showers (including one shower of hailstones and snow) and 30 mph wind gusts and high waves as we crossed a few of the lakes. You ask, "Why did you cross in such rough conditions?" Well, we needed to seek a camp site for the night. These paddles absolutely required seasoned and strong paddlers, and thankfully we were all up to the task. There were no flips. Amen.

The Water
The Boundary Waters and Quetico lakes are pure, clear and pristine waters. Given the fact that the lakes were gouged out by the movement of mile thick glaciers thousands of years ago, the water depth frequently dropped off close to shore as the lakes were carved within granite mountains.

A question we frequently asked before the trip was "where do we get our drinking water while in the Quetico waters? Certainly boiling or purification tablets are the wisest recommendation for drinking any lake water. However, as we spoke to those who regularly paddle these waters, the feedback was "as you paddle in deep water, push your empty water containers as far down into the water as you can reach and then open the cap. Replace the cap before you bring the filled bottle back up. This became our choice, and along with boiling this water for cooking and hot beverages, we drank directly from the bottles in which we stored our water.

Start a Campfire with Flint, Steel, Tinder – and Practice
One evening we played "survivor man" and started our campfire solely by use of flint and steel. A shower of sparks is needed to start a fire along with proper tinder (http://survivalcache.com/fire-tinder/) and - practice, practice and practice. I had brought a **FireSteel Scout** tool (www.lightmyfire.com) composed simply of flint and steel.

It's about as basic a process as you can ask for... people have been lighting fires with flint and steel for many, many years. But, again, it does require practice and the use of both hands.

I did start the fire with this tool, but I won't be throwing away my lighter and hand washing alcohol until I practice some more. The **FireSteel** makes a handy item in my pack for emergency situations. It does work in wet weather, but, it does take a knack.

Paul was the expert in the group and below Paul demonstrates to how to start a fire with flint and steel. As Paul pointed out to us, the key is proper tinder (dried leaves, wood chips, or preferred if available, birch bark) – and practice, practice and more practice.

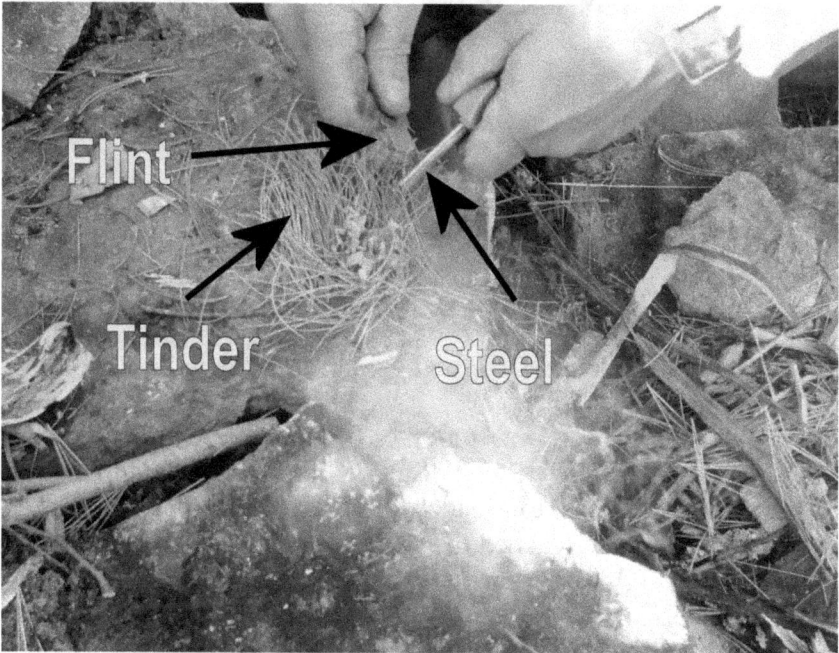

Flint, Steel and Tinder – and Practice

Trip Preparation

We entered the Canadian waters at the Prairie Portage location into Quetico Provincial Park via a water taxi tow on Moose Lake from Ely, MN. To assure the entry date we wanted we needed to apply for an entry permit five months before our preferred date. There is a limited number of entry permits for each day. Piragis Northwoods Company in Ely coordinated our permit application, outfitted us with two We-no-nah canoes, maps, food backpacks, and a large Duluth type backpack that could handle what I had originally packed into three dry bags. No motored vehicles or power boats are allowed within the Quetico wilderness area.

Our Paddling Route

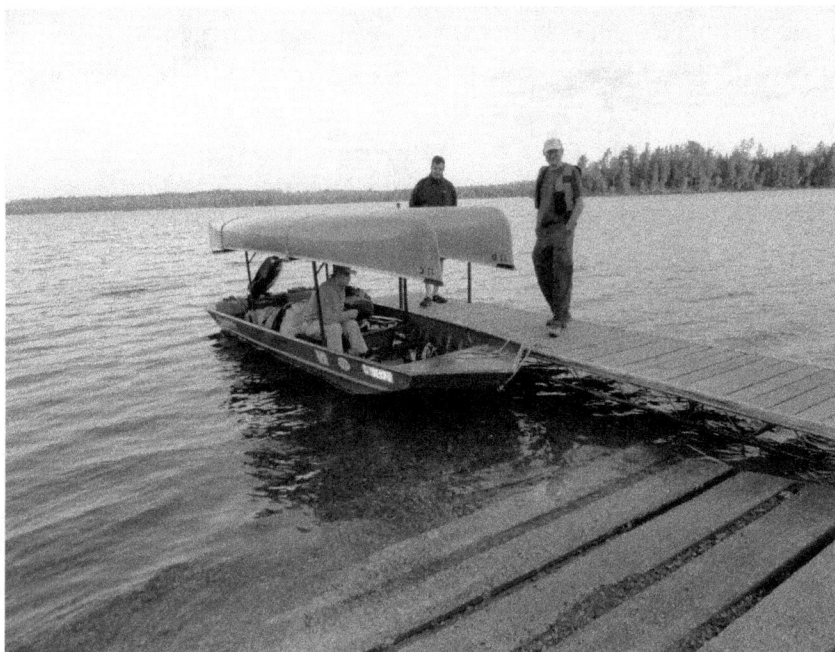

Piragis Outfitters Dropped Us Off at Prairie Portage

Our six day water route was a loop of fifteen lakes within Quetico. From the Prairie Portage Ranger Station entry, we paddled north to Sunday Lake, then east to Meadows Lake, and then north on Agnes Lake until we reached the portage to Silence Lake. We looped back to Prairie Portage via the lake route known as the "S" chain of lakes: Silence, Sultry, Summer, Noon, Shade, West, South, and then to Basswood, Burke and Bayley Bay.

Although we passed through the northern Minnesota Boundary Waters Canoe Area (BWCA) as our canoes were towed with the motorboat, technically we did a Quetico paddling trip.

A Trip for the Physically Fit with a Planned Route

Our experience in the waters of Quetico taught us:

(1) You need to plan your portage route in agreement with the physical condition and paddling experience of your group.

Develop your route considering portage length and portage frequency;

(2) This trip is for the physically fit outdoor enthusiast;

(3) You need strength and endurance paddling skills to handle long mileages and paddling amongst heavy wind and rough waves;

(4) A strong back for heavy, lengthy, and rough portages;

(5) Have at least one member of your group with map and compass reading skills. Remember Quetico has no trail signs or markers;

(6) Outdoor menu planning and cooking skills (at least one person);

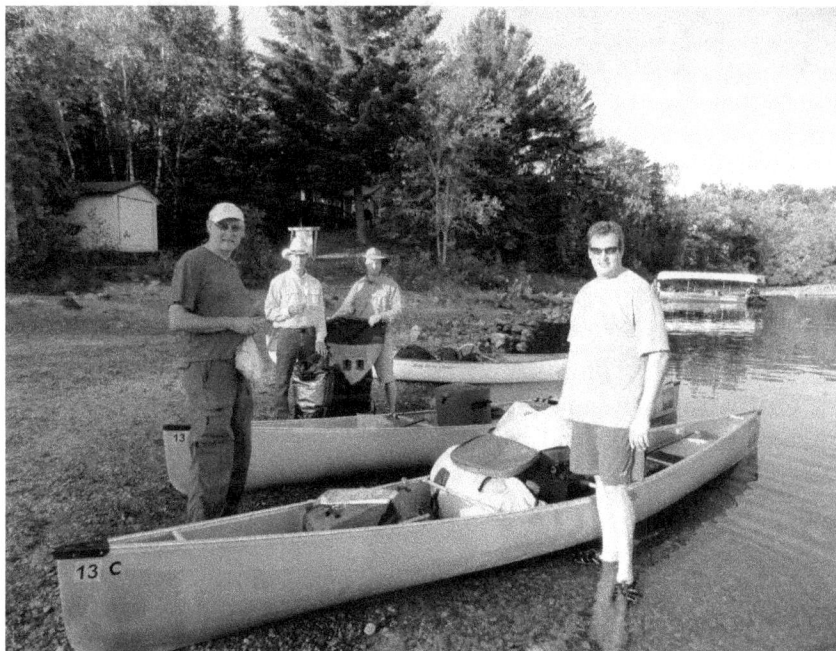

Our Take-out at Prairie Portage

(7) An ability to set up a campsite, start a campfire in different weather conditions (at least one person);

(8) A team mentality to work together in grinding and varying terrain and weather conditions and with camp setups;

(9) In our late September trip we went swimming one day – and the next day had to take shelter because of a snow and rain storm. Bring clothing appropriate for the time of year and any unpredictable changes in weather extremes;

(10) A sense of humor and enjoyment of the wonderful outdoors.

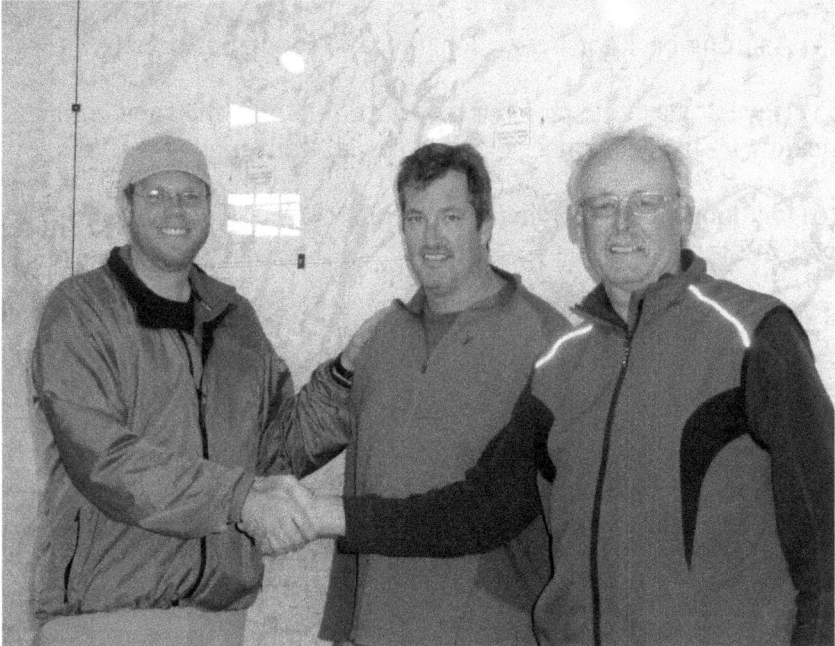

A Heartfelt "Thank You" to Drew, Piragis Northwoods Outfitting Manager, for his outstanding advice and gear.

We all gained an appreciation for the beauty, tranquility and isolation of the Quetico area. Will we return? Yes - absolutely!

Now, I never have to say, "I wish I had paddled the boundary waters of Minnesota and Canada."

References

- Piragis Northwoods Outfitters http://www.piragis.com/

- Canoe On Inn http://www.canoeoninn.com/

- Bearwise http://www.mnr.gov.on.ca/en/Business/Bearwise/

- Boundary Water Canoe Access http://www.bwca.com/

- Boundary Waters Canoe Area & Quetico Provincial Park Canoe Trip Routes
  http://www.canadianwaters.com/boundary-waters-canoe-area-quetico-provincial-park-canoe-trip-routes/

- Mckenzie Maps http://www.bwcamaps.com/

- Quetico Provisional Park
  http://en.wikipedia.org/wiki/Quetico_Provincial_Park.

Video References Paddling Boundary Waters of Minnesota and Ontario
- **Blog: Paddling the Waters of Quetico Provincial Park in Ontario**
  http://outdooradventurers.blogspot.com/2011/09/paddling-boundary-waters-of-minnesota.html

- **Video of Boundary Waters Portages**
  http://www.youtube.com/watch?feature=player_embedded&v=mfqM0oK88zA
- **Spreadsheet of lake sequences, portages and portage distances**
  http://www.professorsteve.com/2011Sept16_BWCAW_MN/2011Sept19_SpreadsheetQuetico.pdf

---

Peak Foliage Paddling and Camping in the Green River Reservoir of Northern Vermont

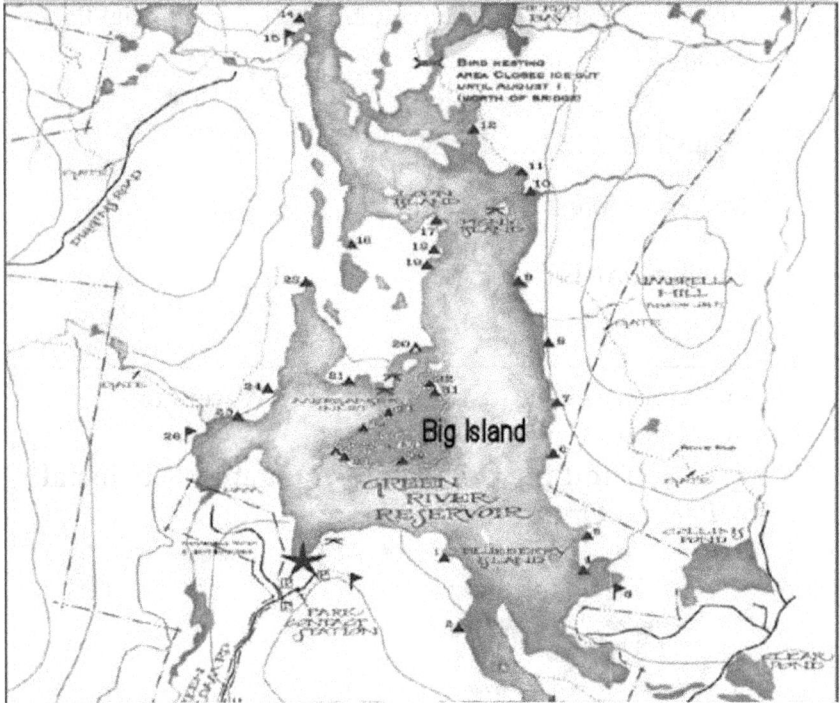

Enjoy the below video and pictures of the magnificent foliage colors of northern Vermont.

In late September, five outdoor enthusiasts and I, using five kayaks and one canoe, did three days of paddling and two nights of tenting in the Green River Reservoir of northern Vermont.

Green River Reservoir became a state park in March 1999 when 5110 acres were purchased from the Morrisville Water and Light Department. This is not your typical Vermont State Park – Green River Reservoir provides camping and paddling experiences in a remote setting. All campsites can only be reached by paddling to them - some a 1 to 2-mile paddle from the launch site.

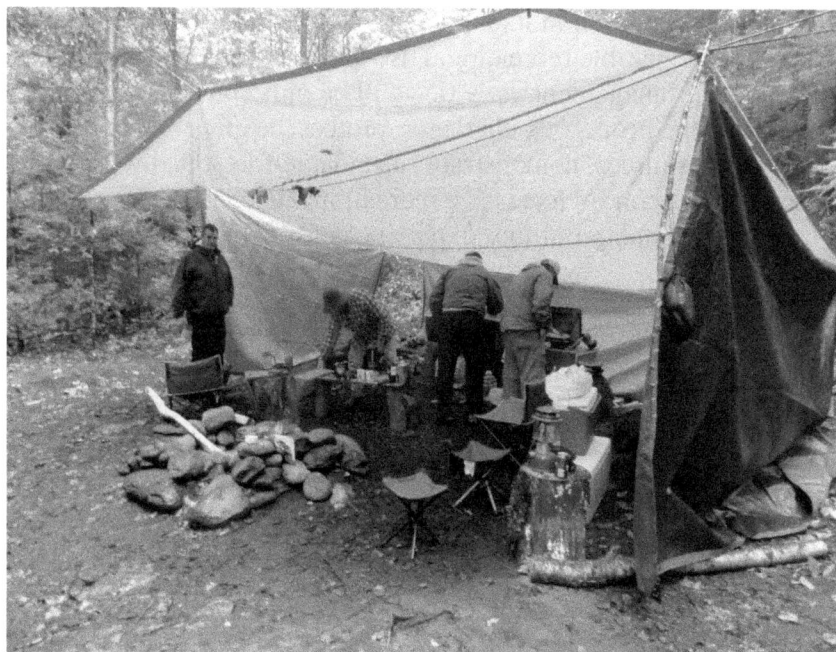

Our Big Island Campsite

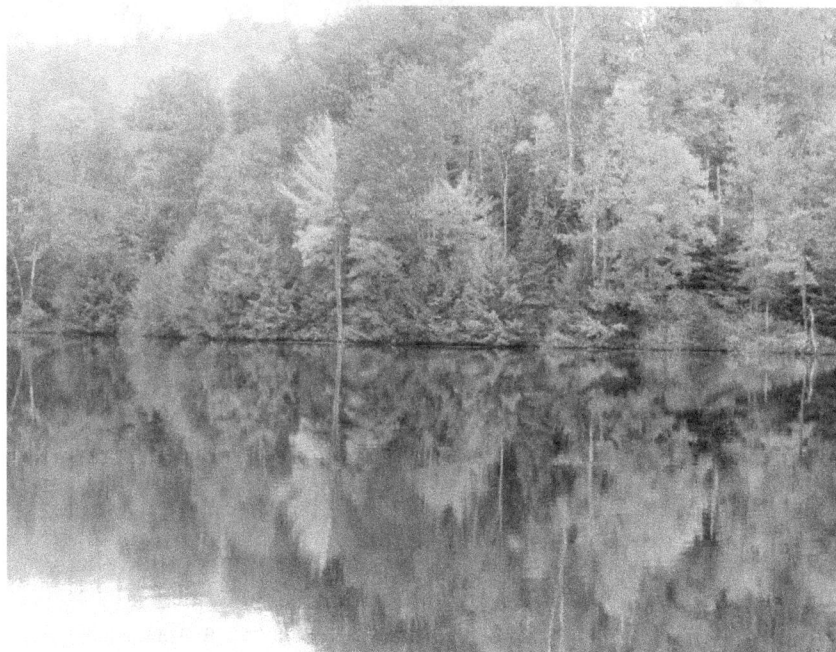

Reflection on the Water. Is This Picture Upside Down?

The park will remain in its wild and undeveloped state, with low-impact, compatible recreational use allowed on and around the Reservoir. Management activities will be only those necessary to maintain the property's character, protect the environment and critical resources, demonstrate sustainable forest and wildlife management, control excessive recreational use, and ensure high-quality outdoor experiences for visitors.

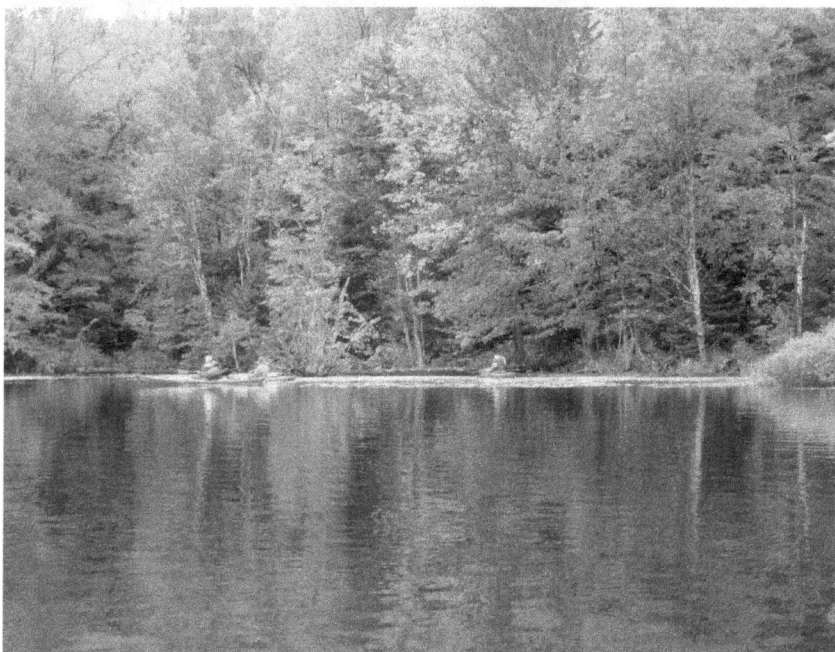

A Gorgeous Fall Day in Vermont

The 653-acre Reservoir includes about 19 miles of shoreline, one of the longest stretches of undeveloped shorelines in Vermont. Access to the park is in the southern part of the Reservoir off of the Green River Dam Road. The Reservoir is designated as a "quiet" lake under Vermont "Use of Public Waters Rules." Boats powered by electric motors up to 5 mph and human-powered watercraft (canoes, kayaks, etc.) are the only ones allowed.

There are 28 remote campsites at various locations around the Reservoir. Camping is allowed only at designated campsites and can **only** be reached by boat. Each remote site has a maximum site occupancy based on the characteristics of the site. There is one designated group campsite that can accommodate up to 12 people.

Some campsites are closed each season and rehabilitated due to overuse through the years.

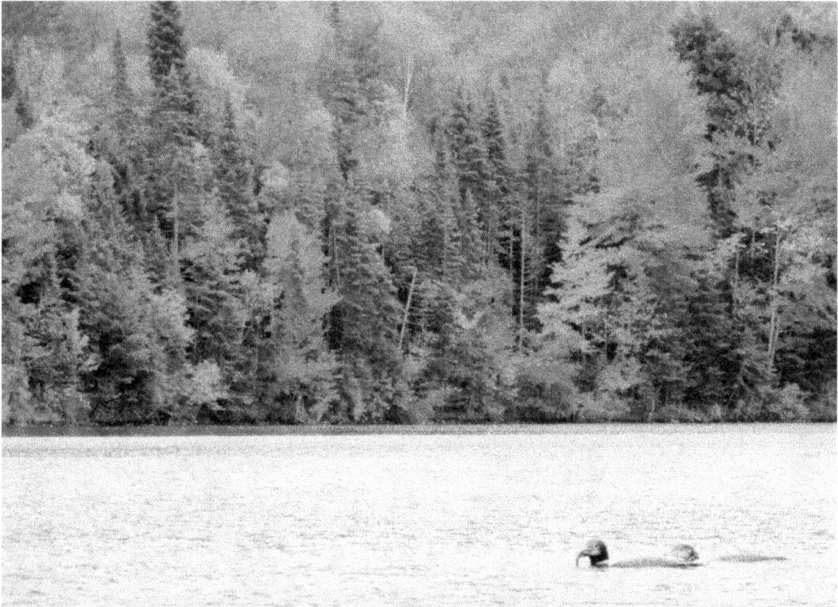
See the Loon Eating a Fish

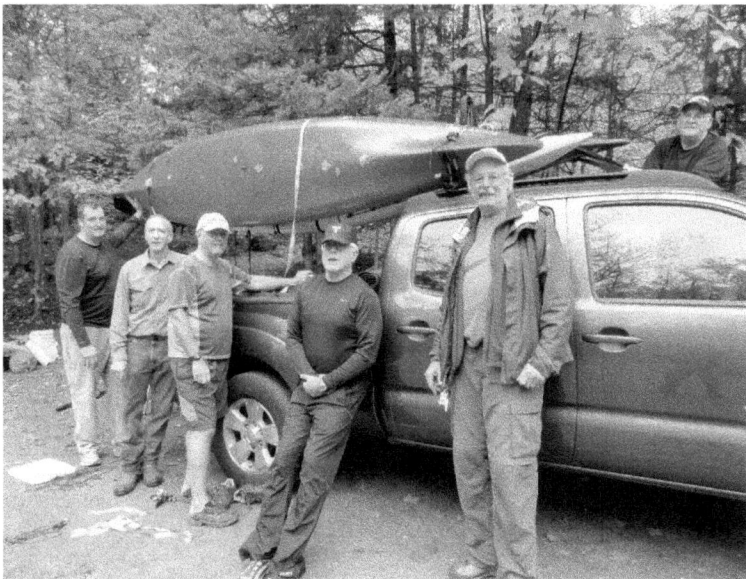
Tired After a Fabulous Three Days in the Wilderness of Vermont

Video Resources Northern Vermont Fall Foliage
- Blog: Green River Reservoir
  http://outdooradventurers.blogspot.com/2012/10
  /peak-foliage-colors-paddling-and.html
- Lasting Memories of Colors in Northern
  Vermont
  http://www.youtube.com/watch?feature=player
  _embedded&v=wC8cLJ49nNQ
- Happy Birthday Linwood from Your Amigos
  http://youtu.be/aajYSMhpbgg

Springer Mountain, Georgia - Southern Terminus of the Appalachian Trail

Along with my sons Shaun and Tim, I visited Springer Mountain, Georgia, the southern end of the Appalachian Trail (AT). The Appalachian Trail Conservatory estimates the AT to be 2,175 miles, but yearly this figure changes with land ownership changes and limitations, and trail section relocations to mitigate foot path erosion. I have no urge to hike all of the AT (at least at this time), but given I was spending a month in Georgia, and I have hiked a great deal of the trail in New Hampshire, Maine, and Vermont, I could not resist hiking the Georgia terminus of the AT to see the two rock-embedded plaques.

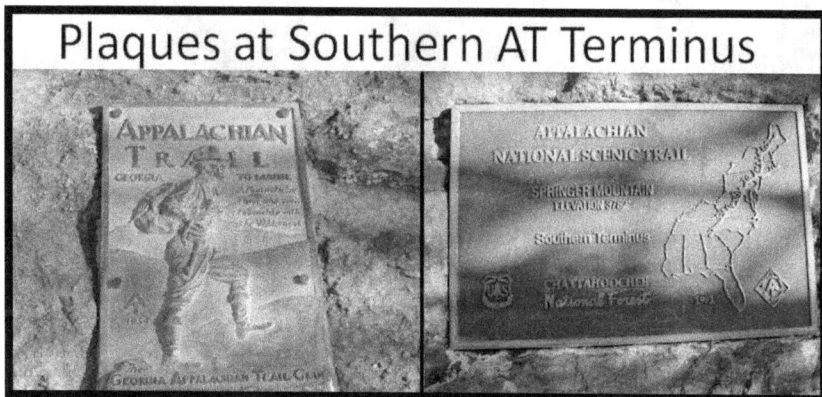

Plaques at Southern AT Terminus

Some folks believe the AT was an Indian trail. That assumption is not true. In 1922 Benton MacKaye, a forester from Massachusetts had the vision of a continuous hiking trail from Georgia to Maine. A single AT was recognized in 1937 and is maintained by thirty-two non-profit organizations.

Less than twenty-five percent of through hikers - those who start from one end of the trail to the other - complete the entire trail. A thru-hiker can start at either of the trail's ends - Mount Katahdin, Maine or Springer Mountain, Georgia.

The final (or beginning) mile of the AT passes through Forest Service Road (FSR) 42 near the top of Springer Mountain. From the small parking lot, you cross the FSR dirt road, locate the AT trail sign (with .9 miles engraved) and follow the vertical white painted rectangular trail (2 x 6 inch) tail markers to the AT's termination atop Springer Mountain. Visitors to the top of Springer Mountain can sign a logbook stored in a metal box encased in a rock holding one of the plaques.

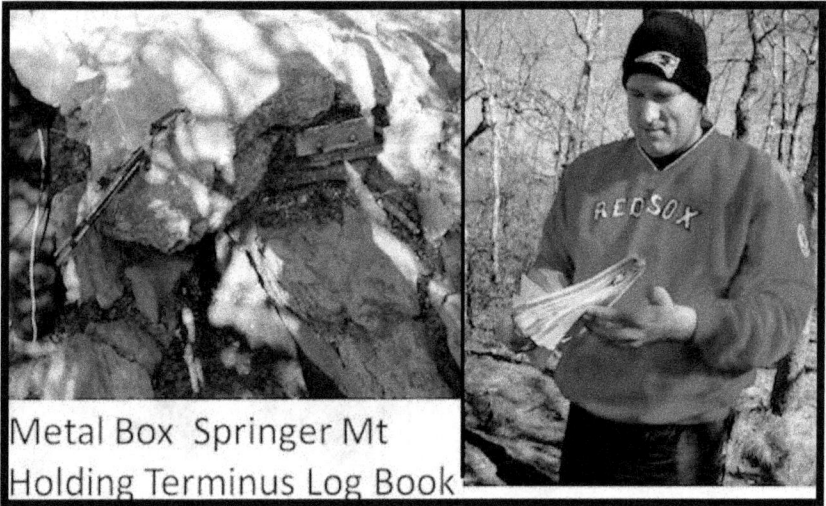

Metal Box Springer Mt
Holding Terminus Log Book

Benton MacKaye Trail
As we returned to the parking lot, we encountered the Benton MacKaye Trail. This is a four and ½-mile spur off the AT that essentially brings you back to the Springer Mountain parking lot. In tribute to Benton MacKaye, we decided to take this trail to return to the parking lot.

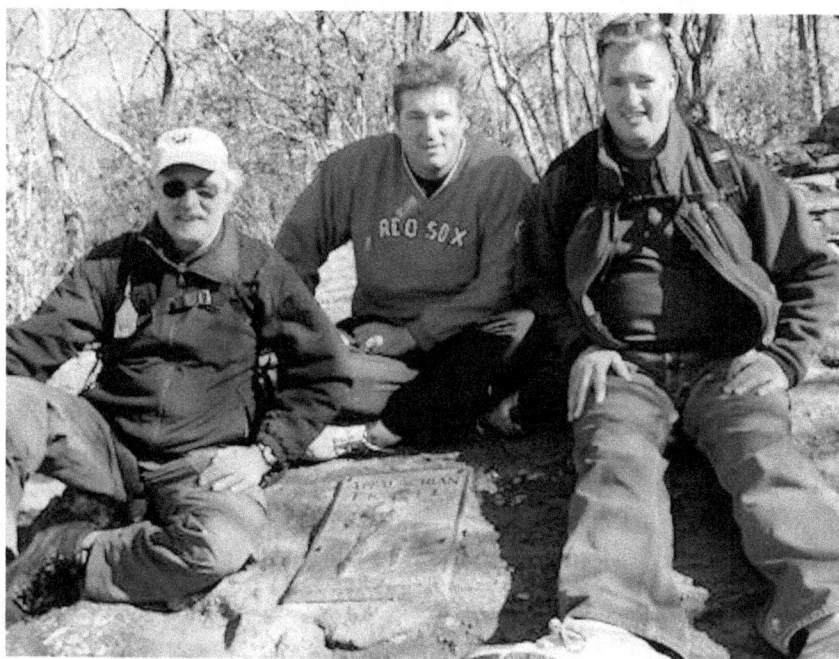

The Southern Terminus Plague of the Appalachian Trail

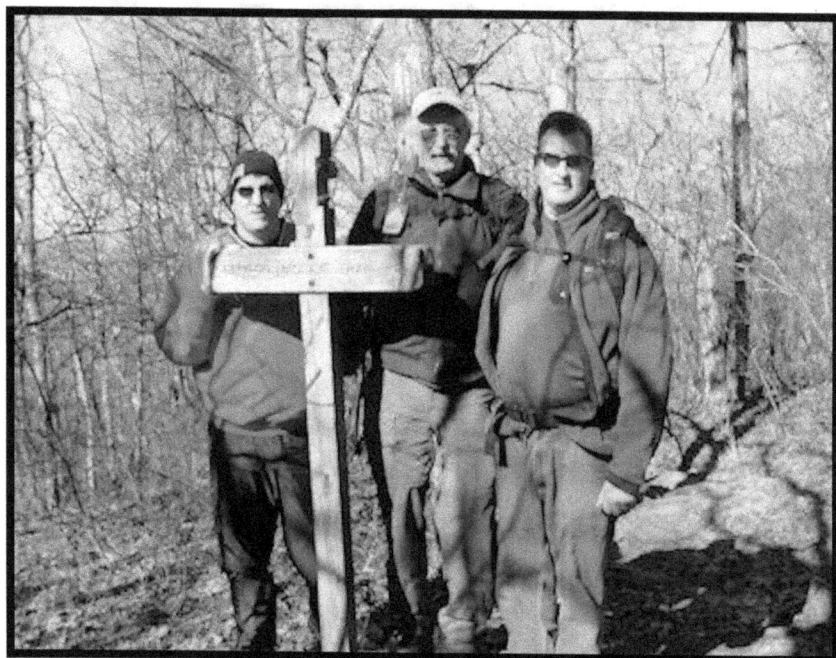

Benton MacKaye Trail Sign

Directions
It took many MapQuest searches, a few Google Earth reviews, and many Google Maps, before I found specific enough directions to Springer Mountain, the southern end of the AT. The Springer Mountain parking lot is located in the Chattahoochee National Forest nine-tenths (.9) miles from the top of Springer Mountain, where two rock-embedded plaques denote the southern end of the AT (note: There are many ways to get to the parking lot.)

Ten point four miles of a Wildness Road
Our last ten plus miles to the Springer Mountain parking lot were on a one-lane rock infested and mud hole red dirt mountain road. Our bumpy ten mile per hour pace was jarring. We frequently had to pull off the road for on-coming cars. The road was literally cut into the side of the mountain with tall Georgia pines on each side. You surely need a four-wheel drive or SUV to use this route.

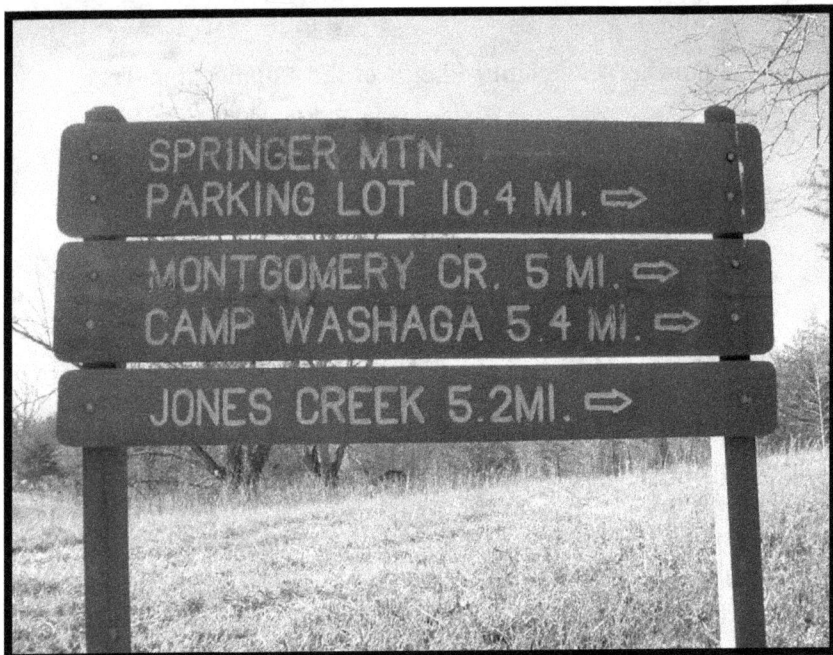

Which Way to Springer Mountain?

Resources for AT Planning and Through-Hiker Experiences

A great resource to learn about the history of the AT, state by state trail maps, and how to plan the hike, can be located at www.appalachiantrail.org/. It takes the average AT hiker six months to finish the entire trail.

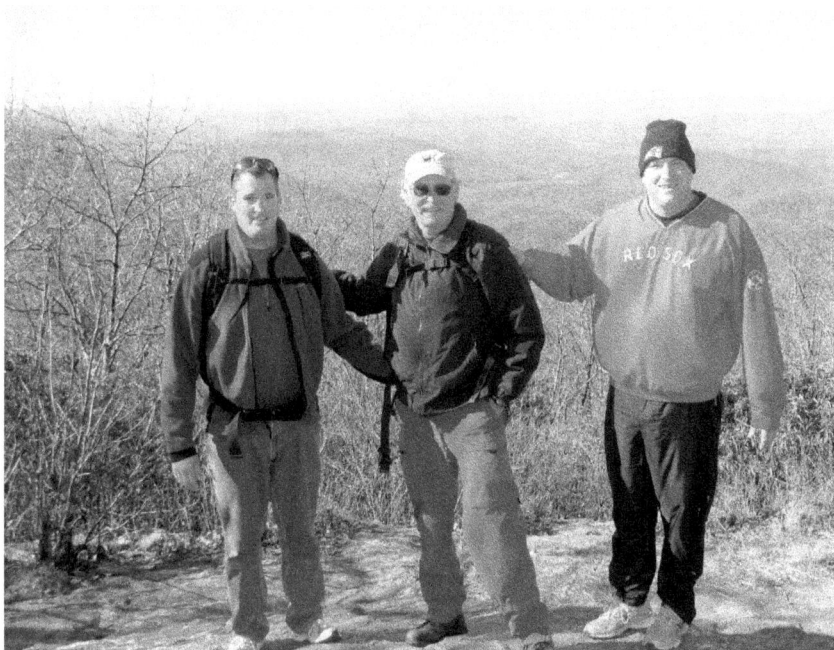

Overlooking the Valley from Southern Terminus of AT

Never Say, "I wish I had…"

Shaun, Tim and I now, never have to say, "We wish we had been to the southern terminus of the AT."

Video Reference Southern Terminus of Appalachian
Trail
Blog: Springer Mountain Georgia
http://outdooradventurers.blogspot.com/2009/11/spri
nger-mountain-georgia-southern.html

A Goffstown NH Giant Pumpkin Weigh-off and Regatta

Giant Pumpkin Weigh-Off & Regatta
Every October

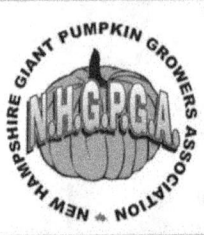

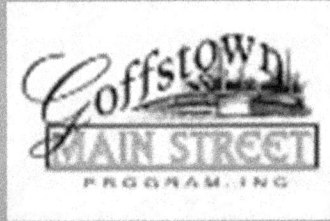

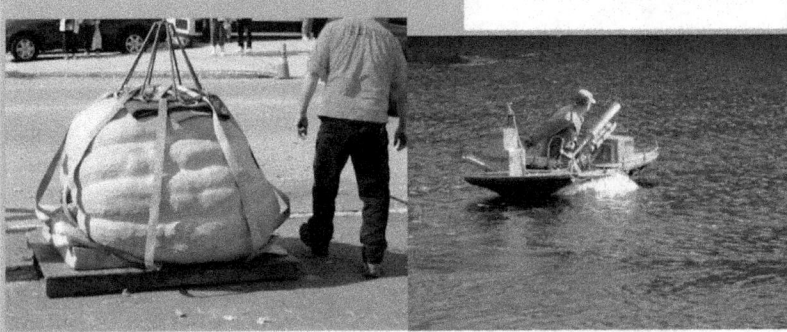

"Pull over, there's a giant pumpkin in the river with a person sitting in it!" my wife said as we were passing over the Piscataquog River in Goffstown, New Hampshire. She had spotted a weird scene. Lo and behold there were several giant pumpkins on the river - and they appeared to be racing each other! We were in the mist of the Goffstown Giant Pumpkin Weigh-off and Regatta.

Jim Beauchemin is a volunteer organizer of the Goffstown Giant Pumpkin Weigh-off and Regatta. I saw Jim's license plate and I asked him, "What does **1,314 LBS** mean?" He enthusiastically told me his giant pumpkin had won first prize at the 2005 Topsfield Fair and his plate number was the weight of his winning giant pumpkin.

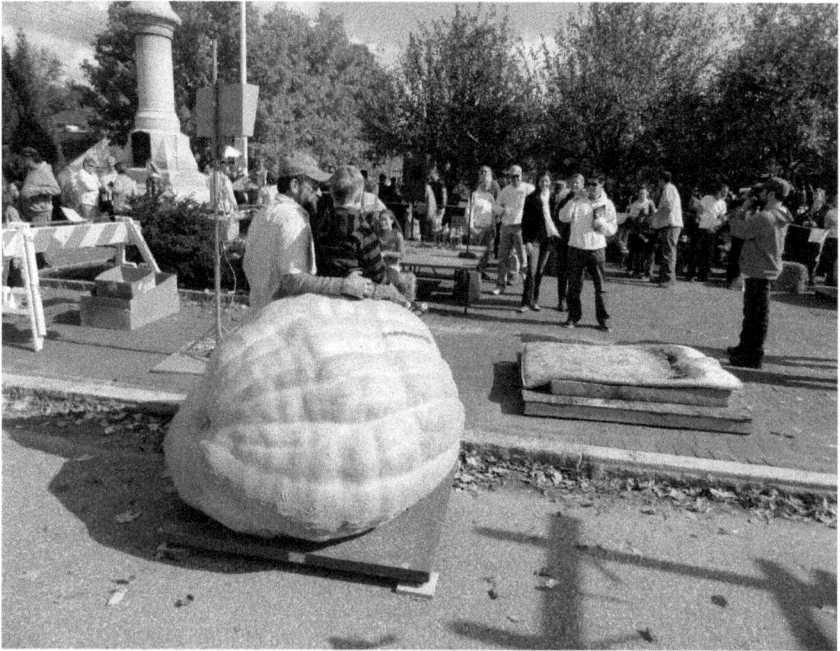

The Winner of the Largest Giant Pumpkin at 1,465 lbs

Because of my prior year glimpse of this unique parade of giant pumpkins on the Piscataquog, and Jim's enthusiasm for this hobby/sport, I made it my quest to see this year's Goffstown Giant Pumpkin Weigh-off and Regatta "upfront and personal."

Here is my whirlwind tour of my two days at the Giant Pumpkin Weigh-off and Regatta:

The New Hampshire Giant Pumpkin Growers Association (NHGPGA) Hosts the Weigh-off

o Front-end loaders carry the giant pumpkins for the weigh-off from their pallets to the scale.

o Jim Beauchemin was the narrator and skillfully kept the crowd's enthusiasm throughout the weigh-off and educating them to giant pumpkin growing.

o Bruce Hooker of Belmont, NH was the winning grower. His pumpkin weighed 1,465 lbs

The Goffstown Giant Pumpkin Regatta is a Boat Race on the Piscataquog River

o Because an excessive amount of rainfall in a short period of time this summer caused many giant pumpkins to grow too fast and split, there was a fear among the Regatta organizers that there would not be enough pumpkins to use as boats this year. Thankfully, several of the growers donated giant pumpkins for use in the Pumpkin Regatta.

At 2 pm the giant pumpkin boat building started

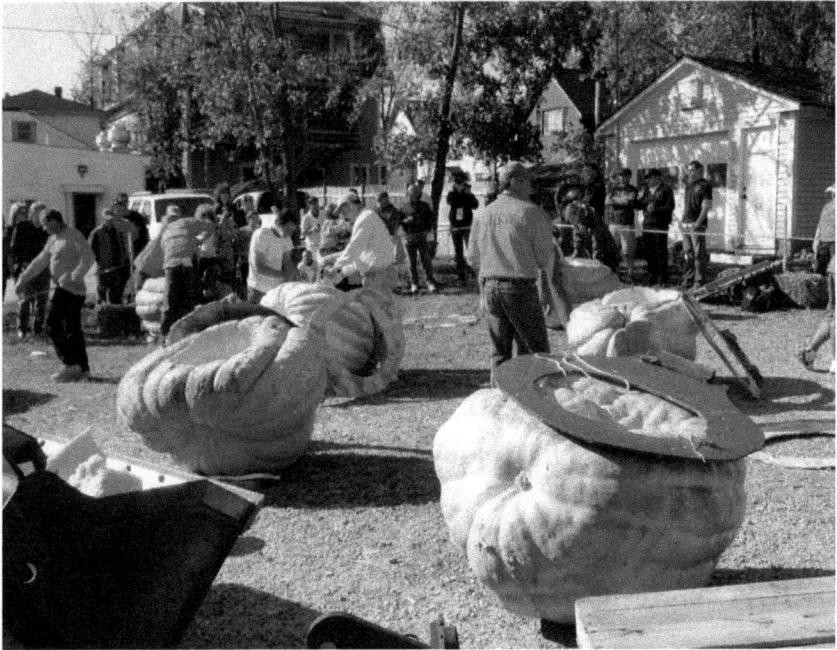

Giant Pumpkins Carved and Ready for Electric Motor

o Bruce Normand expertly guided and supervised the process for "Giant Pumpkin" boat carving and river testing.

o The first boat building task is to use a plywood template and a power saw to cut a two foot or so diameter hole in the top of the pumpkin.

o Only the grower is allowed to remove the seeds from the giant pumpkins, as the seeds can be very valuable. I heard anywhere from $800 to $1,600 per seed from winning giants.

o Bolts attach the plywood around the carved opening and the wood serves as a platform to connect an electric motor.

o Each team has a boat theme. You will see their designs in my video.

Sunday morning each team is assigned a time to test their boats on the Piscataquog River

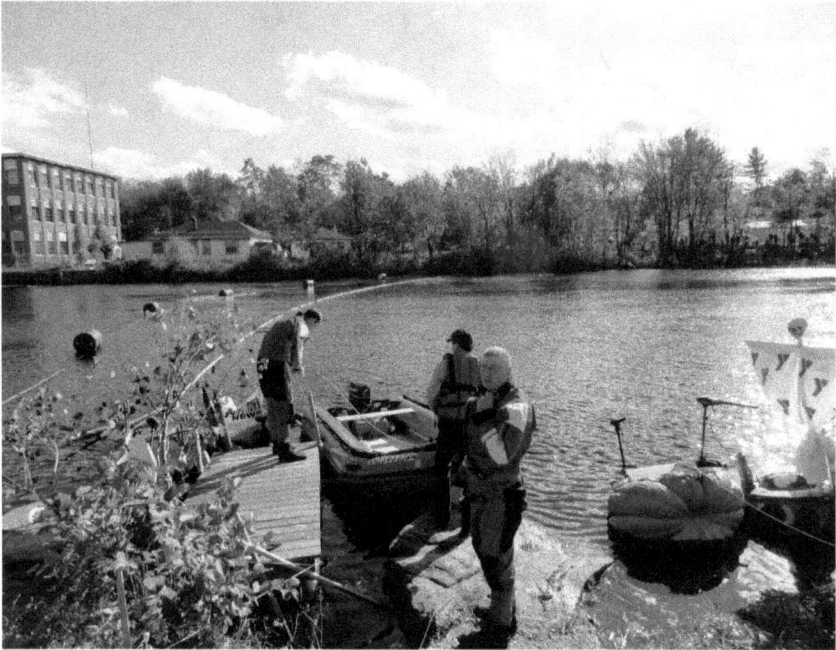

Goffstown Fire and Rescue Readies Safety Boats

o The boats are ballasted with sand. Insufficiently ballasted boats tend to tip, or heel, and can result in capsizing.

o The electric motors and batteries were placed on/in the boat.

o The captains take the boats for a maiden voyage.

o This maiden voyage is as much fun to watch as the actual race itself. Some of the captains had never been in a giant pumpkin before, and you could feel the nervousness in the air.

o The support crews were tremendous with their encouragement and support for all contestants.

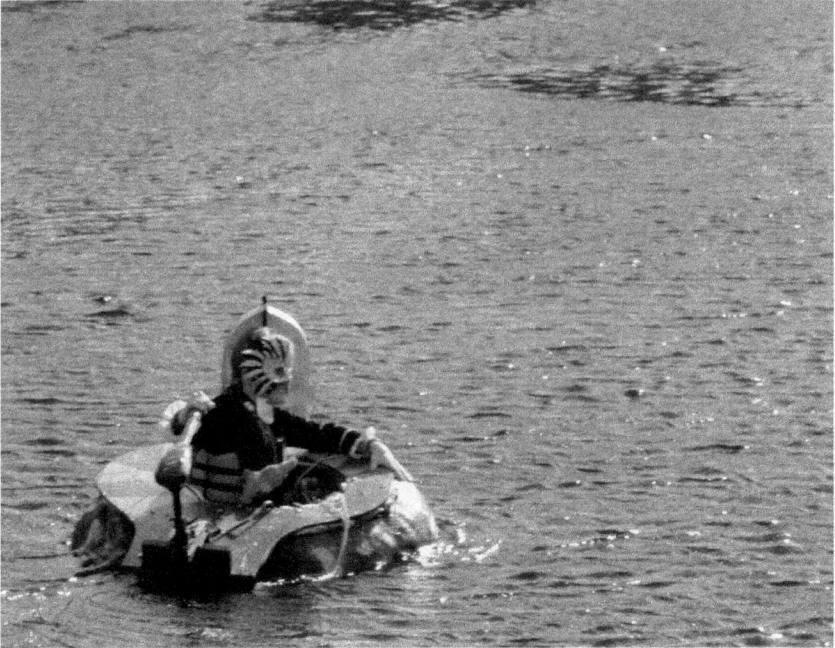

A Captain Takes Her Boat for a Trial Run

o Goffstown Fire and Rescue handled water safety. The Goffstown hydro dam is very near to the start of the race. In case of capsizing, to catch the "captains" of each pumpkin from going over the dam, two safety catch lines were strung across the river just upstream from the dam.

o The Goffstown Chief of Fire and Rescue reviewed the safety issues with all captains.

At 3 pm the Cannon Roared and Nine Giant Pumpkins headed toward the Goffstown Main Street Bridge

o With the Dam at their backs, a breeze in their face, and heading into the strong current, the boats targeted the bridge finish line.

Some of the boats swirled in circles, others seemed to be going downstream with the current, and a few, specifically the Goffstown News Harry Potter theme boat, kept river left aiming straight at the bridge.

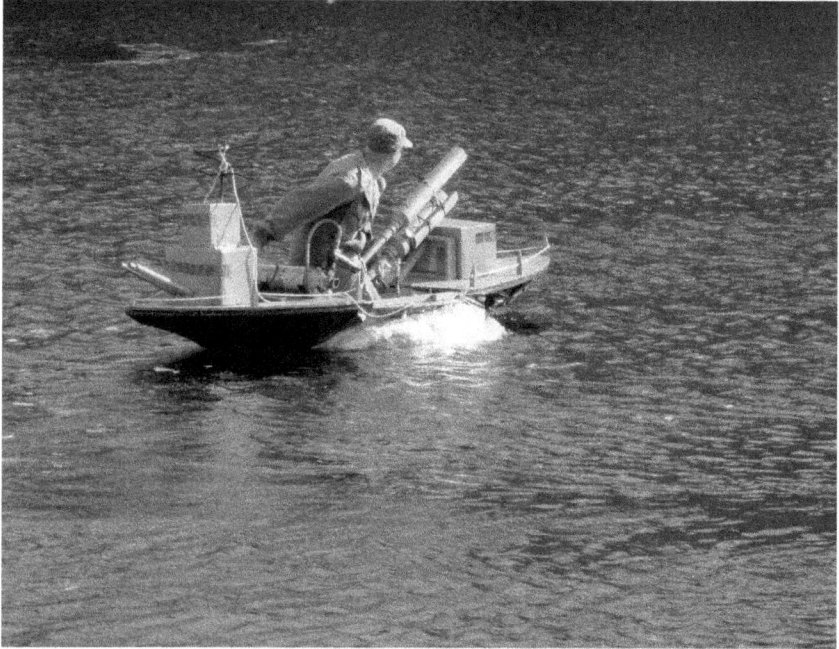

A Boat Captain Fires T-Shirts to the Crowd

o The Giant Pumpkin Eater suddenly appeared upstream honking its horn with water hoses spraying the boats. Indeed some of the boats reciprocated with their own hoses. We had a Regatta "Battle on the Piscataquog" – all in fun.

o To fire up the river-bank spectators, some of the boats used air-cannons to shoot Goffstown Regatta monogrammed t-shirts into the crowd.

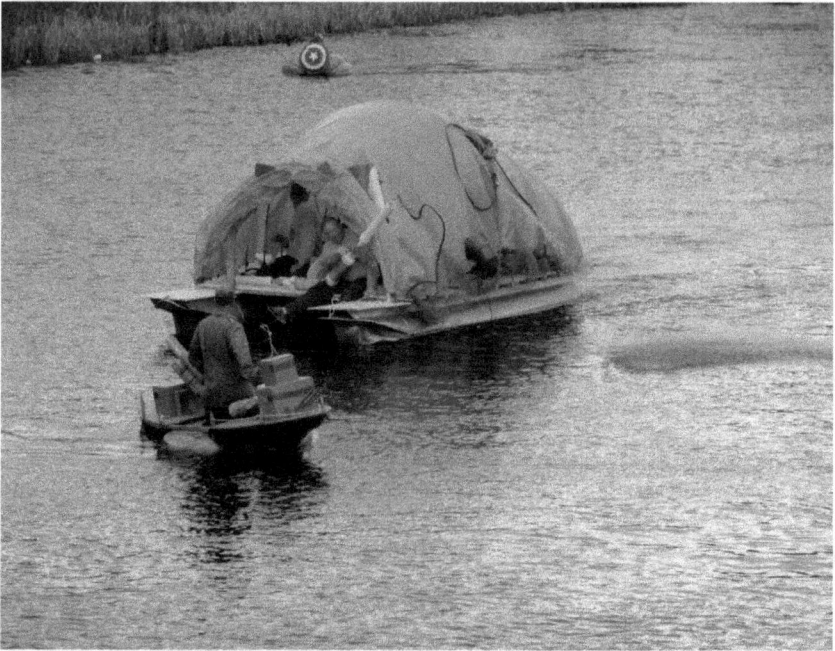

The Giant Pumpkin Eater Puts the Fleet Under Attack

o The winner of the 2011 Giant Pumpkin Regatta was the Harry Potter themed boat of the Goffstown News. Actually, all the boat captains are winners. Meeting the challenge of steering a near-thousand pound pumpkin, seated on their battery with knees up, and reaching back in an awkward position to steer and throttle – showed me that there should be nine trophies awaiting all finishers of the Giant Pumpkin Regatta.

An international flare was present throughout the two days as a TV crew from Germany did interviews and videos.

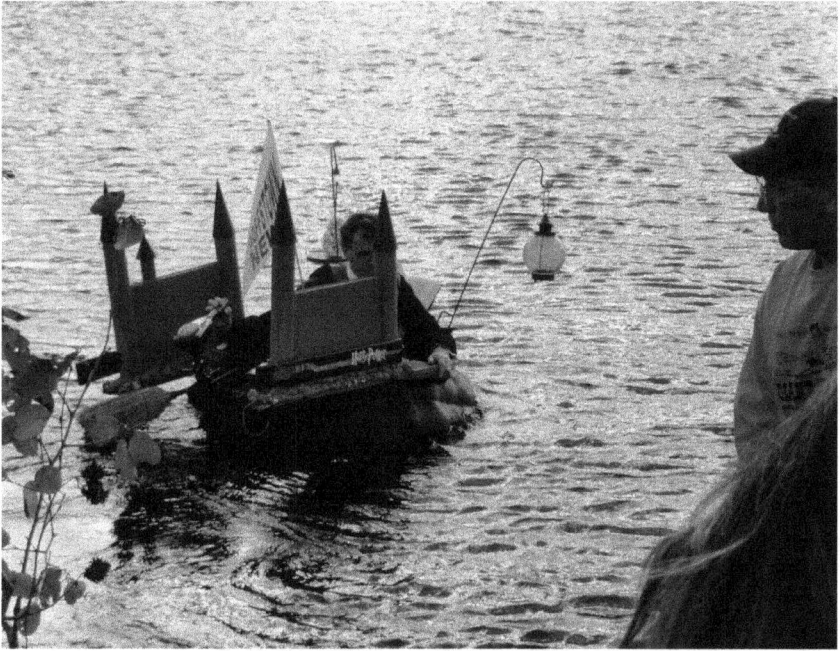

And the Winner is Harry Potter!!

- Thanks to the support of the New Hampshire Giant Pumpkin Growers Association and countless sponsors and volunteers throughout Goffstown, the Giant Pumpkin Weigh-off and Regatta has become the signature event for Goffstown Main Street. I can't wait to attend next year.

I now will never have to say, "I wish I had watched the Goffstown Giant Pumpkin Weigh-off and Regatta".

References

o Jim Beauchemin's Discovery Channel DVD, "**The Secrets of Growing Champion Giant Pumpkins**", is available at https://www.createspace.com/209048. It is an entertaining presentation with a wealth of information on growing giant pumpkins.

o http://www.facebook.com/notes/the-goffstown-news/excess-rain-lack-of-growers-cause-giant-pumpkin-shortage/10150410710915505

o
http://www.unionleader.com/article/20111017/NEWS15/71
0179961

o New Hampshire Giant Pumpkin Growers Association
http://www.nhgpga.org/

o Goffstown Main Street
http://www.goffstownmainstreet.org/

o World Record Giant Pumpkin is 2,009 lbs as of October
1, 2012 held by Ron Wallace of Greene, RI.

> **Video Reference Goffstown Giant Pumpkin Regatta**
> - **Blog: Giant Pumpkin Regatta**
>   http://outdooradventurers.blogspot.com/
>   2011/10/goffstown-nh-giant-pumpkin-
>   weigh-off.html
> - **Video Giant Pumpkin Weigh-off and Regatta**
>   http://www.youtube.com/watch?feature=
>   player_embedded&v=upw0o6B9JBo

Do Mountain Lions Live in New Hampshire?

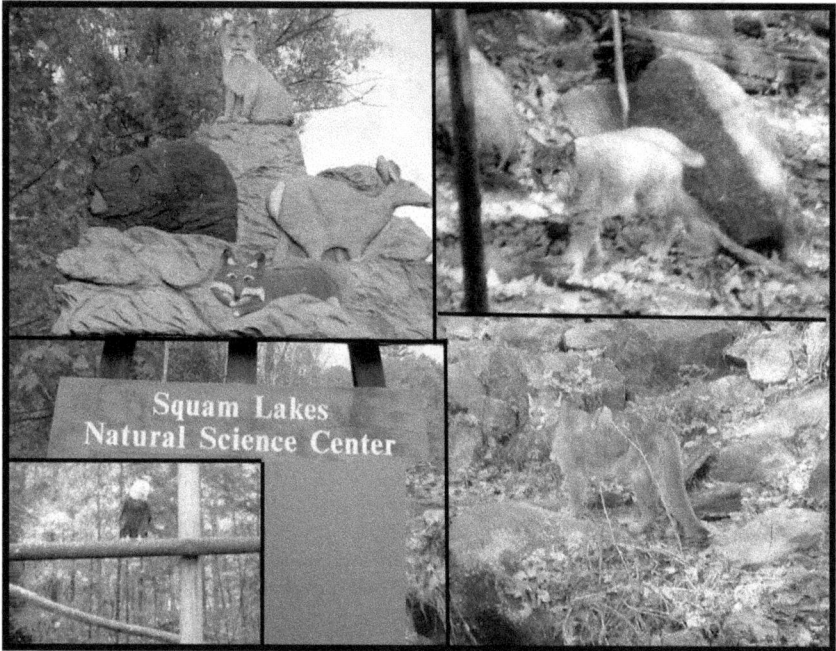

Can You Spot the Mountain Lion, Canada Lynx and Eagle?

Squam Lakes Natural Science Center (http://www.nhnature.org/) in Holderness, NH is the place to go to see New Hampshire's wild animals "up close and personal".

The Sunday Union Leader announced a lecture at Squam Lakes on New Hampshire's large wildcats. Certainly, a topic of interest to all outdoor enthusiasts.

My wife Cathy and I arrived two hours before the 1 pm lecture so we could hike the ¾ mile Gephart Exhibit Trail. The Trail features live native New Hampshire wildlife in natural settings.

Yes, I had seen many of the animals and birds previously in their native habitat, but it was always for a fleeting moment. Now, Cathy and I are in awe seeing the same wildlife in their natural settings, and in an area where we can take pictures at our leisure, and read all about their traits.

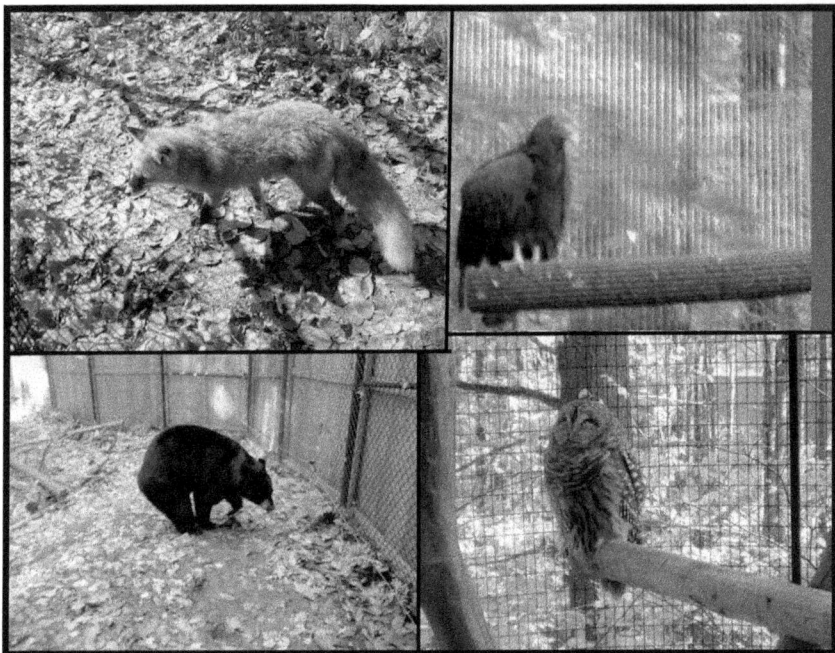

See the Red Fox, Black Bear, Barred Owl and Turkey Vulture

All the animals are in captivity, but in an environment close to their natural habitat and space needs. The animals were orphaned or injured before they came to the Center. Essentially, the Center is now their home.

Never say, "I wish I wish I had seen and learned more about wildlife of New Hampshire."

So, are there mountain lions in NH? Hmm, maybe yes – maybe no. Plan a day at the **Squam Lakes Natural Science Center**

Video References Mountain Lions in NH
- Blog: Are Their Mountain Lions in New Hampshire? http://outdooradventurers.blogspot.com/2009/10/do-we-have-mountain-lions-in-new.html
- Squam Lakes Natural Science Center http://www.nhnature.org/

Winter

There are three kinds of people in this world. Those that watch things happen. Those that make things happen. And those that wonder what happened. Which kind are you?

– Author Unknown

A Winter Swim Clinic for Triathletes

The Breast Stroke or the Freestyle?

Do I learn to swim the freestyle or continue the breast stroke? As a triathlete, I have faced this decision many times. I dare say I have done close to a hundred triathlons over the years, and with each swim I have used the breast stroke. My breast stroke with swim distances a half mile or longer, usually puts me in the middle of my age group.

With the breast stroke I am able to maintain a straight course, whereas many swimmers doing the freestyle (the term *freestyle* is sometimes used as a synonym for *crawl)* on a long swim begin to tire and start zigzagging. A tired swimmer often swims a further distance than me. In a long swim I am the tortoise (with my breast stroke) going slow, BUT steady and straight. I am competing against the hare treading water to rest, and usually weaving along the course. In the long swim I have a chance to finish ahead of some of the less conditioned swimmers.

During the past few years I have focused only on the shorter triathlon distance (usually called the Sprint triathlon) with swim distances between a quarter and third of a mile. In the Sprint triathlon swim I most always find myself last in my age group. Everyone ahead of me uses the freestyle.

In essence, in short distance open water swims the freestyle hare most usually beats the breast stroke tortoise.

The year 2013 made me face my breast stroke decision once again. In 2012 I qualified for the National Senior Games Triathlon to be held in July 2013 in Cleveland. This means I will be representing New Hampshire – and accepting last place is not something we do in New Hampshire. I keep asking myself, "Will the freestyle stroke make me more of a competitor in my age group?"

The Blue Steel Triathlon Club Swim Clinic

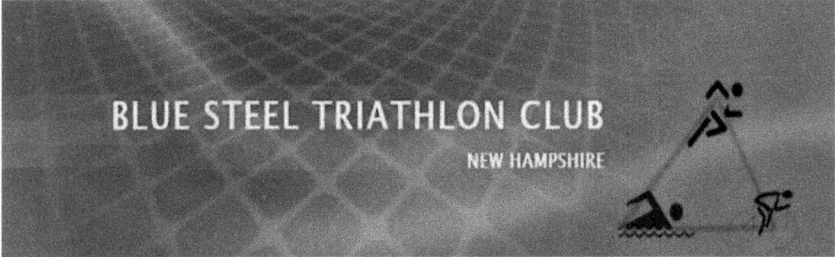

I am a proud member of the Blue Steel Triathlon Club. The Club offers a variety of triathlon oriented Clinics and Events for its members to improve performance as well to encourage teammate camaraderie: We have bike time trials on summer evenings; fun runs for members to enjoy non-competitive group runs; transition clinics for tips and practice to minimize the transition time from swim to bike; and bike to run; and early morning open water group swims at local lakes.

This past October, one of our teammates, **Stacy Sweetser**, an all-American college swimmer with a reputation of being an outstanding swim instructor, offered to put on a Blue Steel swim clinic at the Allard Center YMCA in Goffstown, NH.

The Club would rent two swim lanes, and sign-up would be a first-come first served with a maximum of ten triathletes for each of the two sessions offered.

There was no procrastination this time. My mantra of **Never say, "I wish I had ..."** came to mind, and after receiving the email notice I immediately registered.

Let me describe the class attendees. Indeed, I felt like "a turkey trying to fly with eagles." Most, if not all, of the students were the Club's top triathletes with their attendance at the clinic aimed to further refine their freestyle stroke.

My goal was to see if I could learn and feel confident with the freestyle to make the freestyle my swim stroke for Cleveland.

We started the first class with each of us doing the crawl back and forth in the 25 yard pool. Stacy observed our individual strokes. She then explained how our next five weeks would go –basically a variety of training drills with increasing intensity that would include using hand paddles and training fins. She would also be emailing us YouTube training films and suggestions for each of us she had identified in our practice swims as needing improvement.

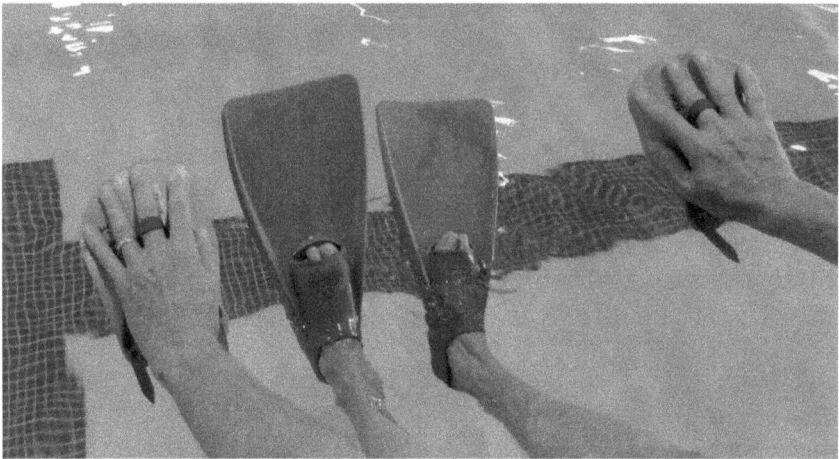

Hand Paddles and Feet Fins Used as Training Devices

Admittedly, my freestyle technique was close to non-existent with my kick, breathing, and arm stroke meeting all criteria for a "Do Not Do This" film.

Over the course of the five weeks, besides drills we did together, Stacy would have us do individual drills to re-enforce each triathlete's specific freestyle technique in order to make it better (i.e. stronger and more efficient).

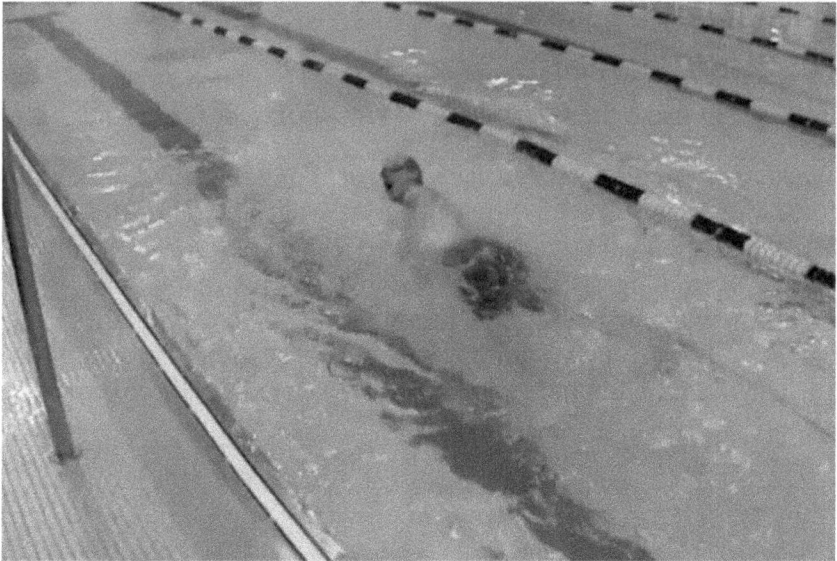

Breathe on both Left and Right Sides

What was so impressive in this clinic was Stacy herself. Her clinic preparation, her ability to focus on us as individuals, as well as a group, made every one of us feel we were each getting special attention. So no matter what the skill level we each started with, Stacy improved us all.

I am not going to describe how the reader can do the freestyle stroke, but some of the impressive things I gathered from Stacy were:

- The high elbow stoke versus my old way of a complete underwater arm pull. Stacy calls it **EVF, Early Vertical Forearm underwater.**

- Bi-lateral breathing. Previously I always breathed only on my right side. An open-water triathlete swimmer breathing only on one side can hinder you swimming straight as well as be an issue with waves.

- Immediately Stacy saw I held my breath underwater. She had me take each breath on my side, and then exhale (blow bubbles) into the water. My breathing and stamina immediately improved.

- With every class Stacy emphasized:

  o Technique over speed

  o The 5th Stroke is to streamline your body

  o Front quadrant focus meaning that you have one or both arms out in front of your torso for most of the stroke cycle.

  o Bilateral Breathing

- Read the below referenced article by Gary Edson, titled, Normal People Do Not Do Deliberate Practice

- Getting comfortable with freestyle on your side. The 6 kick switch drill was great. You can keep your face up/out breathing the whole time until you switch to the other side. You can even turn over on your back so your face never goes in the water, if you would rather.

The Lane Gainer Stretch Cord – Never say, "I wish I had …"

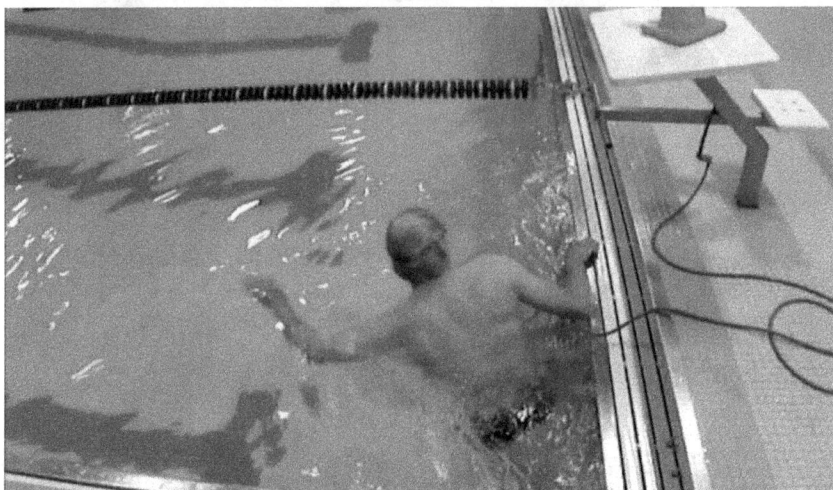

Start of Swim with Lane Gainer Stretch Cord

Near the end of the third week's class, Stacy asked if we wanted to try the Lane Gainer Stretch cord. Immediately the class responded, "What is that?" In a few words, this stretchable nylon cord is tied at one end of the pool. The other end of the cord is tied to a waist belt. The swimmer puts the belt on and starts swimming with the goal of reaching the other end of the pool. As the swimmer nears the center of the 25 yard pool, the cord reaches its natural length and begins to hold the swimmer. This is where the strength/power/technique of the swimmer comes in.

Stacy asked for a volunteer, and one of the better swimmers was ready to go. As he neared the 2/3rd mark you could see him begin straining a bit and his stroke pace increased – the cord was at its normal length and now his power stroke was needed. We yelled encouragement and roared when he finally touched the far end of the pool.

I was the least accomplished of the students, and no way was I going to embarrass myself with the lane gainer cord. Of the six students present that week, only I did not do the cord.

During the week I kept saying to myself, "**Never say I wish I had**

..." when I thought of the lane gainer cord. Come week four, when Stacy asked for volunteers for the cord, I was the first to volunteer with a joking remark, "Let me set the standard for today." I did manage about two-thirds of the pool, and felt remarkably proud.

On week five we again were offered an opportunity to try the lane gainer cord. When it came time for my turn, Stacy suggested to me, "When you think you can go no further, do another ten strokes".

As I passed mid-pool, I started to feel the cord's pull. I kept Stacy's words in my mind, and when I thought I was at my last exhausting stroke, I counted and managed ten more dying strokes. I had swam about three-quarters of the pool's length – further than I had gone on Week 4. Surely not assurance I would quality for a spot on the USA Olympic team, BUT enough to make me delighted.

This winter I will practice the freestyle at indoor pools, and in the spring do as many open water swims as I can.

Make the outdoors and exercise a daily component of your life. **Never say, "I wish I had taken a swim clinic"**

Stacy's Clinic Material:

- As you watch this video, notice the swimmer's hand position under the shoulder area while the elbow is high (but still under water). We did a variety of drills to learn and feel confident with the high elbow stroke. http://www.theraceclub.net/videos/secret-tip-how-to-pull-underwater-drills/

- The below video shows a high elbow sculling drill we did both swimming backwards and then forward. http://www.theraceclub.net/videos/secret-tip-how-to-pull-underwater-drills/

- This is a video that discusses an efficient underwater pull. Highlights... shallow pulling w/ high elbow creates less

frontal drag, still a powerful pull. Great underwater coverage.
http://www.slowtwitch.com/Training/Swimming/How_To_Pull_Underwater_2009.html

References

- Normal People Do Not Do Deliberate Practice
  http://tiny.cc/v88usw

- Freestyle Swimming

- Blue Steel Triathlon Club

Video References Triathlon Swim Clinic
- **Blog: Blue Steel Triathlon Club Swim Clinic**
  http://outdooradventurers.blogspot.com/2013/01/a-winter-swim-clinic-for-triathletes.html

---

A Winter Hike to Carter Notch Hut on the Appalachian Trail

My friend John called and asked me to join him on a winter hike into Carter Notch Hut. John's son Ryan would be hiking with a friend and John wanted to meet them at their overnight stay at the Appalachian Mountain Club hut located on the Appalachian Trail. John and I are life-long members of the AMC.

Mount Hedgehog – a warm-up hike

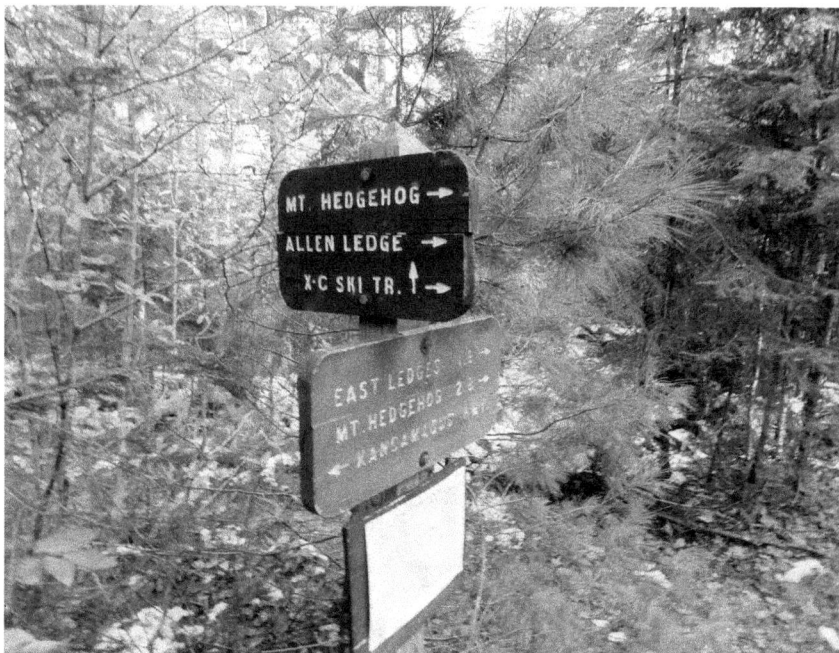

Which Way to Mt Hedgehog?

To prepare for this 3.8 mile hike into the winter wilds of the snowy and icy White Mountains, John wanted to go to the White Mountain area a day earlier for a day hike.

On Friday morning we were at the Kancamagus Highway trailhead for the Mount Hedgehog (2520 ft.) loop trail.

The five mile loop trail was moderately difficult, meaning upward switchback trails, crossing small brooks, over and under a few downed trees across the trail, and a reasonable grade with only the final sections a bit steep and requiring climbing up and over granite ledges.

The AMC trail guidebook suggested this hike could be done in three hours. We did the loop in a respectable three and a half hours. We paced ourselves stopping every fifteen minutes or so to drink water and chew trail mix. As we approached the top, wind and cold caused me to don my winter gloves. We paused at the top for magnificent views of Mt. Passaconaway, the Presidential range and Mt Chocorua (see more on Mt Chocorua in the Summer section of this book).

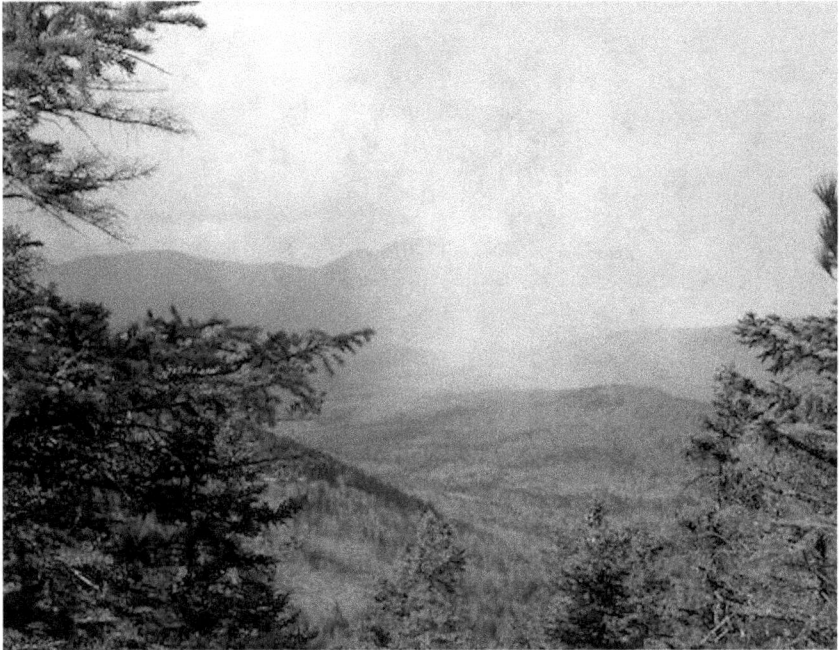

Can you see the Squalls of Snow Below Us?
Looking down from the peak over the tree-studded valley and north toward Mt Washington, we saw dark clouds blowing our way with squalls of snow sowing seeds beneath them – and we quickly picked up our pace, not wanting to be caught on the top of

the mountain. John took this picture from the top of Hedgehog and you can see the fast moving snow squall as a white-looking cloud spiraling to the ground in the valley and quickly heading our way.

The loop back to the trailhead was steep from the top and I could feel my quads aching. All in all, Mt Hedgehog was a good day hike and certainly helped prepare us for the next day's four mile hike into Carter Notch Hut.

Carter Notch Hut

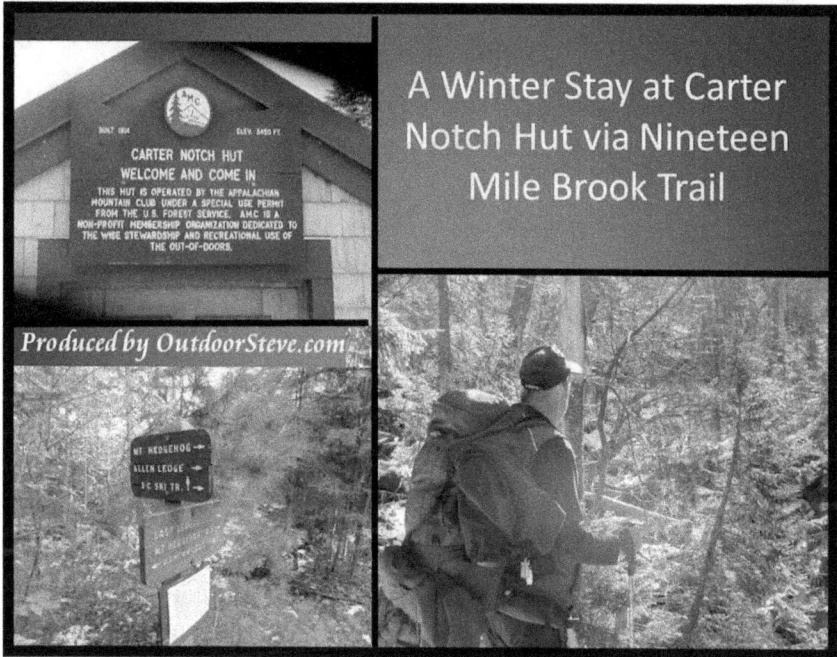

A Winter Stay at Carter Notch Hut via Nineteen Mile Brook Trail

CARTER NOTCH HUT
WELCOME AND COME IN
THIS HUT IS OPERATED BY THE APPALACHIAN MOUNTAIN CLUB UNDER A SPECIAL USE PERMIT FROM THE U.S. FOREST SERVICE. AMC IS A NON-PROFIT MEMBERSHIP ORGANIZATION DEDICATED TO THE WISE STEWARDSHIP AND RECREATIONAL USE OF THE OUT-OF-DOORS.

Produced by OutdoorSteve.com

Carter Notch Hut, elevation 3,450 feet, is the most eastern of the eight AMC huts. In winter the hut is self-service, meaning a caretaker stokes the wood stove at the hut from 5 pm until 9:30 pm (unless extreme cold dictates otherwise). Self-service includes self-cooking and hikers bring their own food and use the hut's utensils and gas stove for cooking.

Water Carried to Hut from Lake

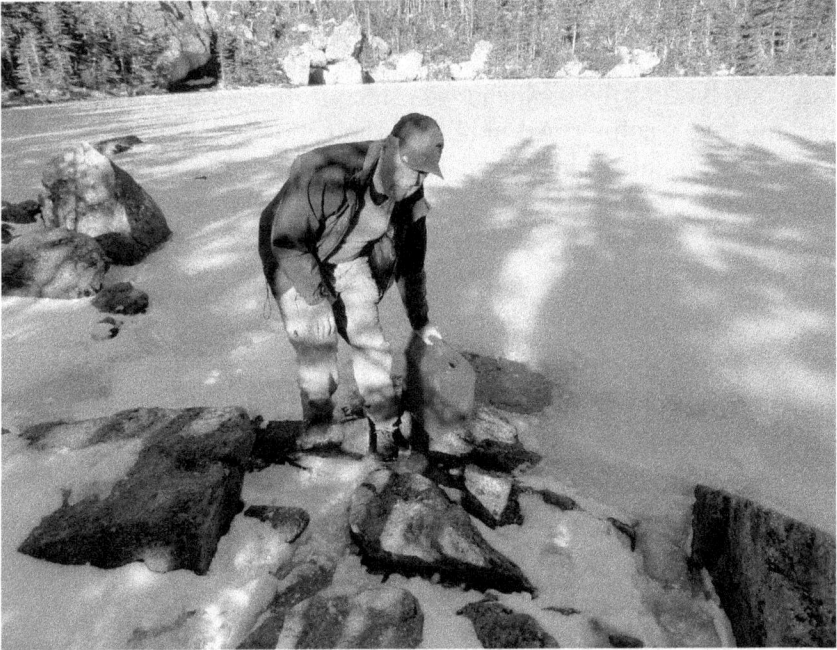

Winter Drinking Water Taken from the Pond and Boiled

There is no running water inside Carter Notch hut in winter, but water is carried into the hut in five gallon jugs as needed for potable water (after boiling). Hikers share responsibility for getting the water through a hole in the ice from a lake near the hut.

Two bunk houses are separate from the hut, and are unheated. The bunkhouses essentially provide bunk beds and protection from rain, snow and wind. Temperatures may reach way below zero in the depth of winter, so a winter sleeping bag is advisable, if not mandatory, such as one rated to -20 degrees F and preferably even lower.

The Master Maine Guide I have often traveled with in summer adventures uses a bag rated for 35 degrees below zero whenever he ventures out into the North Maine Woods during the winter months on guided 5 day cross-country ski trips across Maine's Baxter State Park. Staying warm during the night makes your outing much more enjoyable. Being cold during the night not only saps your energy, but leaves a bad taste in your mouth for ever getting out and enjoying those special scenic vistas and quiet solitudes that only a visit in winter can provide.

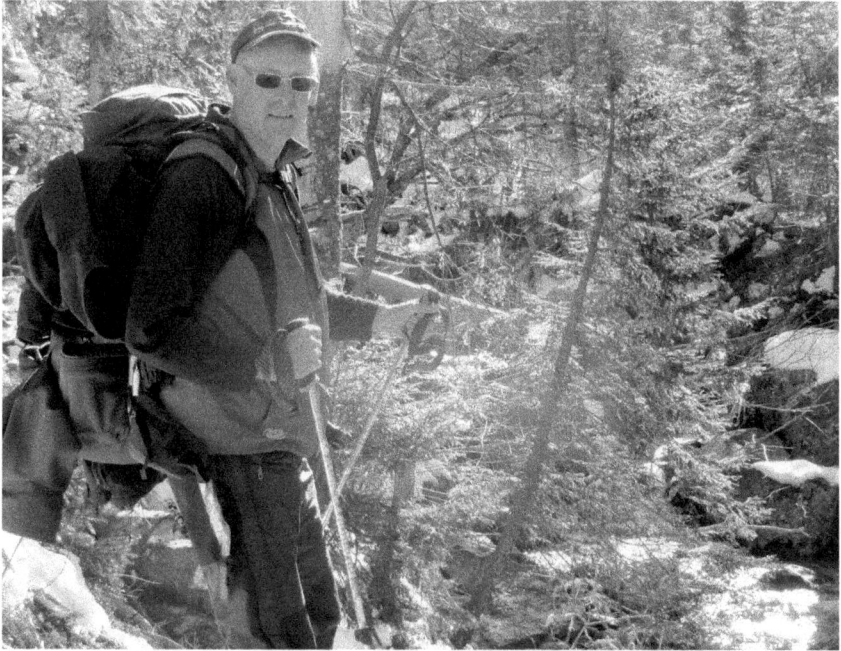

Trekking Poles are like have two extra feet to make it easier to balance and carry that 50 lbs backpack!

John and I used trekking poles to reach the hut, which were important for balance and saving our knees as we poled and stepped over and up on icy covered boulders. As we neared the Hut, the snow began to get deeper, maybe a foot or so in depth.

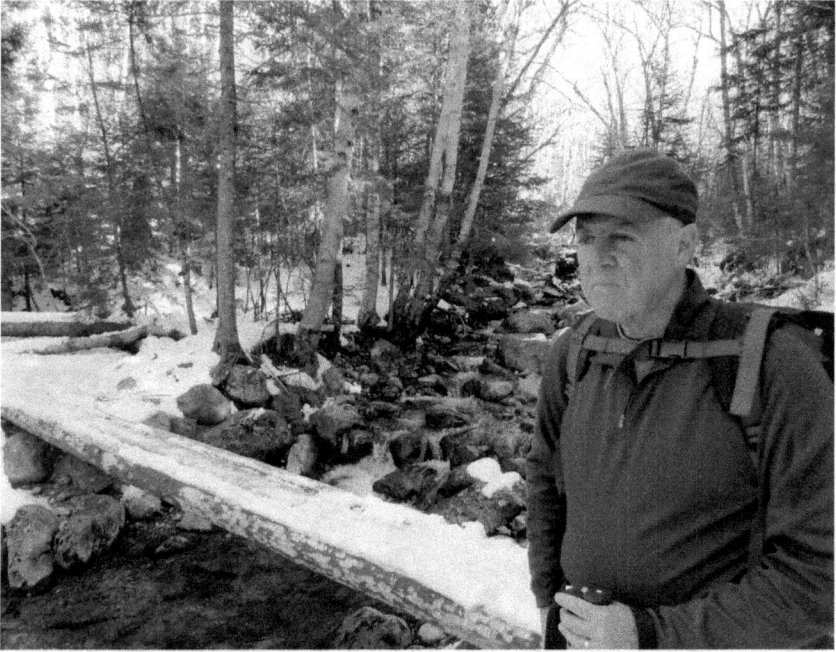

John Just Crossed Over the Ice/Snow Plank Bridge

We crossed four wooden planked bridges of which one had obviously been washed out, most likely in last month's northern NH flood, and in its place was an eight inch ice covered plank. You will see our balancing acts in the video as we warily crisscross three to four feet above the waters of Nineteen Mile Brook and the mountain run-offs.

The Hut Experience

We shared conversation with hikers from Littleton, NH, Maine, and Canada.

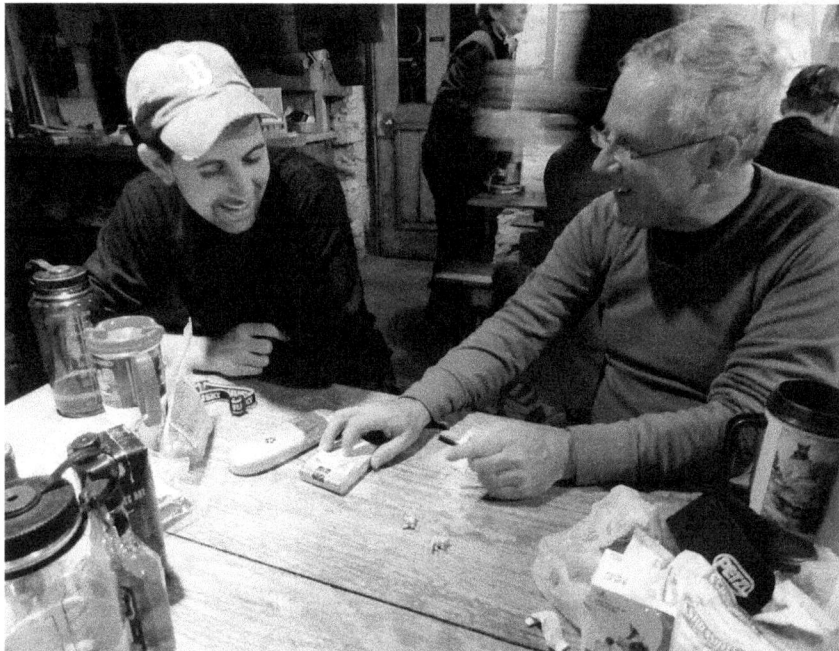

Ryan teaches his Dad a new game at the hut, "Pass the Pigs".

For dinner at the Hut, John made a delicious entrée of chicken pot pie. Ryan made an apple crisp that was to die for! The next morning's breakfast was at the hands of John with bacon and eggs enjoyed with hot coffee and chocolate to prepare us for the hike out.

Ryan and Peter decided to hike the Carter Dome and Mount Height trail back to the trailhead. This is a strenuous hike, but the rewards are magnificent views from the barren peaks of four-thousand footers. John and I returned via Nineteen Mile Brook Trail with a bit of regret for not bringing our crampons.

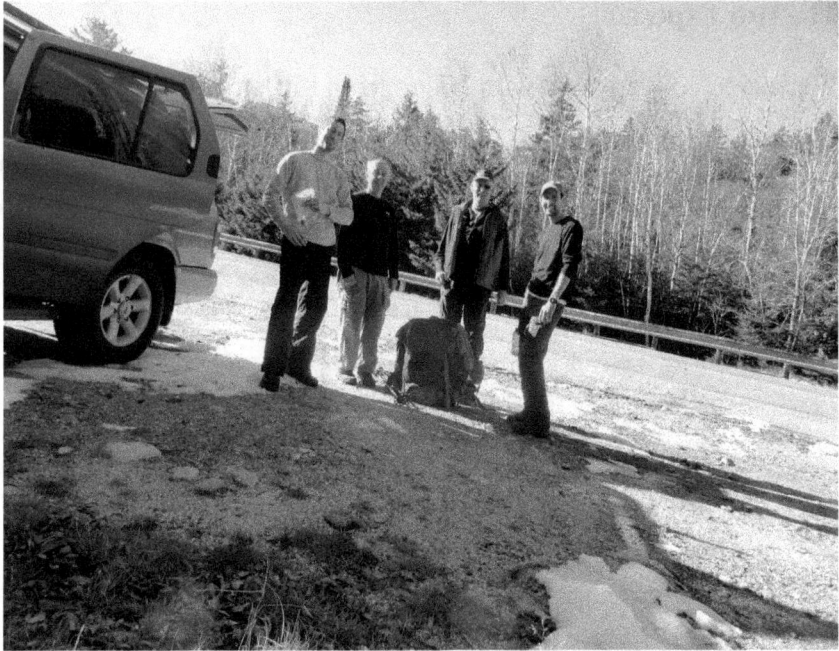

Back to Nineteen Mile Brook Trailhead on Route 16

Enjoy the video as John and I never have to say, "We wish we had joined Ryan and Peter at Carter Notch Hut."

Video of Hike to Carter Notch Hut
- **Blog: A Winter Hike to Carter Notch Hut**
  http://outdooradventurers.blogspot.com/2011/11/winter-hike-to-carter-notch-hut-on.html
- **Video of Visit to Carter Notch Hut via Nineteen-mile Trail**
  http://www.youtube.com/watch?feature=player_embedded&v=kd8JaqvVUfMotch Hutch

Blue Steel Triathlon Club - Bicycle Indoor Time Trials

What do New Hampshire outdoor enthusiasts do on a cold blustery day in March? We ride our bikes indoors! On Sunday March 27th in Milley's Tavern alongside the roaring Merrimack River in Manchester, the Blue Steel Tri Club coordinated a 10K bike race on an indoor course using dynamic bicycle trainers that allows athletes to ride their own bike while pedaling a challenging course simulated with an interactive computer interface.

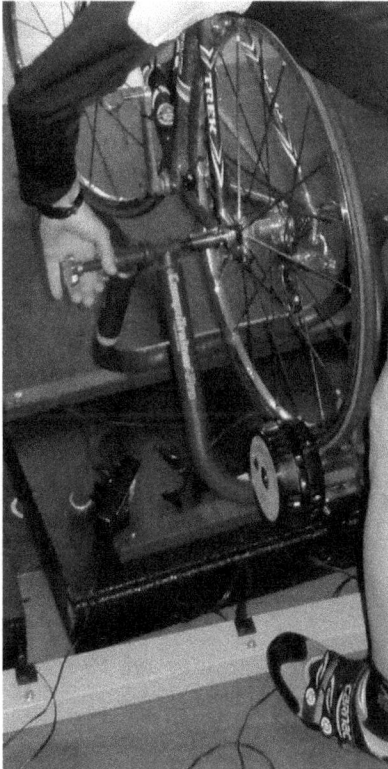

Locking My Bike's Rear Wheel in Place. Notice the Wires from the Spinner (and me) to Transfer Data to the Computer and then to the 8 x 8 Screen in Front of Eight Racers at a time.

Sound easy? Nope! Riding your bike up steep hills mixed with going all-out on flat raceways has you shifting constantly to maintain your cadence and watts.

(You may now be asking yourself, "What is cadence" and "What are watts?" Cadence is the number of revolutions of the crank per minute; roughly speaking, this is the rate at which a cyclist is pedaling or turning the pedals. Watts is longer to define for this book, but in general watts is the amount of power that you are generating by pedaling. It is the latest thing when it comes to cycling. Much like heart rate, watts do not lie. Now go to the Internet and ask, "What are bicycle watts?")

The Fast Splits Company provided the Computrainers, computer software, hardware and peripherals (interface meters between the computer and the rider's trainer).

This was my first indoor simulated bicycle time trail, and I did not know what to expect. Frankly, given the cold weather of our New Hampshire spring, I had only been riding outside twice along with one indoor spinning session three days before the race.

Let's enter the room where the race time trial takes place. There is a computer control station centered in back of eight trainers. In front of the trainers is a 5x6 foot computer screen image (below) with the name of each of the eight riders, and race specific information for each rider to see their race position and effort: how far behind/ahead of the others; distance traveled; time into the race; speed; watts (calculated by rider/bike weight, velocity in mph, amongst other variables.)
(http://bikecalculator.com/veloUS.html.)

We had sixty-four men and women cyclists ranging in age to 70 years young.

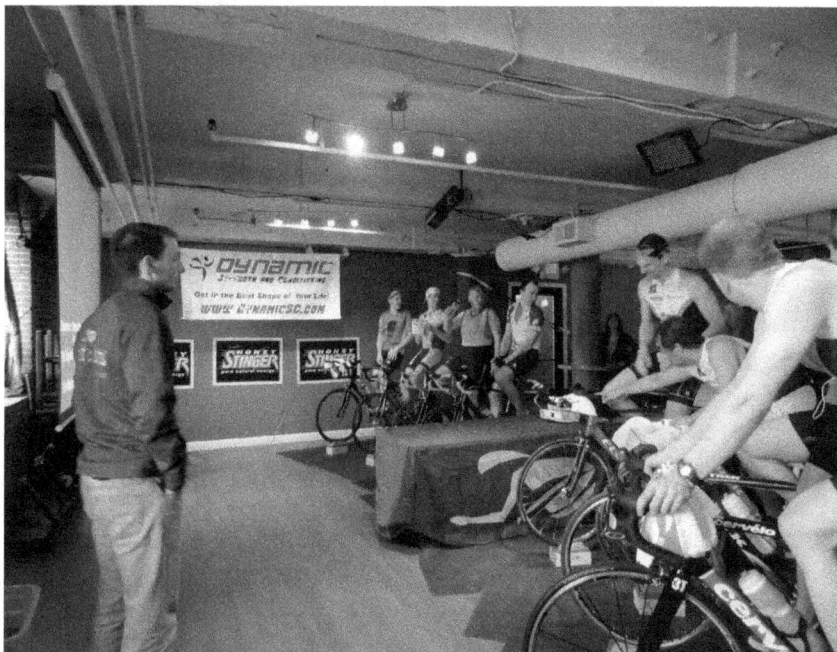

Get Set – Ready Go!

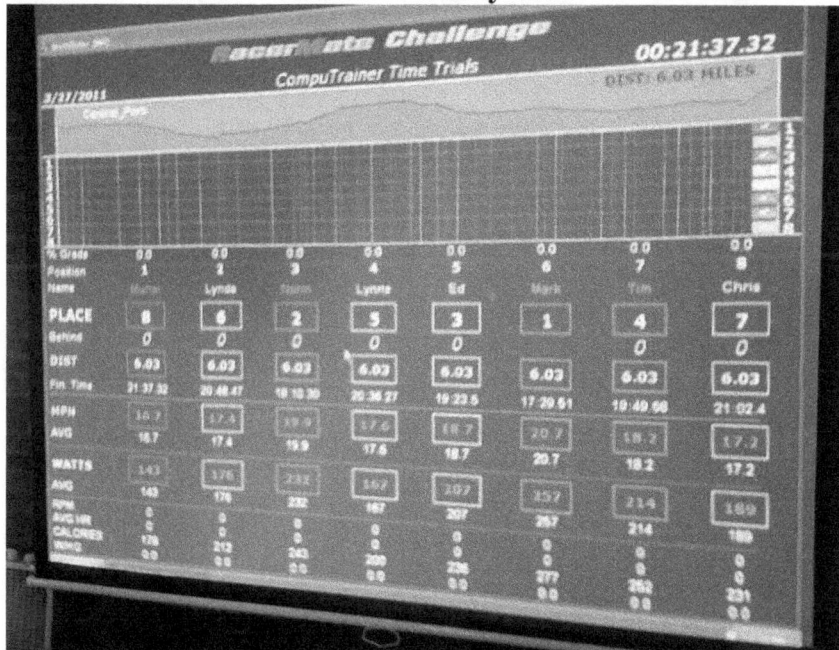

Watch Screen During Race While Pedaling to See How I am doing in the Race Compared to my Competition

A race like this cannot exist with just athletes. Three behind the scenes people made this event happen. Jeff Litchfield and Mike Bradford of Blue Steel Tri Club organized the event and worked throughout the day handling issues to make sure things went smoothly. Johnny from Blue Steel Cyclery, our Gold Sponsor, helped athletes set up their bikes, checked air pressure, inserted skewers if needed (a skewer is the rod for securing the rear wheel on the training stand, if the bike is not compatible with the trainer), and other maintenance items as requested by the athletes.

The selected interviews in the **Video References** below go beyond asking the traditional, "How did you feel while racing?" Instead I, as a fellow competitor, wanted to hear and learn - "What parameters from the race screen were important to you during the race?" Many of the responses are humorous as they show the competitiveness of friendly rivalry.

Video References Indoor Cycling Time Trials

- Blog: Blue Steel Triathlon Club – Indoor Cycling Time Trials
  http://outdooradventurers.blogspot.com/2011/04/blue-steel-triathlon-club-bikes-indoor.html
- A Peek at Indoor Cycling Time Trials
  http://www.youtube.com/watch?feature=player_embedded&v=8ihu4XZdZ_U

Training for Winter Wild in New Hampshire

Winter in New Hampshire offers unique and exciting opportunities for outdoor enthusiasts. In this month's blog I share my training and research in preparation for running a race up the ski slopes of Mt Sunapee in the middle of the winter. The race is called "Winter Wild" (http://www.winterwild.com/) is held March at Mt Sunapee Ski Mountain, Newbury, NH (http://www.mountsunapee.com/).

The rules for this race are pretty simple. Whatever you carry up the hill is what you must descend the hill with. You cannot leave anything stashed anywhere on the mountain! Whatever you go up with, you must return with to the bottom of the hill. Acceptable devices are downhill skis, XC Skis, Telemark Skis, snowboards, snowshoes, crampons or just plain running shoes.

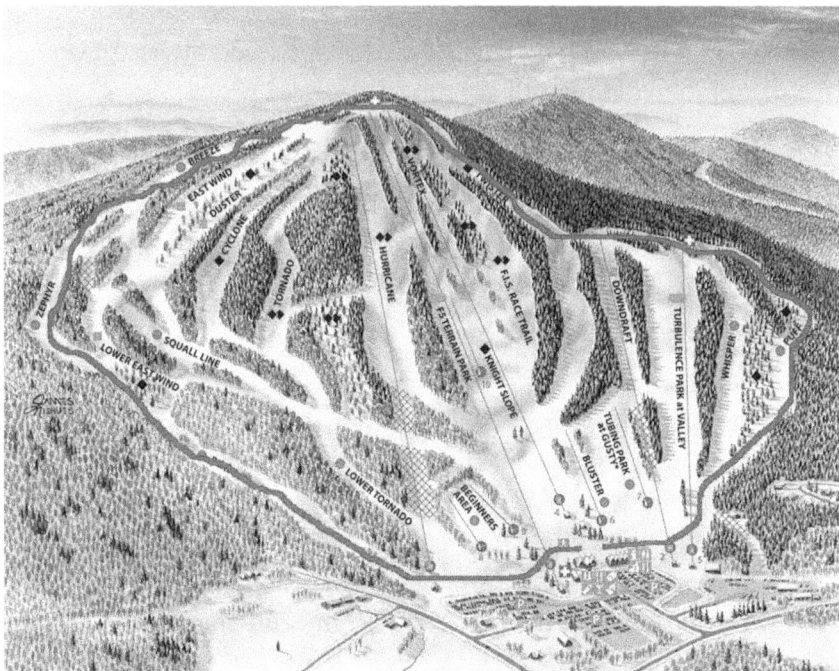

Pats Peak Ski Trail Map with Winter Wild Course Outlined

The first **Video Reference** below describes my winter training run at Pats Peak (http://www.patspeak.com/). The second video is my practice run on the Mt Sunapee course – one week before the race.

Both courses are marked on the video's maps in red and follow the perimeter of their ski areas. The courses start at the bottom of the mountain at the ski lodges, and finish on steep downhills that rush you back to the lodge. The Pats Peak course is counter clockwise, and the Mt Sunapee course is clockwise.

The Mt Sunapee course starts up Elliot Slope to the access road where you begin ascending the Williamson Trail to Stovepipe and up to the Mount Sunapee summit. You descend the Upper Ridge trail all the way down to the Lower Ridge trail and finish in front of the Spruce Lodge.

The learning experience:
Since this was be my first time doing this type of winter event, my practice runs at both Pat's Peak and Mt Sunapee would help me decide:

- Was I in good enough physical shape to do my first ever uphill and downhill ski run?

- Do I wear running shoes or hiking boots? Or, do I carry my back country skis up the hill, and ski down? Or do I carry my snowshoes uphill and use them downhill?

- Do I wear crampons? I had never run in crampons before so I was concerned about their feel.

- What clothing should I wear for a run up a mountain in a New Hampshire winter at below freezing temps?

- After the Pats Peak run I experienced a sore right calf. My remedy was to use a wooden dowel to massage my calf on the days before the race. Would my calf stand up under race conditions?

- During my Mt Sunapee training run, I was half way

through the two mile downhill when I felt an ache in my quads. I walked for a minute and then continued my run. That evening I started using my wooden dowel to massage both quads. Was I really ready for Mt Sunapee?

- The Sunapee training run also produced a blister on my left middle toe. I suspect the uphill trek in my hiking boots caused this. Would a Band-Aid two days before the race be enough to cure the blister?

- In preparation for this grueling uphill/downhill run, I began two days before the race to drink lots of water as a preventive for possible cramps. Did I start my hydration soon enough?

- Did my running base of twenty to twenty five miles a week have me at a good cardiac level for this unique winter ski mountain run? The lesson here is before you do a ski mountain race be sure to get in good physical shape.

The section after this, **Winter Wild at Mount Sunapee New Hampshire,** describes the day of the race results.

Enjoy the below videos for this unique winter event, and never have to say, "I wish I had run the Mt Sunapee Winter Wild race".

Video Reference Winter Wild in New Hampshire
- **Blog: Mt Sunapee and Pat's Peak Winter Wild**
http://outdooradventurers.blogspot.com/2011/02/winter-wild-in-new-hampshire.html
- **Pat's Peak**
http://www.youtube.com/watch?feature=player_embedded&v=wCzj8hWdbuI
- **Mt Sunapee**
http://www.youtube.com/watch?feature=player_embedded&v=G4n_NgzyF8g

---

Winter Wild at Mt Sunapee New Hampshire

MOUNT
SUNAPEE

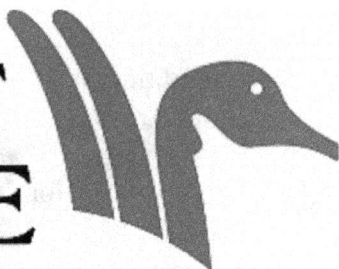

Winter in New Hampshire offers exciting opportunities for outdoor enthusiasts. The **Winter Wild** is a unique ski area race (http://www.winterwild.com/) and is held at Mt Sunapee Ski Mountain, Newbury, NH (http://www.mountsunapee.com/).

The section prior to this, **Training for Winter Wild**, describes the training and concerns I had with preparing for the **Winter Wild at Sunapee.** Fitness level, type of skiing equipment, injuries, and other concerns are shared. If you have a desire to experience an exceptional NH winter experience – be prepared physically and mentally.

The rules for this four mile snow-covered uphill/downhill race at Mt Sunapee are pretty easy. You cannot leave anything stashed anywhere on the mountain! Whatever you go up with you must return with to the bottom of the hill.

Oh, did I mention the temperature was ten degrees with a slight "cooling" breeze?

The 133 athletes wore a mixture of ski attire and their warmest winter running clothing. Some wore their alpine, telemark, or cross-country skis and did a combination of skiing with mostly herringbone "walking" up the steep ski slopes with the expectation they were going to reach the top and go "screaming" down on those same skis. Others backpacked their skis to the top. Many skiers used climbing "skins" on the bottom of their skis for traction uphill on the icy and snowy slopes. Quite a few wore crampons on their hiking boots or running shoes.

My choice was my hiking boots with my ice crampons.

The Mt Sunapee course is marked on the map in red and follows the clockwise perimeter of the ski area. The course begins at Spruce Lodge and then proceeds up Elliot Slope to the access road down where you ascend the Williamson Trail to Stovepipe and on up to the Mount Sunapee summit. You descend the Upper Ridge trail to the Lower Ridge trail returning to the lodge.

Mount Sunapee Trail Map with Winter Wild Course Outlined

Some Winter Wild moments:
• We had a 6:30 am start in order to have all the participants off the mountain by the time the Mountain opens at 8 am for the general public.
• Half way through the two-mile uphill I felt a cramp coming on in my right calf. I slowed to a walk until I felt the cramp was not returning, and then continued my run and walk pace.
• It was foggy as the athletes ascended the 2,726 foot mountain with its three secondary peaks - and at the uppermost peak it was snowing hard. The temperature at the top was in the mid-teens.

Enjoy **Video References** as you join me in this unique winter event.

Oh, I had an enjoyable run. I was thrilled to have participated in this unique winter race.

I never have to say, "I wish I had run the Mt Sunapee Winter Wild. race".

Video Reference Mt Sunapee Winter Wild Race
- Blog: Mt Sunapee Winter Wild
  http://outdooradventurers.blogspot.com/201
  1/03/winter-wild-at-mt-sunapee-new-
  hampshire.html
- Mt Sunapee Winter Wild
  http://www.youtube.com/watch?feature=pla
  yer_embedded&v=1jQpVHUg3q0

A Winter Sleigh Ride

One winter on a snowy February day at Dixville Notch, New Hampshire I had the pleasure to interview sleigh ride owners Dennis and Tina Willey (hitchhorses.com). The Willey's took Cathy and I "over hill and over dale" on a romantic sleigh ride at The Balsams Grand Resort wooded property.

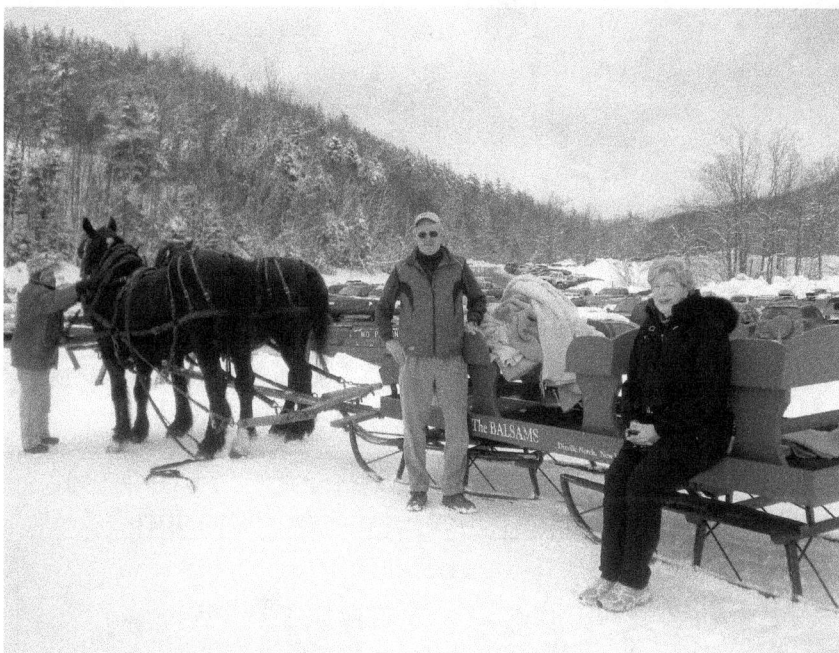

A Sleigh Ride at "The Balsams"

Attending our **Enjoying the Great North Woods** presentation were the two Inn-Bedded Resorters of the Balsams, Alexandra and Luke (alexandluke.com), Canadian social media travel superstars. Alex and Luke have spent the past year crisscrossing North America, sharing their traveling adventures through social media tools like Facebook, Twitter, and more. As guests of the Balsams, the pair tries all of the fine dining and outdoor adventures The **Balsams** has to offer, and then shares them using social media.

The next day we took a two hour cross-country ski on groomed trails through more hills surrounding Dixville Notch. Later we entertained guests of the majestic Balsams Grand Resort (thebalsams.com) with videos of our XC and sleigh memories.

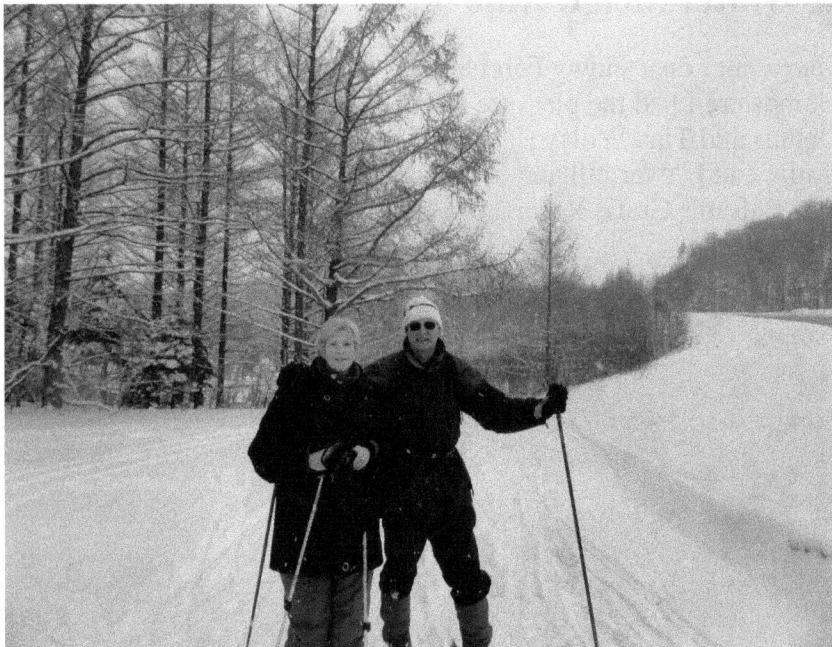

The Balsams Groomed Cross-Country Ski Trail

See the below **Video Reference** and **Never say, "I wish I had enjoyed unique winter experiences in New Hampshire"**.

Video Reference A Winter Sleigh Ride
- Blog: A Unique New Hampshire Winter
  http://outdooradventurers.blogspot.com/2011/02/enj oy-winter-experience-in-new.html
- XC Skiing in Bedford, NH
  http://www.youtube.com/watch?feature=player_ embedded&v=zhtnvjLhq-A
- Enjoy a Winter Sleigh Ride
  http://www.youtube.com/watch?feature=player_ embedded&v=zu9z3dVaiYk

An Alligator Golfing Challenge at Forest Glen Golf and Country Club, Naples, FL

Cathy and I spent five days in Naples, Florida with our friends John and Donna. We had the pleasure of playing golf as their guests at the Forest Glen Golf and Country Club.

As we approached the Tee of the tenth hole, we had a surprise. Enjoy our wildlife **Video Reference** below as we meet a ten foot alligator infringing on our t-time.

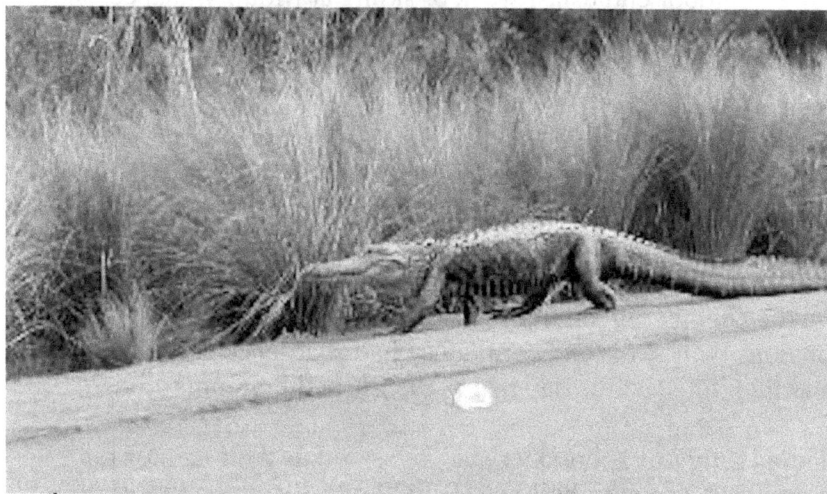

10th Tee Box at Forest Glen Resort, Naples, FL. This 10 foot Gator is Walking Away from where he was Resting Between the Two Tee Markers Where I am about to T-off!

Video Reference Alligator on 10th Golf Hole
- Blog Post Forest Glen Golf Resort Florida
  http://outdooradventurers.blogspot.com/2011/02/wildlife-golfing-experience-at-forest.html
- Video of alligator on 10th Hole of Forest Glen
  http://www.youtube.com/watch?feature=player_embedded&v=aWMiVhEhEec

A New Hampshire Winter of Ice Boating, Alpine Skiing, XC Skiing, Snowshoeing, and Fenway Park

Last week our two grandchildren (Madison 13 and Carson 10) from Kennesaw, Georgia, joined their Uncle Tim, Nana and Papa for an outdoor enthusiast week of skiing at Mount Sunapee, snowshoeing to a beaver dam at Perkins Pond, and a tour of Fenway Park in Boston, MA.

Madison (alpine skier) and Carson (snowboarder) skied last year for the first time. Both took lessons, and had three days of "falling, getting back up, and then trying it again".

Day one this year was on Mt Sunapee's South Peak Learning Area on the beginner green trails. As the day progressed it became obvious their skills and confidence had sharpened from last year, and they finished the day taking the lift to the Summit Lodge.

Tim is truly an expert skier, and he served as their mentor for confidence and skill building. Days 2 and 3 were on the intermediate blue trails of the full mountain.

To get a sense of their skill level see the below video of Carson, Madison, and Tim making their way down South Peak. The end of the video has a brief snowshoe hike to the Perkins Pond beaver dam.

Ice Boat and Snow-shoeing through the Woods

Our friend Dundee called. He wanted to show us his custom made ice boat on Perkins Pond. In addition, he wanted company snowshoeing though the woods visiting a beaver dam on the pond's outlet stream. This was an opportunity outdoor enthusiasts could not turn down.

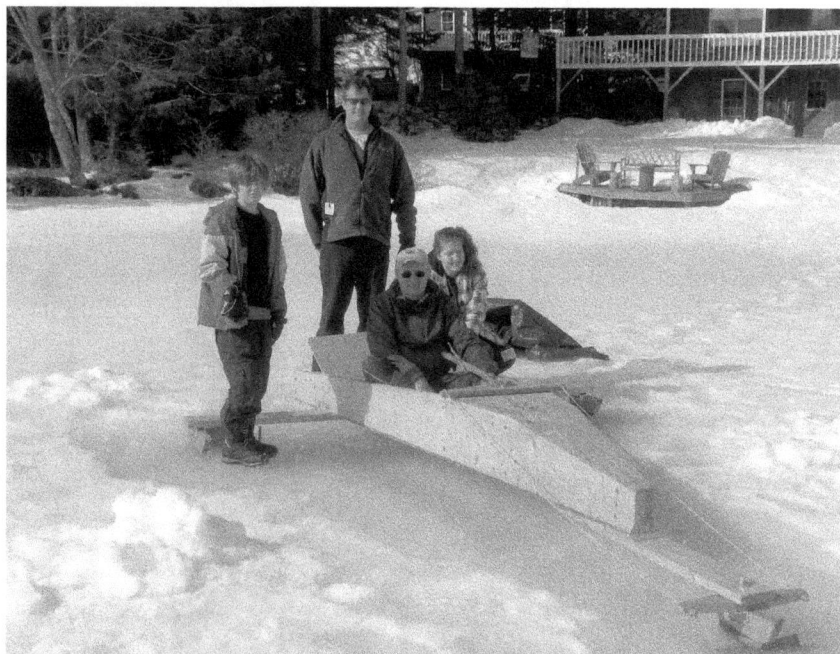

Getting Ready for an Iceboat Ride

Yes, snowshoes are essential tools for anyone whose life or living depends on the ability to get around in areas of deep and frequent snowfall. In addition, snowshoes are used for winter recreation. Snowshoeing is easy to learn, and is a relatively safe and inexpensive recreational activity. As a source to more information on snowshoeing go to http://en.wikipedia.org/wiki/Snowshoe.

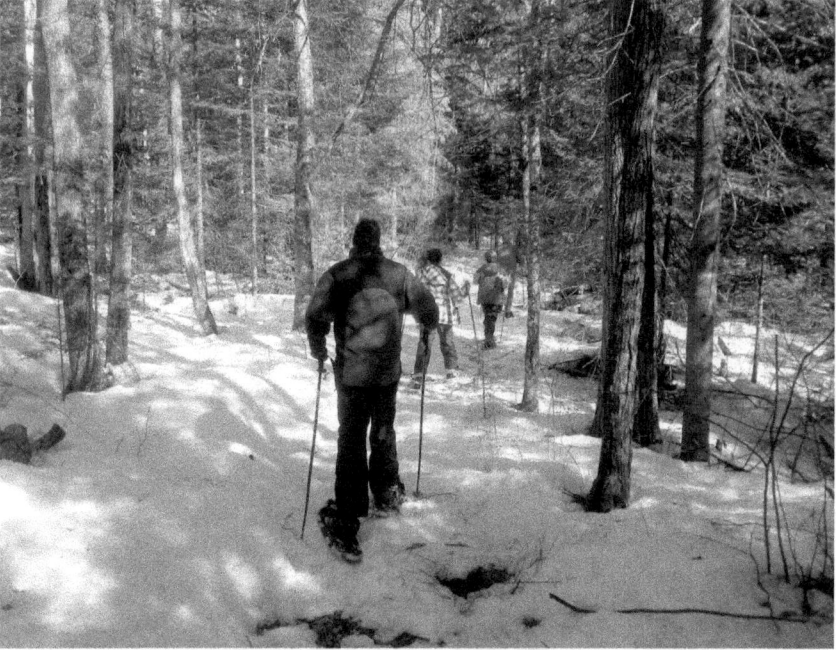
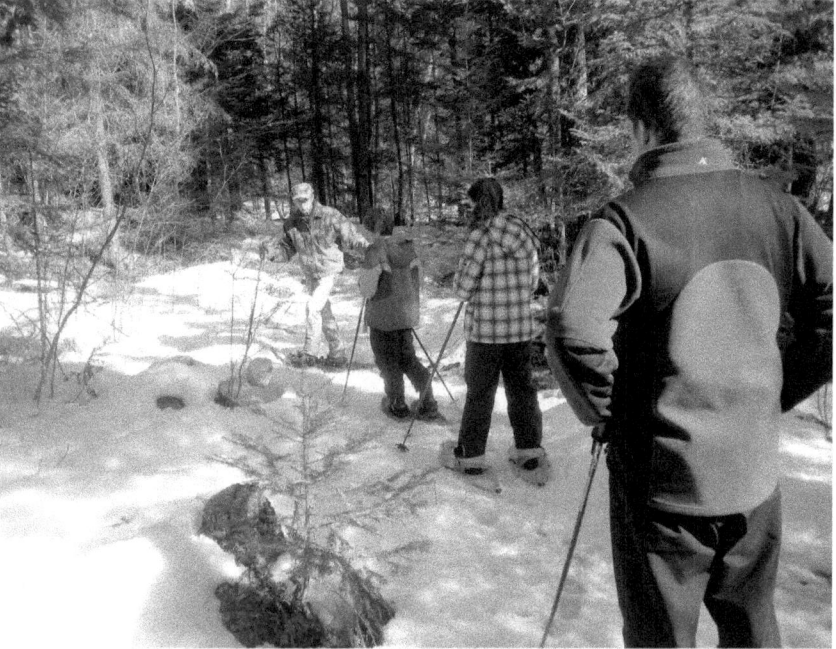

Snow Shoeing and Looking for Animal Tracks

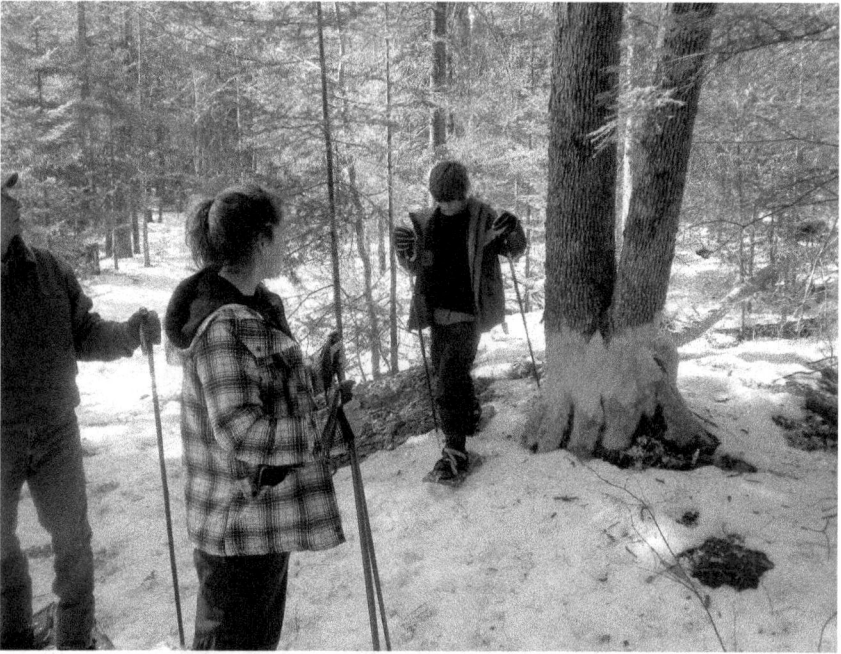
Inspecting the Beaver Tree Damage

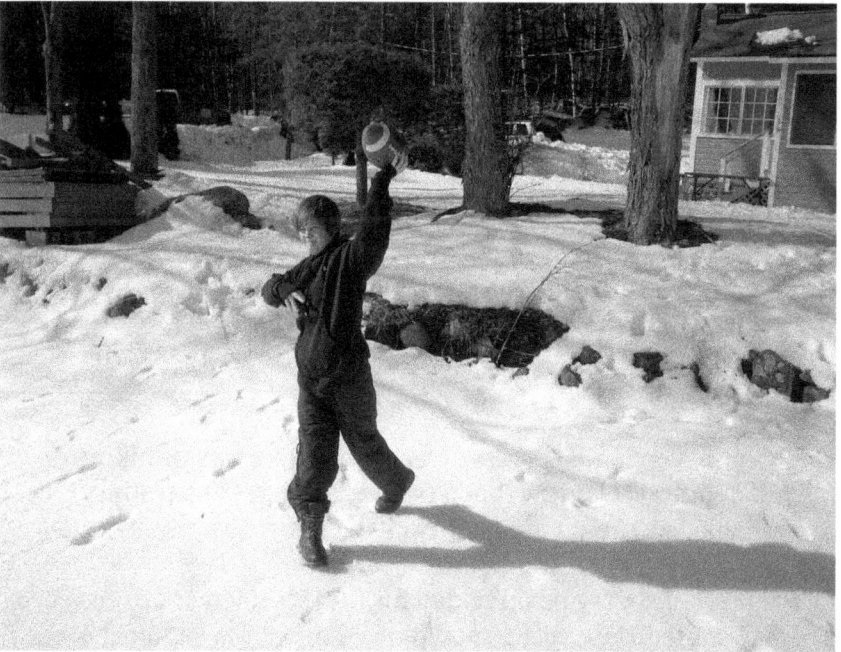
Football on a Frozen Pond

Telemark/Backcountry Practice and Lessons

Outdoor Steve was not to be denied from getting on his backcountry skis. Steve had not tried telemark skiing nor cross-country skied this season. To never say, "I wish I had telemark skied this year", he decided to practice his telemark turns on the "bunny hill".

Telemark skiing, also known as "free heel skiing", is a form of downhill skiing using bindings where the boot is attached only at the toe, similar to those of Cross-country skiing – thus my interest in both as my cross-country and telemark skis are one in the same! I have been told there is a difference, but for me things are close enough with one pair of skis. A good reference is http://en.wikipedia.org/wiki/Telemark_skiing.

Telemark skiing has a style of turn where one ski is advanced in front of the other and the heel is raised on the rear ski, and with the skier in a very bent knee position. It is a form of downhill skiing using bindings where the boot is attached only at the toe like Cross-country skiing, allowing the heel to come up from the ski. Because the heel is free, it allows the skier to go into a lunge position in order to turn. The act of lunging while turning is a technique called the telemark turn. Some see it as genuflecting or almost kneeing on one knee, just like in church.

Admittedly Steve is still in the telemark "beginner" stage.

Day one was OK, as he began to feel comfortable after being off his skis for over a year.

Day two was trying, and at the end of the two hours of hiking up the hill and then telemark down (snow plowing to be truthful), Steve managed a few turns that "felt" like he was a telemarker.

Day three was a very positive day for Steve's telemark experience. The day started slow, as he snowplowed down the beginner's hill, as he tried to get the "feel" of a telemark turn. Finally, after much contemplation of whether to join Cathy in the lodge, he saw a

Sunapee Ski instructor on the slope, and asked him about instruction. It turns out the instructor taught telemark lessons. It was Steve's lucky day as Mike was the only telemark instructor at the Mountain.

Telemark skiing has been called "the world's oldest new sport". Telemark skiing (or "tele") has also been called "the most rhythmic and flowing way to descend a snow covered mountain or backcountry trail." One thing I do know with absolute certainty: tele skiing is all about the stroke, the sensation, that feeling and exhilaration that comes from getting into the groove of the tele turn.

To paraphrase John Muir, "Telemark skiing gives access to places to play, places where nature may heal and give strength to body and soul, to interact with wildlife, to feel the forces of gravity, the energy of a gathering storm. A lot of tele skiers find a big part of the stroke to be in the friendships they develop with other members of the tribe, and for some a big attraction is the challenge of learning a new approach to skiing their local resort or terrain park. And then there are the philosophical, almost "Zen-like" aspects to the sport."

While all of these things add to the fun of tele skiing, the true stroke is hard to describe. It can be an almost ethereal experience in those moments when everything comes together: form, function, time and space. Yet it is almost uncanny how something as intangible as this stroke can come to dominate a large part of so many of our lives. Frankly, I have yet to learn the tele stroke (http://www.telemarktips.com/WhatsTele.html).

Telemark Instruction
Mike had me try a few of my tele turns, and he immediately diagnosed one of my (many) major flaws – I was using my uphill ski to "grab" the hill when turning, and I thus crossed my skis. Opps, away I fell. He demonstrated "my" snowplow, emphasizing its deficiency. He then demonstrated the turn with the uphill ski being kept flat through the turn. Now it was my turn to see if I learned from Mike. Walla, I made a decent snowplow. I practiced a few turns with Mike's additional comments. I immediately felt a

comfort level with Mike's instructions – and certainly my turns. I was now ready to be shown the proper tele turn.

Mike had me parallel the hill as I slid one ski in front of the other while keeping both skis parallel. Mike quickly pointed out I did not raise my left heel. I could have sworn I had it raised, but when I looked down, it was only in my imagination. Mike certainly has excellent observational skills – and a very wonderful teaching manner.

My hour was up, and it was time to leave the hill. I doubt if I will make it back on snow this year, so hopefully this blog post will remind me of the instructions of Mike. If you want a wonderful telemark instructor, you can reach Mike at the Mt Sunapee Learning Center or at Eastman 's Recreation Center.

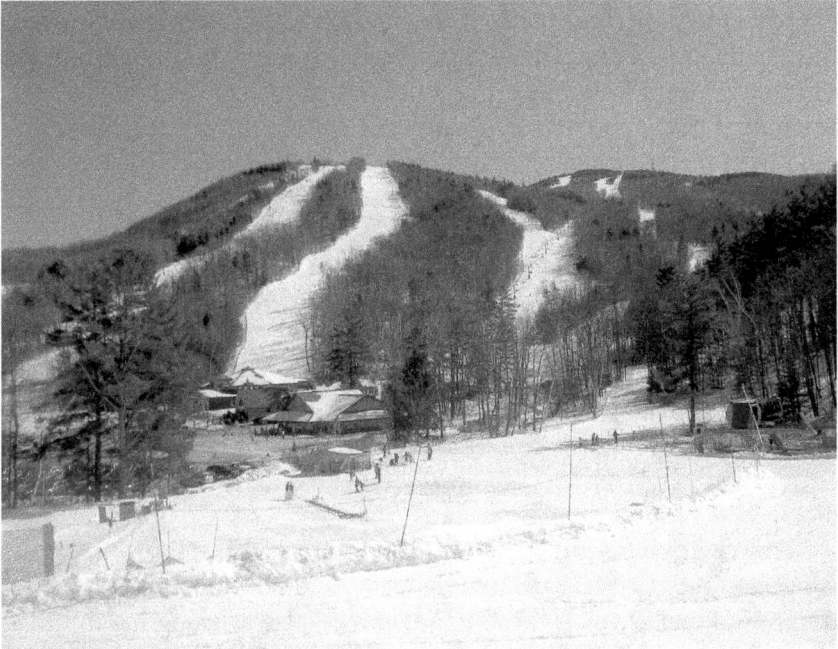

The Ski Slopes of Mt Sunapee

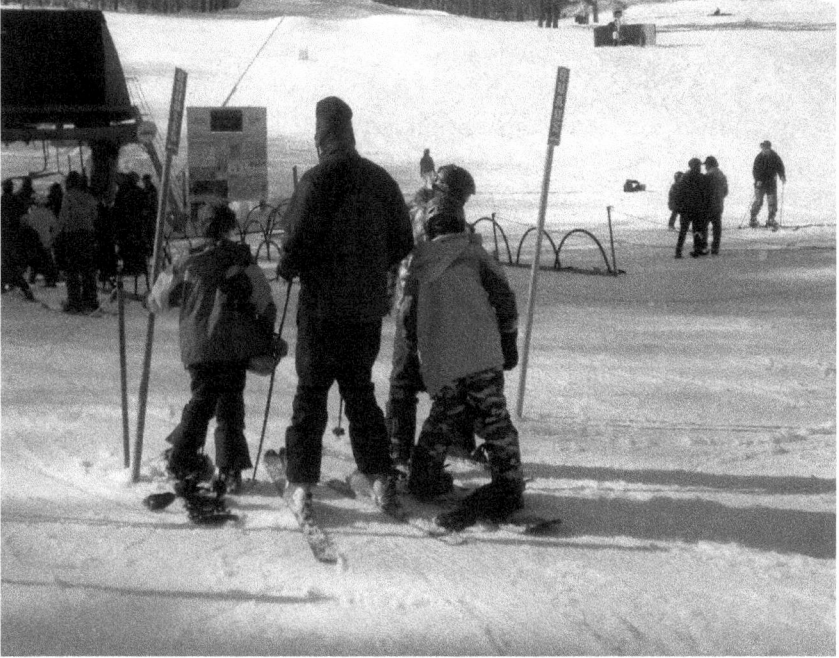

Alpine and Snowboarding

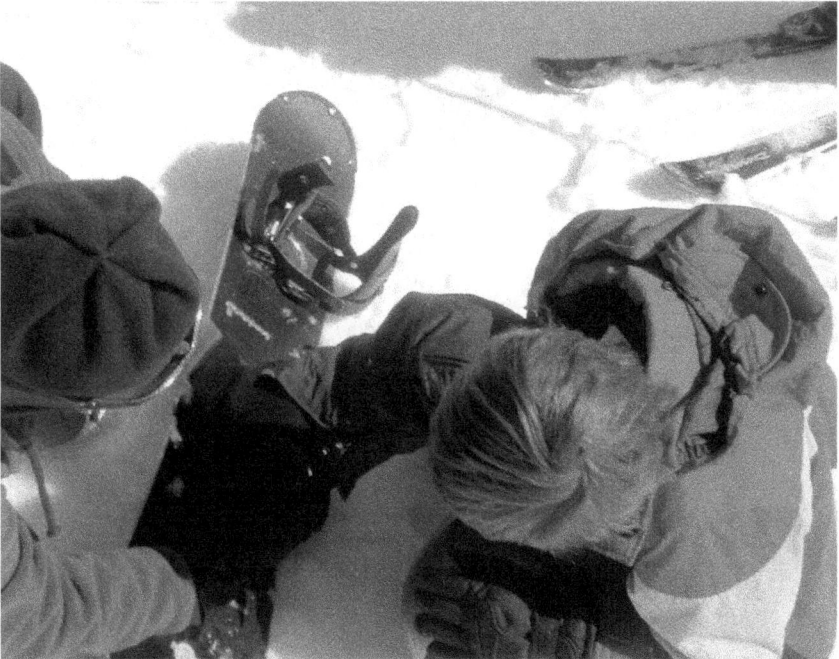

Snow Boarding Repairs

Fenway Park

My grandson, Carson, is a left-handed pitcher, and an avid Red Sox fan. He wanted to tour Fenway Park. Fenway is being prepared for the Red Sox April 4th opener. The field this year needed sod due to the ice hockey games Fenway hosted this winter.

See the below brief video of the Fenway Park tour. Note the wolf-like animal in the outfield. Of course, this is a stuffed animal, and when asked, our tour guide explained that stuffed animals are used to keep the geese from eating the newly sown seed.

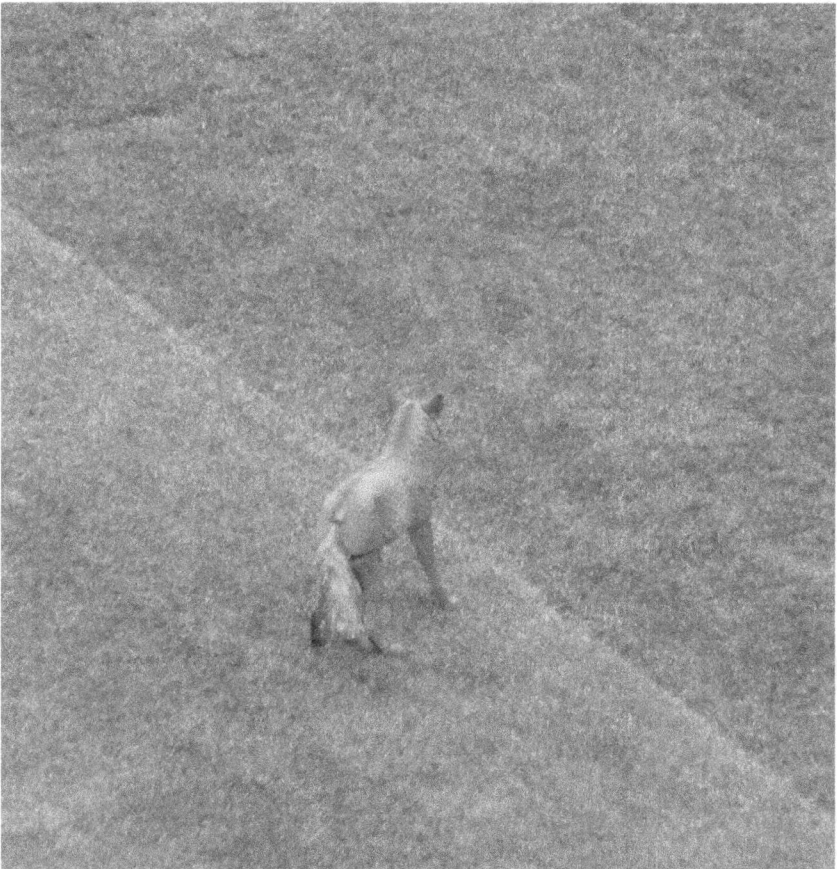

Keeping the Birds Off the Turf. Does this Wolf Really Work?

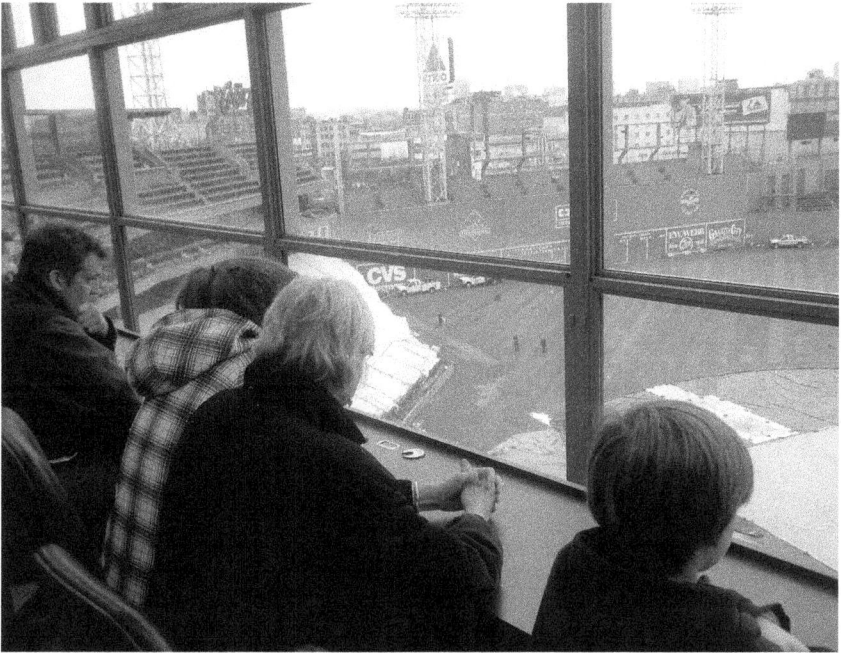

A Look from Fenway Park's VIP Seats

I now never have to say, "I wish I had offered to my grandkids the outdoor winter fun in northern New England".

Video Reference NH Winter Vacation of Snowboarding, Downhill Skiing, Snow Shoeing, Celtics and Fenway Park
- **Blog: NH Winter Vacation**
  http://outdooradventurers.blogspot.com/2010/03/family-that-enjoys-winter-together.html
- **NH Skiing Mt Sunapee and Snowshoeing Video**
  http://www.youtube.com/watch?feature=player_embedded&v=dRm1mZdHrxk
- **A Winter Tour of Fenway Park**
  http://www.youtube.com/watch?v=RQHHCibZUWo&feature=player_embedded

Deep Travel and Way Down Upon the Suwannee River

I am preparing to paddle the Suwannee River!

I posted a blog on my hike along the Suwannee River, **Paddle Florida - Get Down on the Suwannee River, and Go with the Flow!** I received a phone call shortly after announcing my post from my friend Dundee saying he wanted to paddle the Suwannee. My response was, "If you organize it, I will go". Well, in the middle of March the following year, Dundee, John, Shaun and I were paddling the Suwannee River.

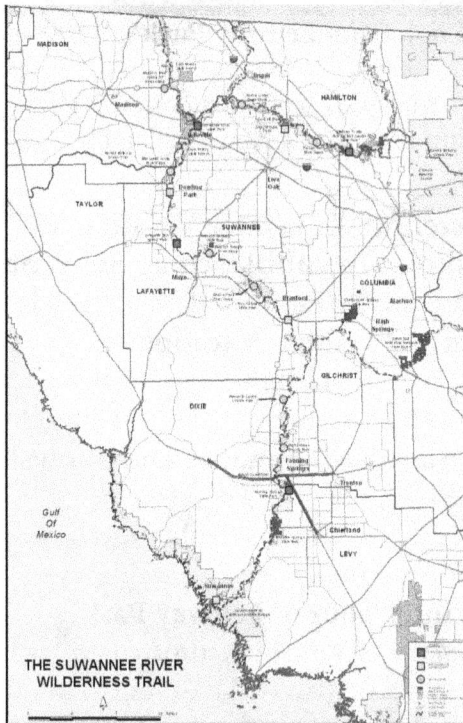

The Suwannee River Wilderness Trail

In five days we will kayak and canoe 70 of the 246 miles of the Suwannee River starting in Florida close to the Georgia border where the Suwannee flows under Rte 6. We will pull out five days later at Suwannee River State Park in Live Oak, FL after camping 4 nights along the River.

Planning the Trip

In preparing for the trip under Dundee's leadership, we Googled the "Suwannee River", read William A. Logan's, Canoeing and Camping 213 miles of The Beautiful Suwannee River, and watched Logan's DVD. My sister Barbara and husband Larry introduced me to the lore of the Suwannee River - and Barbara will provide contacts and maps from the Suwannee River Management District Department of Land Acquisition and Management. The White Springs water level is used to determine the water conditions. In my email correspondence with Edwin McCook, SRMD Land Management Specialist, he says, "I like to paddle the river between 50' and 60' above sea level as shown by the White Springs marker", pictured in an earlier section of this book.

As part of our planning Dundee and I took a day trip to Vermont in the summer to visit with his cousin Arthur. Arthur is a retired biologist who had responsibilities in the Suwannee River area, and he readily shared sights of interest, warnings, and camping suggestions (i.e. firewood is plentiful, check the water level at White Springs before you start, "alligators will not bother you", etc.)

Deep Travel

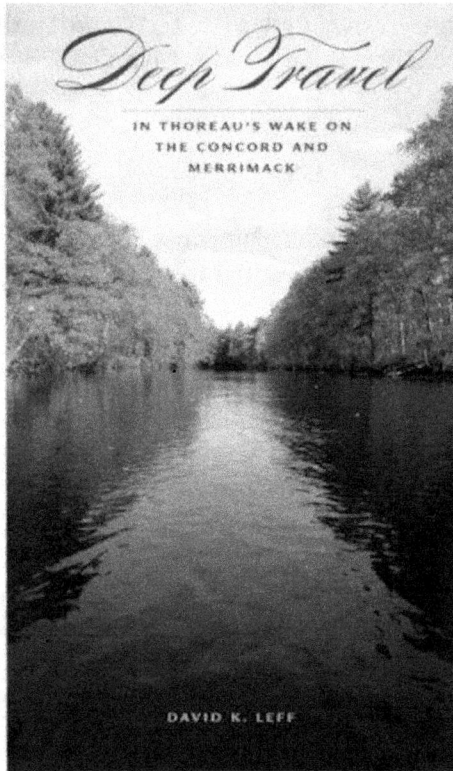

My Deep Travel Inspiration

A response from my friend Doug to my Dreaming the Appalachian Trail blog post in January suggested I look at David Leff's web site http://www.davidkleff.com/. I checked David's web site, emailed him, and I now have an autographed copy of his book, **Deep Travel: In Thoreau's Wake on the Concord and Merrimack**.

So how does **Deep Travel** relate to my Suwannee paddle plans? Let me share a few paragraphs from David's **Deep Travel**:

"At its simplest, deep travel is about heightened awareness. It is careful looking. It is paying attention to what is around you. Deep travel demands that we immerse ourselves fully in places and realize that they exist in time as well as space. A deep traveler knows the world is four-dimensional and can't be experienced with eyes and ears only.

Deep travel is not so much a matter of seeing sights as it is sight seeking. It is a searching for the patterns and juxtapositions of culture and nature and delighting in the incongruities left by the inexorable passage of time. Deep travelers revel in the wild, inspiring call of a kingfisher as it flies over a couple of trolling anglers with Bud longnecks in one hand and rods in the other. They savor the sight of a tree shaded burial ground squeezed between big-box retailers on a traffic choked commercial strip.

Deep travelers look not so much for scenery or enchanting objects as for a tapestry of comprehension woven from stone walls, retail establishments, street and topographical names, transportation networks, building styles, plant and animal assemblages, advertising signs, and other artifacts. Each element makes a statement about the landscape as a whole and the relationship of one part to another. Together, they tell a story. Deep travel is an ecological way of looking where everything we see has a function and all the parts are related, no matter how seemingly disparate or contradictory.

Like animals that remain intensely aware of their surroundings and any alteration to them because predation or starvation await the unwary, deep travelers work to be keenly conscious of their environs. They strive for the alertness and acuity of wildland firefighters or soldiers whose survival depends on their knowledge of topography, history, weather, vegetation, and the observance of changes in minute phenomena. Such mindfulness simultaneously enriches experience and makes the voyager worthy of the journey."

David's book, and in particular the above section, made me realized the Suwannee was an opportunity to improve my deep traveler skills. My friend Dundee is a deep traveler and he always "stops to smell the roses" and appreciate the moment of the forests, animals, flora and sky. Me, I need to remind myself to be a deep traveler, and as David says, "At its simplest, deep travel is about heightened awareness. …..A deep traveler knows the world is four-dimensional and can't be experienced with eyes and ears only."

I never want to say, "I wish I had been a deep traveler on the Suwannee River."

Video Reference Deep Travel and the Suwanee River

- Blog: Deep Travel and the Suwanee River
  http://outdooradventurers.blogspot.com/2010/02/way-down-upon-suwannee-river.html
- Suwanee River
  http://en.wikipedia.org/wiki/Suwannee_River
- Deep Travel In Thoreau's Wake on the Concord and Merrimack
  http://www.uiowapress.org/books/2009-spring/leff.htm
- Dreaming the Appalachian Trail
  http://outdooradventurers.blogspot.com/2010/01/dreaming-appalachian-trail.html

---

Let's Go Spinning!

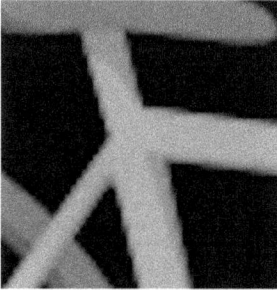

Blue Steel Cyclery

"Do you want to go spinning?" my friend Dick asked. My first response was, "I do not do yarn".

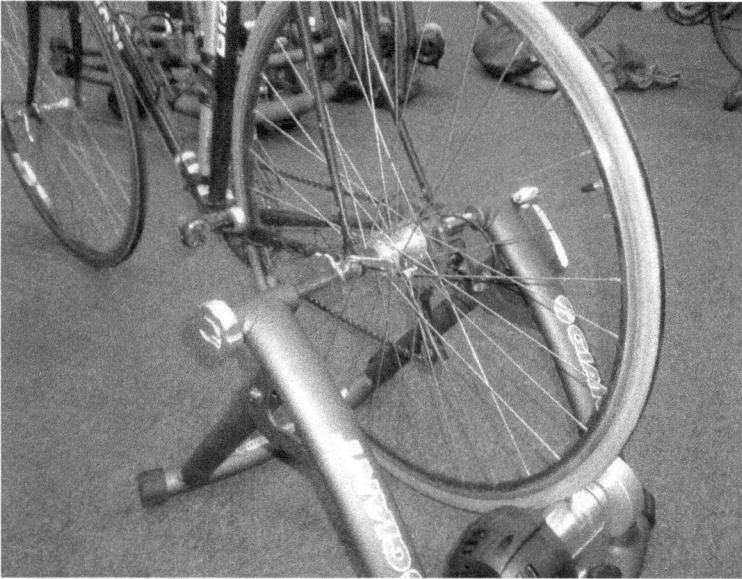

Fixed Rear Wheel of My Road Bike is Locked

So what is spinning? For an outdoor enthusiast, spinning is a bicycle aerobic exercise that can either take place on a specially designed stationary bike-like device called (obviously enough) a spinning bike, or, you can put your own bicycle in a climbing block and stationary trainer, and pedal nowhere. Fixed wheel helps improve your pedaling and bicycle posture technique.

A perfect time for spinning is on a cold, windy, snowy night in the middle of a New Hampshire winter. What a great time to meet friends, get cardio exercise, learn the secrets of pedaling from experts, and adjust your bike's hardware. I attended an evening one hour indoor cycling spinning class at Blue Steel Cyclery in Manchester, NH. (http://www.bluesteelcyclery.com/)

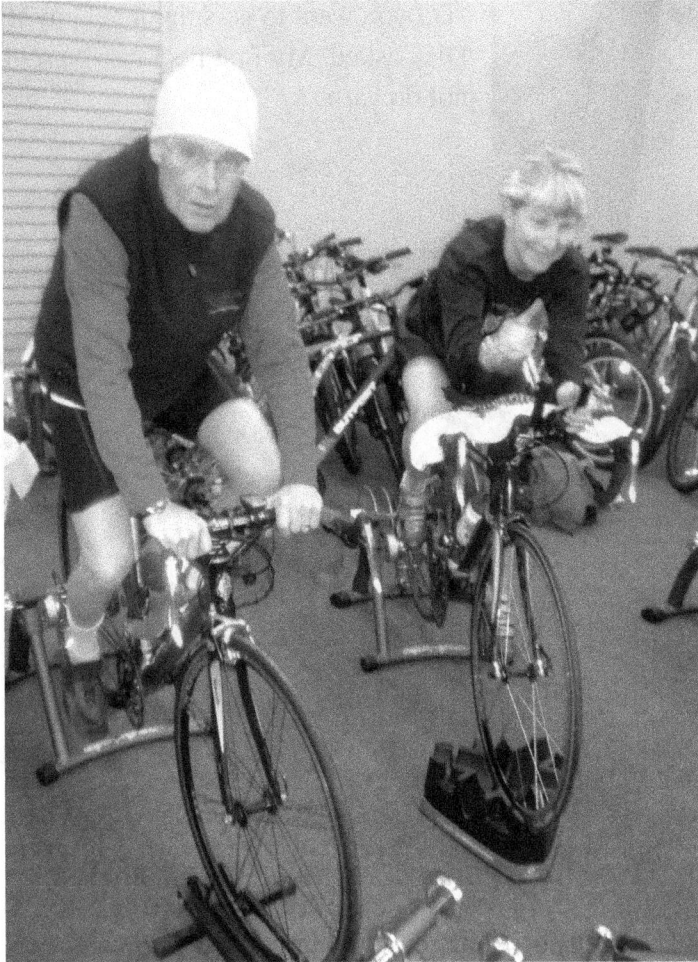

Dick and Kathy Spinning Nowhere

First, let me stress this class is not for the novice bicyclist. The pace of the class is aimed at experienced bicyclists preparing for spring competition and long outdoor mileages. I use this class to be ready for my summer triathlons.

Our Instructor Ready to Put us Through Our Paces (Gears)

The class is led by Jack, a USAC Level III Coach (www.usacycling.org/). As we pedal with motivating beat music in the background, Jack talks us through a visualization of an outdoor cycling workout: "You're going up a long hill now; you can't see the top yet...."

During the class you vary your pace -- sometimes pedaling at a high cadence, other times cranking up the gear level, and even pedaling from a standing position. We do routines that are designed to simulate terrain and situations similar to riding a bike outdoors. Some of the movements and positions include hill climbs, sprints and interval training.

Blue Steel Cyclery bike shop provides space for our twice weekly "bike ride". The staff even helps with minor equipment adjustments, such as helping me when my cadence meter was not registering and assisting me when my handlebars needed a more efficient alignment. Without Blue Steel's continued support this class would not be possible.

Jack hardily encourages us to drink plenty of water. Indoor cycling is very energetic and causes a lot of sweating, and a person can easily get dehydrated. Spinning burns serious calories and offers an awesome aerobic workout that makes your heart pump fast. It also tones your quadriceps and outer thigh muscles. Because you stay in one place with the same basic movement throughout, spinning makes it easier to concentrate on your form than in an outdoor environment.

We follow Jack's encouragement and instruction: "pedal with only your left leg for one minute, one minute slow pedaling with both legs, and then pedal with the right leg for one minute."

To get more information on spinning go to http://yourtotalhealth.ivillage.com/diet-fitness/spinning-101.html and Indoor Cycling Tips and Training

What do I bring to the class?
• My bicycle and my bike shoes
• A bottle of water (I am definitely going to sweat.)
• Hat or sweat band
• Towel for wiping away perspiration
• Power meters and heart rate monitors are encouraged
• Padded bicycle shorts

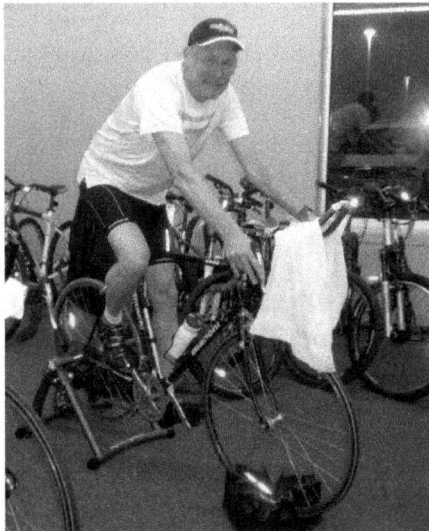

Bike, Hat, Shorts, Towel, Water Bottle, Meters

I now, never have to say, "I wish I had done winter spinning."

Video References A Winter Spinning Class
  • **Let's Go Spinning**
    http://outdooradventurers.blogspot.com/201
    0/01/lets-go-spinning.html

The Outdoors as a Daily
Component of Life

Regret for the things we did can be tempered by time. It is the things we did not do that is inconsolable – Sydney J. Harris

Get Exercised Outdoors

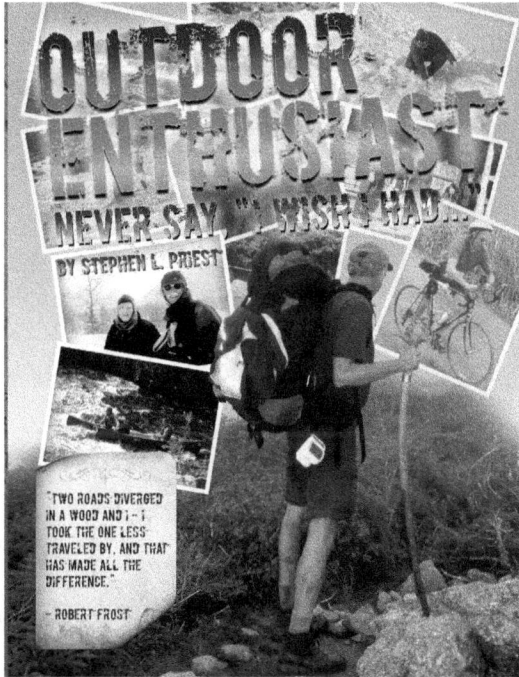

New Hampshire Magazine **Selects** Outdoor Enthusiast: Never say, 'I wish I had...'' **as Bookshelf June 2009 Book of the Month**

Couch potatoes, arise!

Stephen Priest sees his torn Achilles tendon as "good fortune". Without the injury (now years ago) he wouldn't have become an outdoor enthusiast nor written a book about it. When Priest's doctors told him that there was an even chance the tendon would tear again in the future, he set out to prove them wrong. He began an exercise program (starting with walking just the distance between two telephone poles) that led to a lifetime of hiking, biking, kayaking, cross-country skiing, marathon running, swimming and even shovel-sliding.

He wants others to enjoy the outdoors as much as he does. His 242-page book, "Outdoor Enthusiast" (http://www.outdoorsteve.com/, Amazon.com) outlines a plan for getting started (yes, between telephone poles is part of it) and for how to continue living a healthy lifestyle by being outdoors. He uses his own experiences with his outdoor activities to discuss the challenges and cautions of each. He also writes extensively about avoiding injuries (first of all, stretch), being a guest in nature's habitat (watch out for bobcats) and where to go to "play" in New Hampshire, Maine and Vermont. If you're ready to leave your couch or to kick your current exercise routine up a notch, this book can tell you a thing or two about how to do it.

> **Reference NH Magazine Selects Outdoor Enthusiast**
> - Blog: Get Exercise Outdoors!
>   http://outdooradventurers.blogspot.com/2009/06/new-hampshire-magazine-selects-outdoor.html
> - New Hampshire Magazine
>   http://www.nhmagazine.com/

Outdoor Enthusiast Campfire Chat: Starting Your Campfire with Rotten Birch Bark

Most campers know birch bark contains a combustible oil and will burn fiercely even when wet. We also know that it is not appropriate to peel bark from a live tree.

What was missing from my knowledge was if old rotten and damp birch bark will still serve as kindle to quickly start a file.

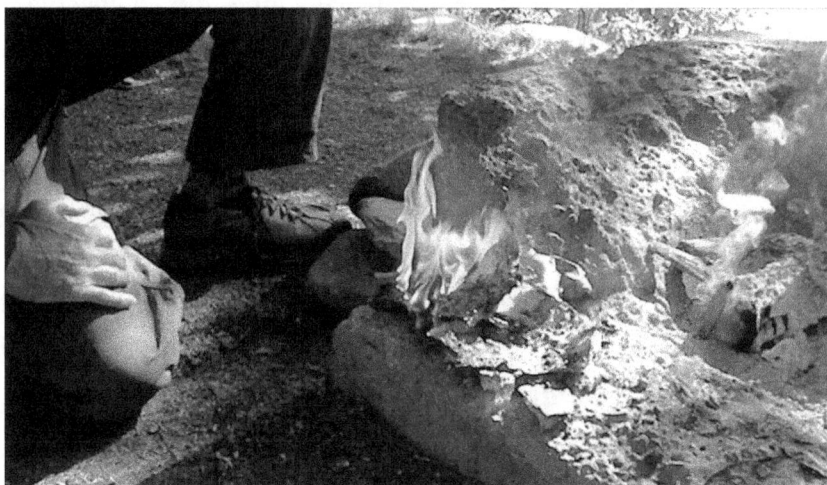

Rotten Birch Bark Good Kindling

During a recent hike in the Great North Woods of New Hampshire we passed through a swampy area with old blown down birches. They obviously had been lying on the floor of this forest for years. My friend thought over time this downed tree had lost its combustible oil. I was not sure, and I never wanted to say, "I wish I had tried using rotten birch bark to start a camp fire". Certainly, rather than wait to test this theory under emergency conditions, we tried it now.

See the below video on using rotten birch bark to start a camp fire.

> **Video References Using Rotten Birch Bark to Start a Camp Fire**
> - Using Rotten Birch Bark
>   http://outdooradventurers.blogspot.com/2010/06/outdoor-enthusiast-campfire-chat.html

Apps for the Outdoors

Bedford Community TV is showing a streaming video of **Apps for the Outdoors: *Smart Phone Technology for Fresh Air Activities*** by Outdoor Steve

----

Let's use smart phone apps with your outdoor activity. Do you know how fast you ran? How many miles did you bike last month? How far did you walk your dog? How many miles did you paddle? Can your friends look at a map and tell where you are on a remote wilderness trek? Smart phone apps can provide a fun and easy way to maintain a chronology of your outdoor activities.

Interestingly, as quoted from **6 Ways to Make Exercise More Fun, Effective and Even Tasty**, *"Multiple studies have found that high-tech gadgets – such as ....., and fitness apps – help people stick to exercise programs. Who wants to disappoint their iphone?"*

Browser Search "Outdoor Enthusiast Apps"

A smart phone with GPS connectivity makes available a wealth of outdoor applications (apps). Enter keywords "outdoor enthusiast apps" in your preferred search engine and you will see a plethora of web sites and blogs for Android, iPhone, Blackberry and other smart phone outdoor apps. Refine your search further with specific keywords such as "Canoe Android apps", "Hiking iPhone apps", etc.

Here are four smart phone Android GPS apps and two desktop/laptop apps I have used for different outdoor activities.

	Map My Fitness	Run Keeper	My Tracks	Google	Where's My Droid
Website	MapMyFitness.com	RunKeeper.com	MyTracks.com	Google.com/Earth & Google.com	WheresMyDroid.com
Questions	✓How far did we hike today?	✓How far did I bicycle and at what speed?	✓How far did I walk my dog?	✓How far to paddle around the lake? ✓Find a campfire breakfast.	✓Where is my ocean paddling friend now?

Browser Search for Our Breakfast Eggs

John assumed responsibility to plan and cook our meals for our Suwannee River paddling trek. He expressed a desire to "do something different" on this trip. Through a Google search he found a site recommending cooking an egg inside an orange over an open campfire. The result was absolutely delicious. Go to the **Video References** box below to see this unique breakfast treat.

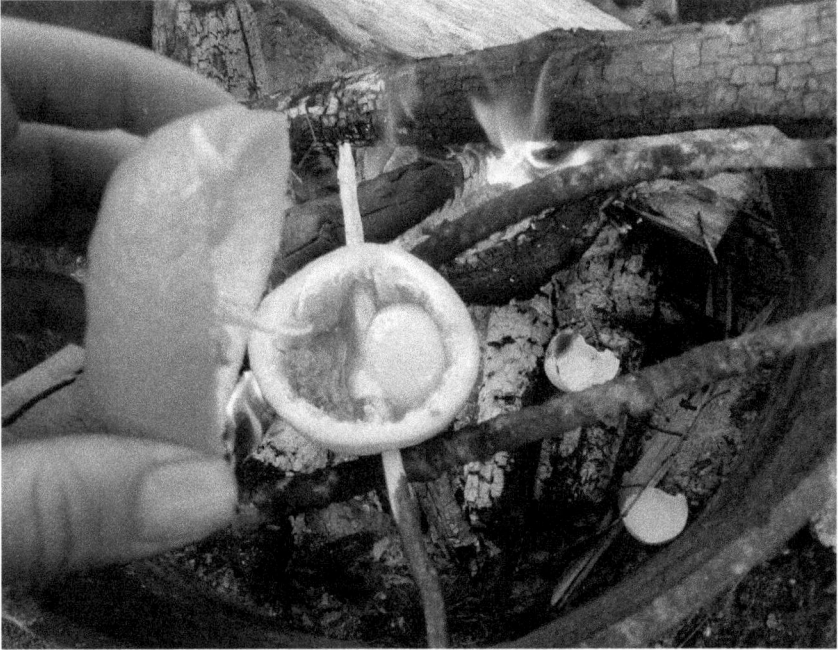

Cook an Egg in an Orange

John further impressed us with his campfire cooking creativity by serving us a banana sundae – a banana with most of the skin left on it. Slice the banana lengthwise, and then put bits of chocolate in the slit. Place the combined desert inside aluminum foil and heat in the campfire ashes for a few minutes. Indeed, it tastes like a banana sundae!

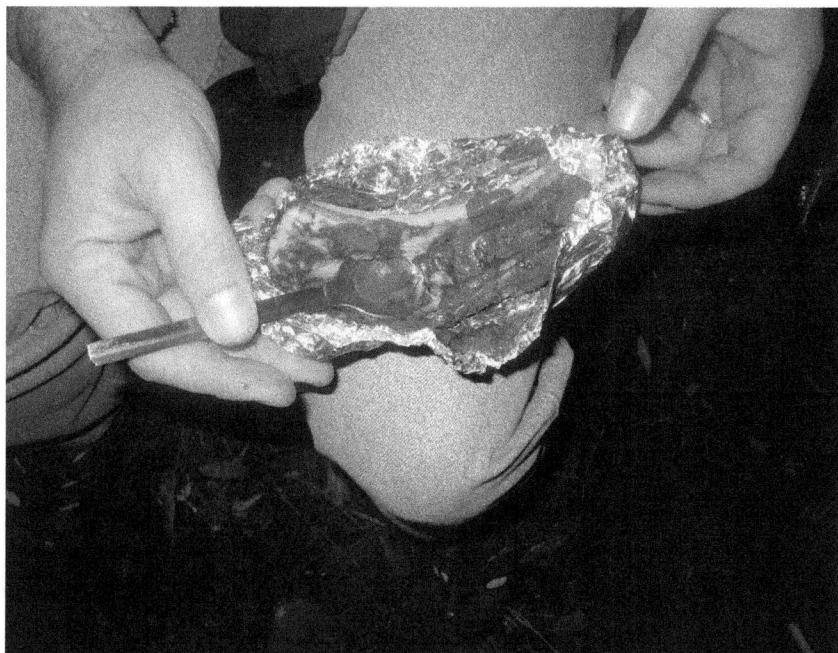

A Banana Sundae Prepared an Open Flame Campfire

On another trip we further tested my outdoor breakfast cooking skills by cooking an egg inside an onion. Outdoor Steve's Fireside Chat: How to Cook an Egg in an Onion. Interestingly as of today I have over 40,000 YouTube views on **How to cook an egg in an onion.**

iMapMyFitness

Recently I used my **iMapMyfitness** app with a fellow outdoor enthusiast who carved a walking and dirt bike trail on his New Hampshire forested property. He asked me if I could give him the total distance of this pathway with all its turns and hills accurately measured.

At the beginning of his trailhead I opened my app, clicked the Start Arrow, and proceeded to walk into his forest trail. The app had a camera feature and we took a picture of a tree where a bear had recently clawed. After meandering for nearly a half hour over this forested trail we arrived at our starting point where I clicked the Pause and the Save button. We then went to his house and his desktop computer, and viewed the statistics of our trek.

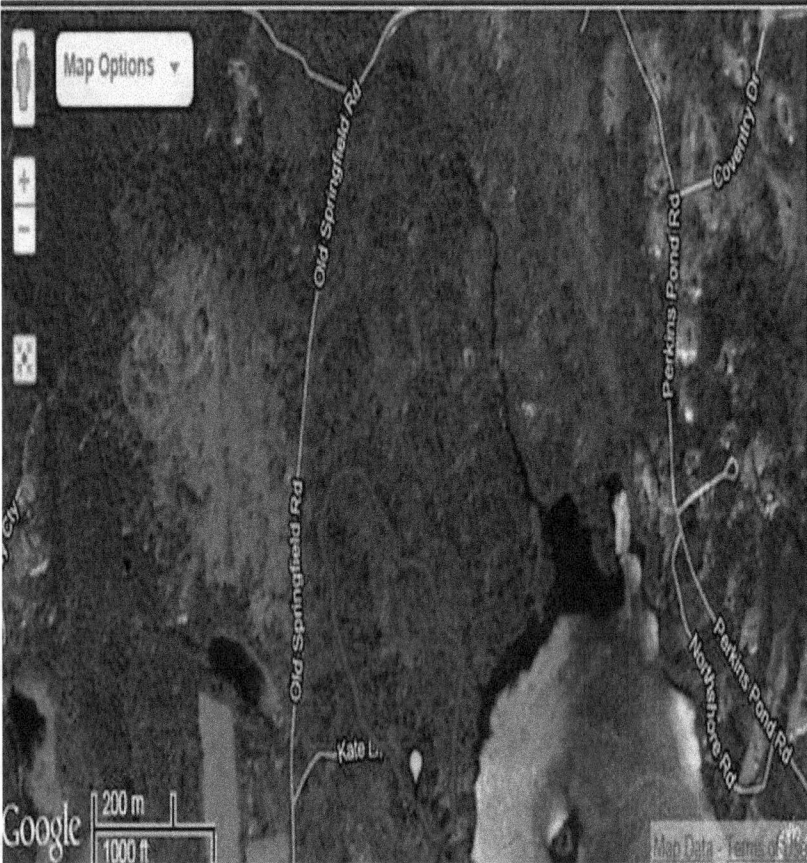

Mapping a Trail with iMapMyfitness

There is no extra step to take the map and stats data from your phone and transfer it to your laptop. All your routes and workouts data are stored in iMapMyFitness online servers and not locally on your phone.

Getting Started with MapMyFitness

Start: **Touch Record Workout**	Select your **activity** type: i.e. walk, run, dog walk, bicycle, etc.	**Pause, Save, Resume**

Where's My Droid

Can your spouse/friends follow you and locate where you are on a remote wilderness trek? Yes, if you have the WheresMyDroid (WMD) app installed on your smartphone.

1. Download the **Where's My Droid** (WMD) app to the cell phone you want to have tracked.

2. Using the Command feature in the WMD app, go to the **Ring Setup** and **GPS Setup** to see the default Attention Words (e.g. **Ring Phone**, and **Find GPS**, respectively)

3. Share the Attention Words with those who will be following you. To follow you, they simply send a text message from their smart phone to your phone. The only text sent is the Attention Words.

4. The sender will get a text message back with your GPS coordinates. Enter the GPS coordinates into Google Earth, and they will see your Droid's location.

5. **Where's My Droid** assisted me when I was kayaking and camping on the Maine Island Trail. Given that my friend and I were off the coast of Maine, we wanted our family to know exactly where we were. I gave them my **Where's my Droid** attention words, and periodically they sent text messages and received our coordinates for Google mapping. A real cool application. But, most importantly, a great safety feature.

6. Click the below **Video Reference** to see how to download an app to your smart phone (I use **Where's My Droid** as an example.)

Similar GPS location apps to **Where's My Droid** are also available for the iPhone and blackberry at http://www.apple.com/icloud/features/find-my.html and http://appworld.blackberry.com/webstore/content/13560/?lang=en.

Google Earth

Google Earth was a valuable tool for me to plan my paddling trek around Lake Francis in the Connecticut Lakes area of northern New Hampshire. Before I went to the area we wanted know the paddling distance around the Lake. Use the below **Video Reference** link to see how Google Earth's Ruler feature was used for this outdoor trek.

MyTracks

My Tracks monitors my distance and speed whenever I do a power walk. As the **Video Reference** will show, a simple press of **Start**, and then away I go. This app has a voice that I can set to announce my distance and speed by minutes, for example or you can set it for none, 1 minute, 2 minutes, etc. It can also be set to announce after 1 mile, 2 miles, or whatever interval you desire.

RunKeeper

Run Keeper maintains logs of my bicycle rides. It is similar to My Tracks in that it also has a voice announcement feature. I must admit however, that while the wind is whistling through my helmet, hearing the voice announcements from Run Keeper was difficult. Like **My Tracks**, the GPS keeps the logs online and so all trips are available on my desktop for historical and comparative viewing.

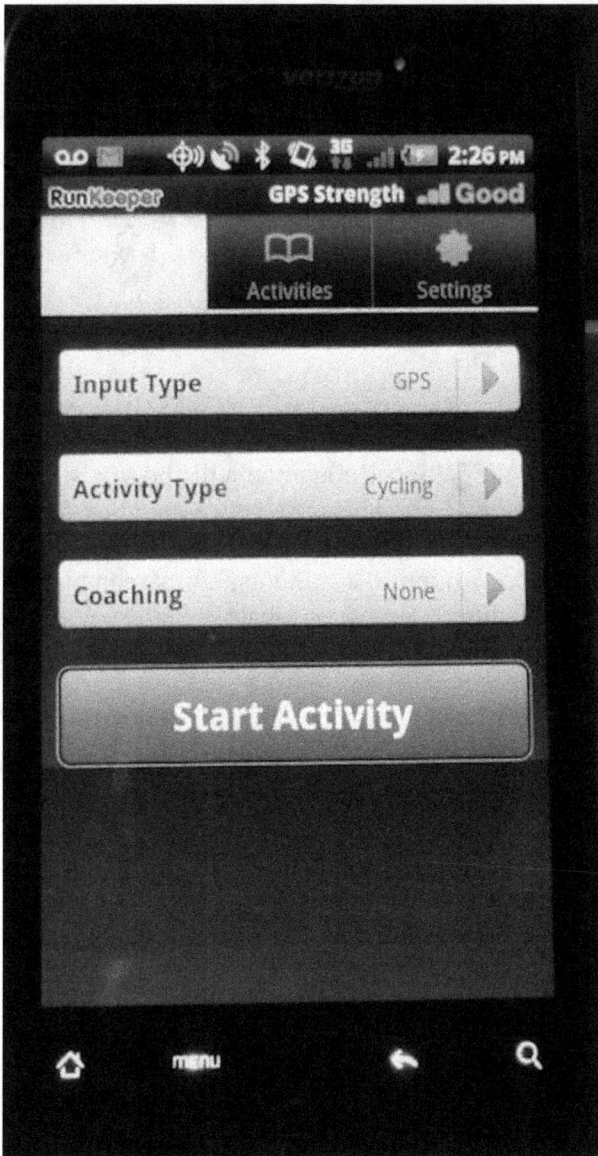

RunKeeper Ready for a Bicycle Ride

Technology for Extended Outdoor Trips Using Solar and Hand-Crank Power for LED Flashlight, Radio and Mobile Phone Charging

Battery life and re-charging has been an issue when using my smart phone on many of my outdoor adventures. As new smart phones are released the length of the battery's operational time before needing a recharge is improving, but even these enhanced charge lengths are still an issue with my overnight treks – unless I carry a spare battery (but this will have the length of charge issue also) or use a solar charger (Hmmn – of course you will need to have sun exposure for an extended period of time, and ideally remain in a so-called steady orientation to the optimum sun angle in order to maximize solar charging.)

I used my browser entering keywords, "**Hand-Crank Powered LED Flashlight with Radio and Mobile Phone Charger**". Lo and behold there are now many companies offering technology to rescue me by extending my smart phone battery life for prolonged treks – as well as power for flashlights and radios. Power sources for battery recharging for overnight and longer outdoor trips is now as simple as turning a crank handle to output stable, voltage-regulated power to my smart phone.

These devices can weigh less than 4 ounces, be smaller than my fist, are water resistant and impact and shock resistant, and need no battery or light bulb. Hand-crank power through technology is a great wilderness piece of equipment, and will shortly be part of my household emergency pack as well. Some manufacturer say not all smart phones are not yet ready for this device, so check the device specifications before you order – and absolutely before you prepare for a trip. Assume nothing, when it comes to your dependence on the smart phone being charged for the first time in the wilderness.

Another outdoor issue I have experienced is losing GPS satellite coverage. Temporary loss of satellite signal can give you weird statistics, such as when running a voice announcement gave me my pace as being 8 minutes per mile for the first mile. I then walked a bit and the next time the voice reported it told me I was at a 7 minute 30 second pace. Is this a satellite GPS issue? Hmm, remember to weigh and consider the statistical results. Satellite reception for GPS receivers will be more of an issue when hiking under a forest canopy than say, paddling in open water.

Apps Recommendation

This discussion shows how an app can be used to enhance your outdoor enthusiasm and accomplishments. It is not a recommendation for a particular app. Some apps are intended for one activity; whereas others serve a variety of activities. Many apps are free, or have a minimal charge. The apps here offer a free version and for a minimal cost you can get an upgrade version.

Share Your Use of Technology for Enhanced Outdoor Activities.

Search for an outdoor app related to your favorite outdoor activity; From within your smart phone, download the app. Browse through its features – and test each one. Challenge yourself with all kinds of questions: Does the app provide you an opportunity to enlighten your outdoor experience? Does the app challenge you in your activity training? Does it offer statistics and opportunities to expand your outdoor experience?

Never say, "I wish I had tried smart phone technology for my outdoor activity"

Videos for Apps for the Outdoors

- Blog Post: Apps for the Outdoors
  http://outdooradventurers.blogspot.com/2012/
  05/using-technology-with-outdoor.html

- Where's My Droid Download and Setup Demo
  http://www.youtube.com/watch?v=aboHdPjV
  fWg&feature=player_embedded
- Google Earth Ruler Demo on Lake Francis in
  New Hampshire
  http://www.youtube.com/watch?v=xtCeDhYY
  un0&feature=player_embedded
- Demonstration of My Tracks and Run Keeper
  http://www.youtube.com/watch?v=uylJAD-
  4x44&feature=player_embedded
- Six Ways to Make Exercise More Effective
  http://www.parade.com/health/slideshows/fit
  ness/6-ways-to-make-exercise-more-
  fun.html#?slideindex=0

Outdoor Enthusiast Campfire Chat: How to Cook an Egg in an Onion

In my March 31, 2010 blog post, **I Never Have to Say, "I wish I had paddled Florida's Suwannee River",** I created a video showing John, our camp chief chef, cooking an egg in an orange over an open campfire.

A Great North Woods paddling and tenting trip to northern New Hampshire's Lake Francis, allowed me to take my campsite breakfast cooking experience a bit further. Paul Tawrell's outdoor enthusiast book, **Wilderness Camping and Hiking**, described a method of cooking an egg over an open campfire in an onion. Being one to never say, "I wish I had cooked an egg in an onion over an open campfire", I decided to try Paul's recommendation.

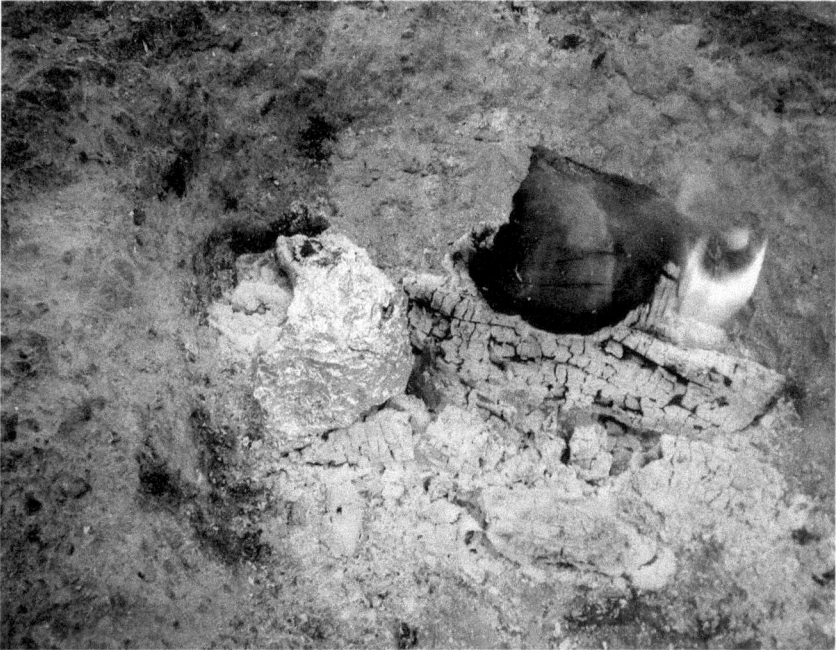

Egg in Onion Wrapped in Aluminum Foil in Campfire Ashes

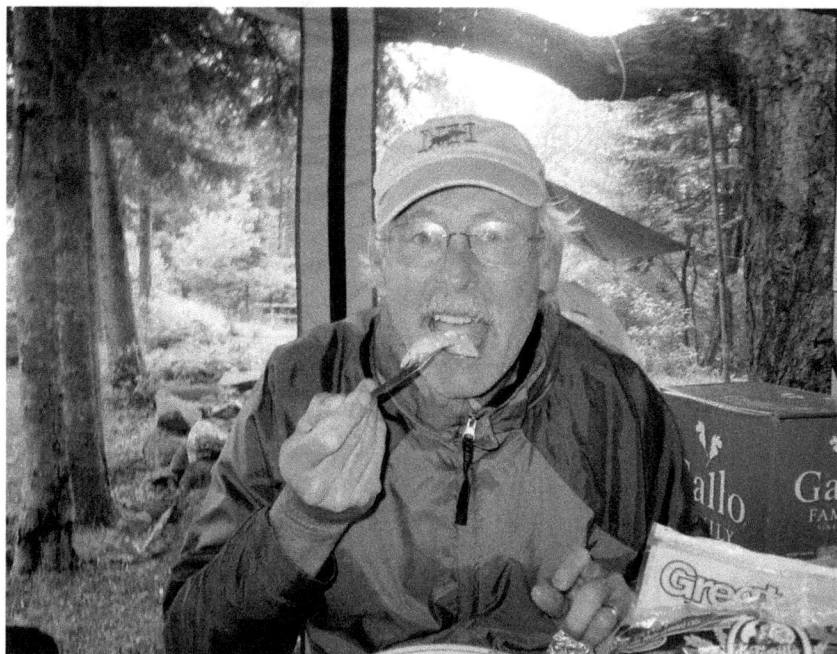

The First Taste of the Egg Cooked in an Onion

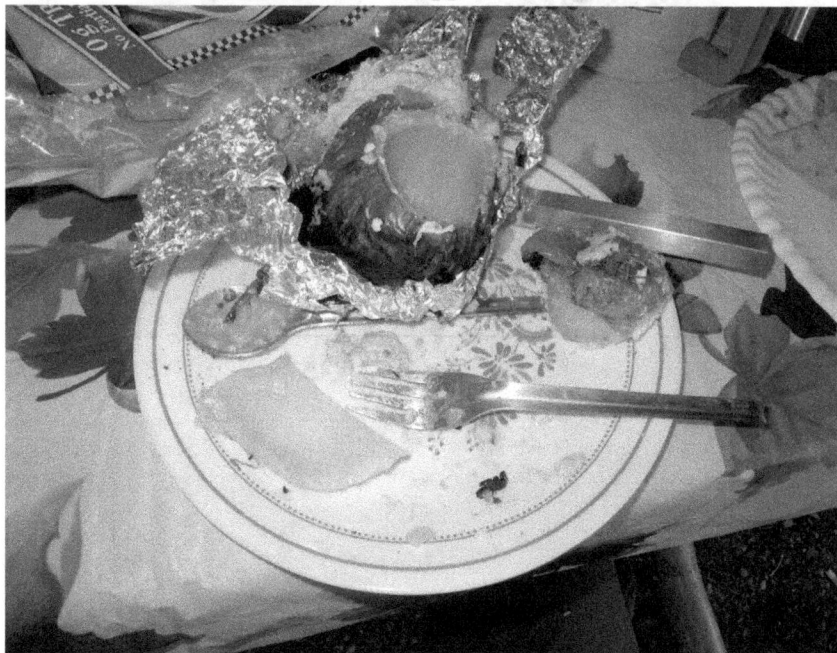

The Egg is Eaten!

Appreciate the below **Video Reference Egg in an Onion** to see Outdoor Steve's experience with an onion, egg, and campfire.

This video has gone viral on YouTube.com and as of the date of this book there have been over 40,000 views of Cook an Egg in an Onion Over an Open Campfire by Outdoor Steve.wmv.

Video References: Campfire Chats
- **Blog: How Cook an Egg in an Onion**
  http://outdooradventurers.blogspot.com/2010/06/outdoor-enthusiast-happenings-how-to.html

- **Cook an Egg in an Onion Over an Open Campfire**
  http://www.youtube.com/watch?feature=player_embedded&v=fkg9tenysmM

The Ottertail Paddle - Pros and Cons, How it's Made, and "Let's Give it a Test"

A Quest for an Ottertail Paddle

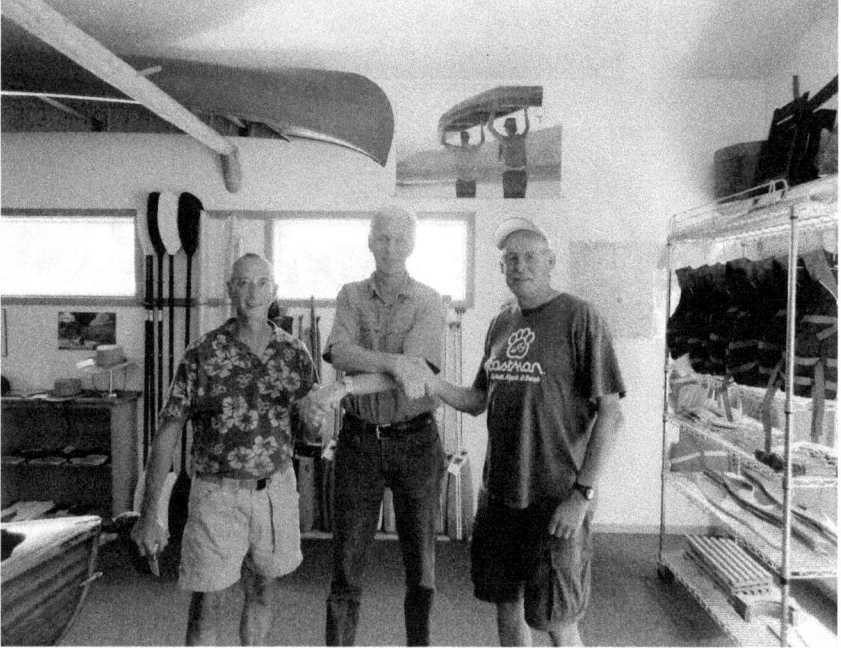

L-R: Dundee, Dick and Steve at Buckhorn Canoe Company

Canoe paddles come in various shapes and styles. I have used square tip, bent shaft, beavertail, and oversized paddles - *but never the Ottertail*. My quest for an Ottertail paddle began this summer on the Trent-Severn Waterway after I met Dick Persson of Buckhorn Canoe Company in Buckhorn, Ontario.

Dick was providing me a tour of his workshop/store, when I asked about the thin blade paddle hanging on his showroom wall. Dick's explanation of the Ottertail caught my attention when he mentioned you could do the J-stroke paddle return without taking the paddle from the water. I have been using the J-stoke when canoeing for the past few years, and his mention of a change in my J-stroke was something I just had to try. Dick shared his use and knowledge of the Ottertail paddle in the video below.

255

What is an Ottertail Paddle - and its Pros and Cons?

The video interview of Dick best describes the use of the Ottertail, but as an introduction here, let me respond to the obvious question, **"What is an Ottertail paddle?"**

The major distinction between the Ottertail and other paddles is its narrow blade. The Ottertail is most often used from the stern. Its distinctive shape is easier on the shoulder for traveling long distances. The Ottertail is popular with canoeists for lake and flat water travel.

Ottertails come in a variety of shapes and materials. The grip has many styles (Maine Guide, t-grip, standard grip, etc.) The Ottertail blade is thinner than most other paddles. Blades can be straight, wider at the top and narrower at the bottom, and thinner at the top and wider at the bottom. Most blades are rounded at the end and allow the paddle to slice through the water easily and gently.

The Ottertail Paddle is similar in design to that of the Beaver Tail but has a longer and narrower blade rounded at the tip and because the blade is narrow and long, it has a shorter shaft length than some other styles when sized properly for the same user.

All canoes should be equipped with an extra paddle, so why not carry an Ottertail for the long trip on flat water. When in whitewater or needing speed to return back to camp for dinner or when trying to outrun an oncoming storm, grab the beavertail or square tail paddle and more speedily head for shore.

A Custom Made Ottertail Paddle

My next step was to try an Ottertail paddle. Interestingly, none of my paddling buddies had an Ottertail, so I turned to my cousin Linwood, a Master Maine Guide. He located a paddle maker, Dri-Ki Woodworking in nearby Patten, Maine where I could have my own Ottertail paddle custom built. An exchange of emails with owner Rick Keim, led to my visit to Dri-Ki Woodworking to watch the hand fabrication of my Ottertail paddle. Rick gave me a tour of his shop and then said, "Let me build an Ottertail for you now".

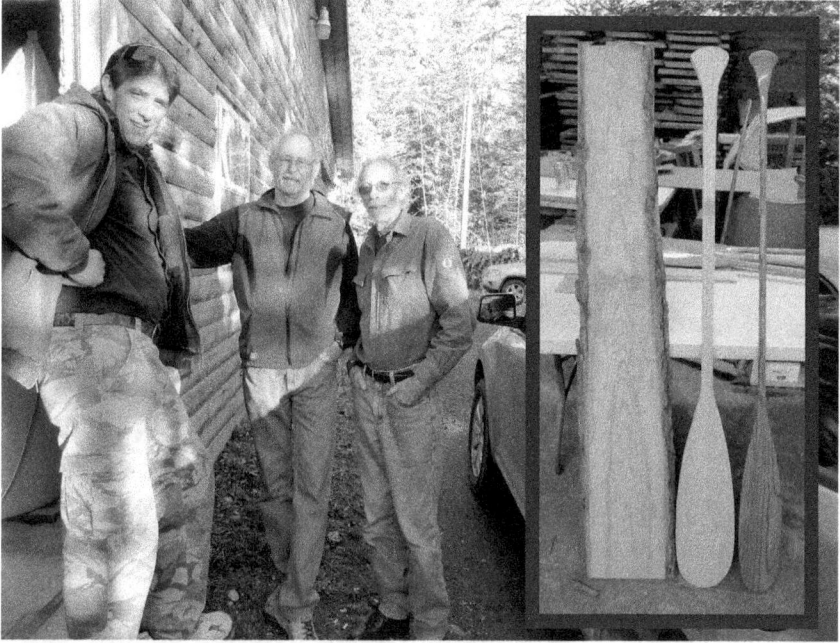

Rick, Steve and Linwood with Plank, Raw Cut and Ottertail

The below Video References show craftsman/artist/ Rick going through the various processes required to build my custom paddle. Rick buys the white ash logs which have a beautiful grain and is a light and strong wood, perfect for canoe paddles. Rick dries and mills the logs himself, then uses the outer part of the log, the straightest grain, for the paddle. The paddle is outlined in pencil on a plank, and a band saw is used to rough cut a rough shaped paddle. Then a variety of planer and sawing equipment are used to obtain the Ottertail shape. Once Rick is comfortable with the paddle, it receives two separate polyurethane dips. The paddle is now ready for the canoeist.

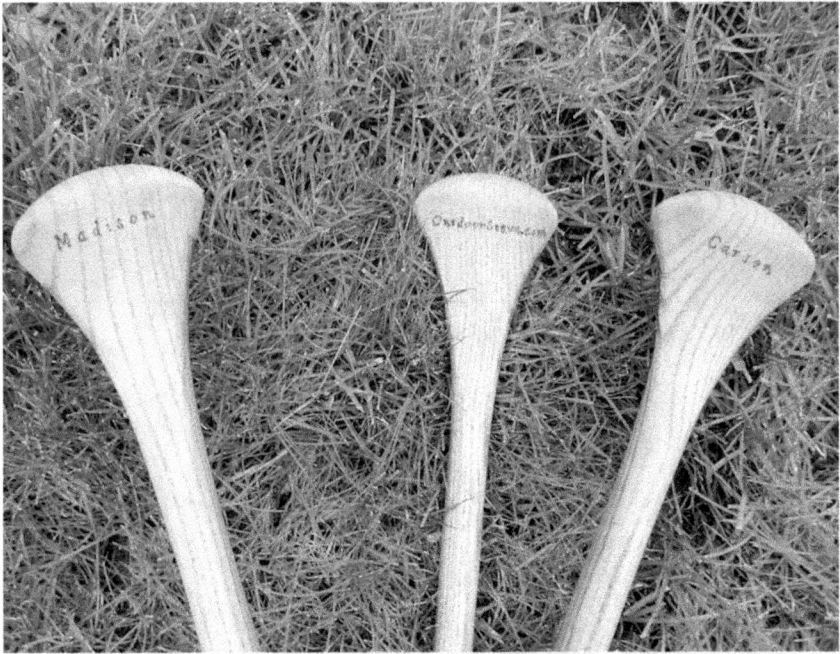

**Three Engraved Hand-fabricated Ottertail Paddles
Can You Read the Inscriptions?**

There are various ways to determine the length of an Ottertail paddle. The method we used was to measure from the floor to the bottom of my chin. And while we were at it, why not make a custom paddle for my grandchildren, Madison and Carson.

Let's Give Our Ottertail Paddles a Test

Our quest for the Ottertail has taken us to two countries and two northern New England states. In August we went to the Buckhorn Canoe Company in Buckhorn, Ontario and Dick Persson compared the pros and cons of the Beavertail and Ottertail paddle designs. Dick explained the use of the Ottertail in the J-Stroke. In November we went to Dri-Ki Woodworking in Patten, Maine for our made-to-order Ottertails, and to see how the Ottertail and Beavertail Paddles are made.

The first paddle with our personalized Ottertails came in Sunapee, New Hampshire on a below freezing December day with ice forming on Perkins Pond. This was no time for a flip!

Enjoy the below **Video References** as my friend Dundee and I test our new custom made Ottertail paddles for their virgin dip in canoeing waters.

Give the Ottertail Paddle a try - it will enlighten and broaden your canoeing experiences.

Never say, "I wish I had canoed with an Ottertail Paddle"

- Trent-Severn Waterway Special Memories of Buckhorn Canoe Company
- Buckhorn Canoe Company
- Dri-KiWoodworking
- Paddling.Net: Up the Creek with the Right Paddle

- How to do the J-Stroke in Canoeing

Video References for Ottertail Paddle

- Blog: The Ottertail Paddle: 1)Pros and Con; 2) How it's Made; and 3) Let's give it a test http://outdooradventurers.blogspot.com/2012/12/the-ottertail-paddle-its-pros-and-cons.html
- What is an Ottertail Paddle by Dick Persson http://www.youtube.com/watch?v=Td2wl_7y860&feature=player_embedded
- The Making of An Ottertail Paddle by Rick Keim http://www.youtube.com/watch?v=kLNFTWFfZJg&feature=player_embedded
- Steve Tests His Ottertail Paddle http://www.youtube.com/watch?v=3qgCpE7SuMw&feature=player_embedded
- The Ottertail Tutorial – Presented by Bedford Community Television (BCTV) – Produced by Stephen L. Priest http://www.youtube.com/watch?v=aPqr1hAJXa0&feature=youtu.be

---

A Hand-crafted Ladder from a Beaver Fell

Enjoy the below **Video Reference** describing the process of making a very unique hand-crafted ladder from a beaver fell hemlock tree taken from the north end New Hampshire's Perkins Pond

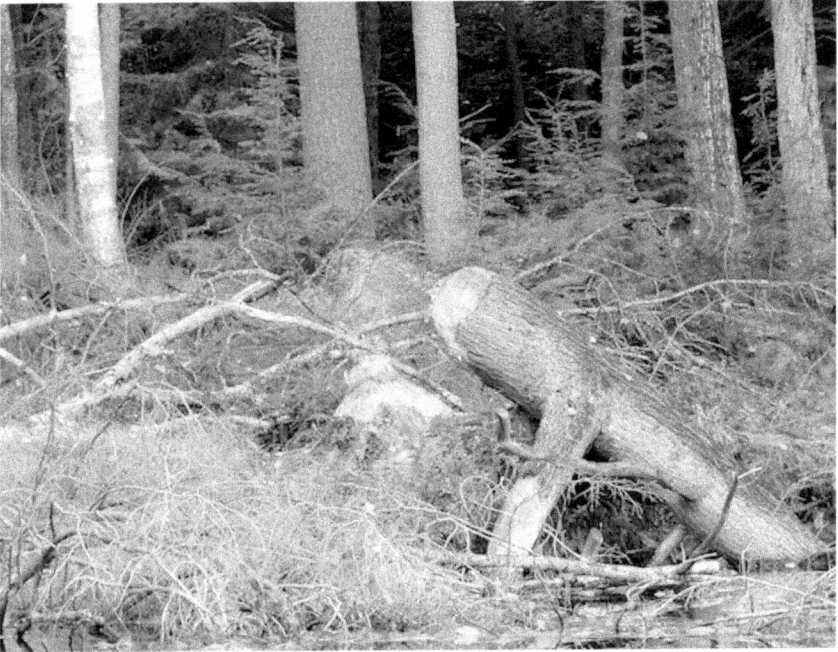

A Beaver Fell Hemlock

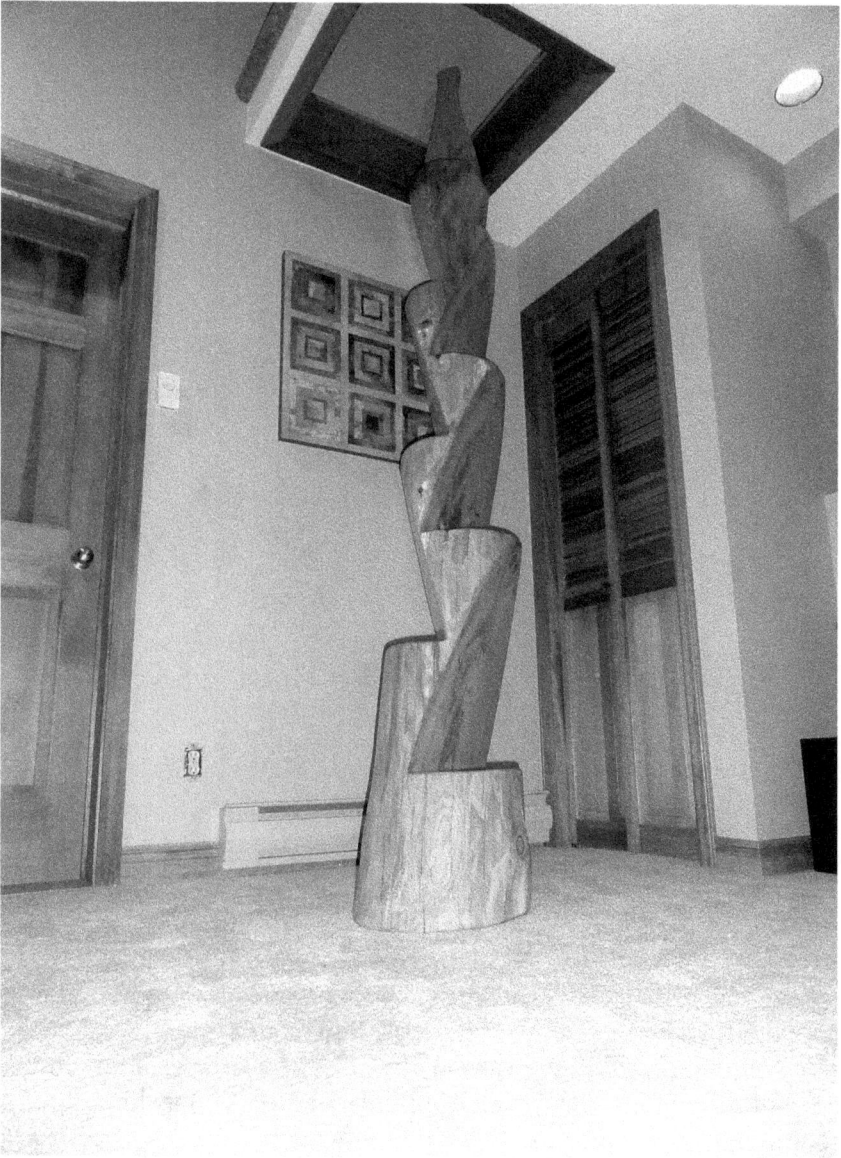

A Master-Craftsman Work from the Above Beaver Fell

Video Reference for a Hand-Crafted Ladder from a
Beaver Fell
http://youtu.be/uwpElEsRq3E

A Friendly Axe Throwing Contest in Northern New Hampshire

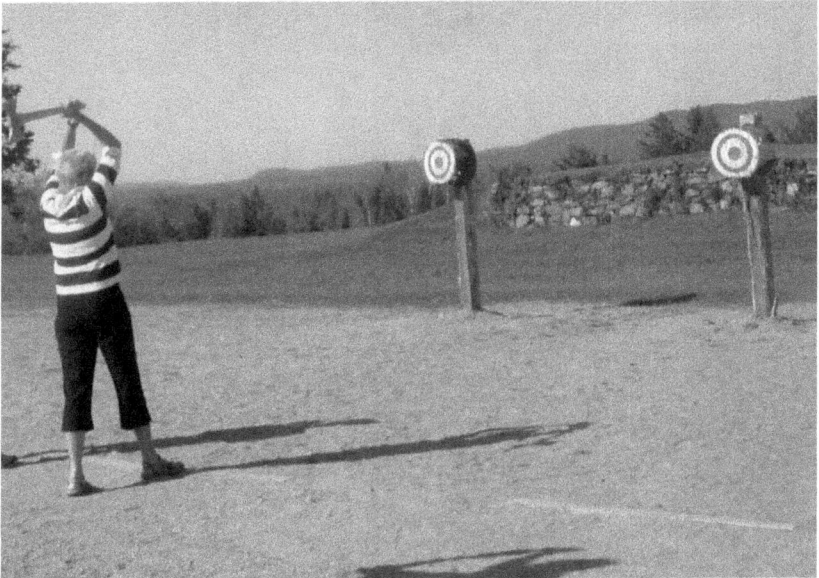

A Mountain View Grand Hotel Guest Axe Throwing Contest

My wife and I, and two friends, spent two glorious days at the Mountain View Grand in Whitefield, New Hampshire (http://www.mountainviewgrand.com/). The MVG, established in 1865, is one of the four grand old hotels of New Hampshire. Its facilities were marvelous with a feel of what it must have been like 100 plus years ago sitting on the large veranda overlooking a panorama of the White and Franconia Mountains sipping a glass of one's favorite wine.

The staff dining, activities, and housekeeping staffs were all friendly and made us feel very much welcomed. The MVG course was nestled amongst the farmland and forests with a feel of historic New Hampshire.

The scheduled activities included an "axe throwing contest". Well, being one to never say, "I wish I had..." I smile when writing "contest" because it really was a brief orientation to this northern New England sport. All attendees were gently superbly coached by Jeff of MVG on how to "throw the axe", and we then had a friendly "competition". We had a very unique experience to talk about forever.

We ate all our meals in three different dining areas. I feel like a salesperson, but in all honesty, each was distinctive. I was really awed with the way the scallop and lobster stew was served.

First came a saucer with one scallop and a piece of lobster meat. Opps, I thought I ordered a stew? As I was about to question the server on my "stew", he arrived with a separate pitcher in hand and poured stew and spices into the saucer. It made the most unique presentation -- and the stew was "to kill for".

On another evening, we decided to dine in the "Wine Cellar". Guess what? Indeed we were seated in the wine cellar of the MGV with wine cabinets everywhere. What a very special atmosphere. Wow!

I think you get my drift of this wonderful grand hotel. We look forward to returning soon.

Never say, "I wish I had stayed at the Mountain View Grand Resort & Spa."

Video of Friendly Axe Throwing Contest
http://youtu.be/8hrn2nHwOAM

Eclectic Sharings

Don't judge those who try and fail, judge those who fail to try. - Unknown

---

Dreaming the Appalachian Trail

The Man - Brad Viles

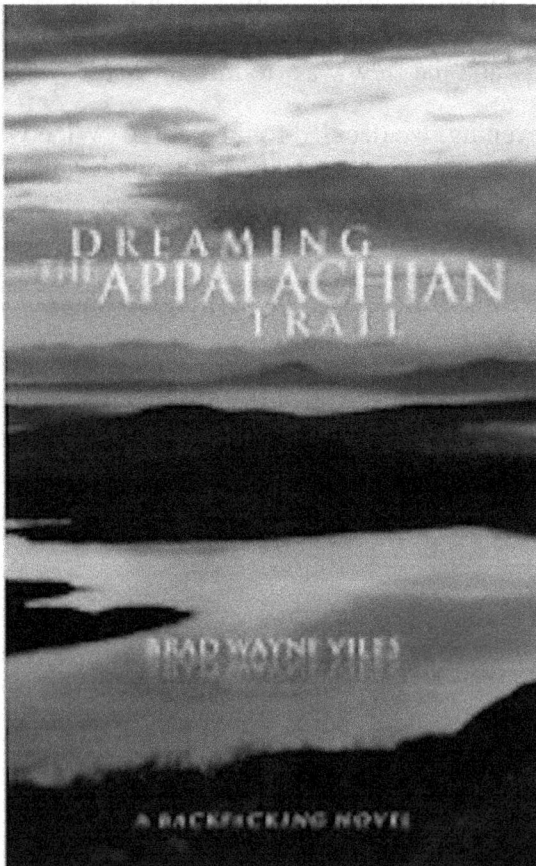

I encourage you to read Brad Viles's book, Dreaming the

Appalachian Trail. I write this blog in admiration for a man I have never met in person. We have corresponded via email, have chatted on the phone, and have exchanged books. Indeed, I have read many of his writings in the **Bangor Daily News**. Brad was a weekly freelance writer for this Maine newspaper with articles focused on the great outdoors from a person who made the outdoors a daily component of this life.

I was so enthralled with Dreaming … that I just had to have my wife Cathy listen as I read her two chapters of beautiful prose that reminded me of reading Robert Frost's, *"Two roads diverged in the woods, and I took the one less traveled by"*. I pictured Brad reading to an intent group of outdoor enthusiasts by a campfire next to a river in Maine.

Snippets from Contents of Dreaming
Dreaming the Appalachian Trail is a fictional account of Brad's Appalachian Trail (AT) hike from Georgia to Maine. Along the way he encounters violent storms, strange people, spectacular scenery and events that change his life. The trail itself is major character in this story of imagination and wonder.

I absolutely loved the **Dreaming the AT** characters, and in particular Non-stop's frog/tadpole metaphor. *"A frog can't explain to a tadpole what he will become when grown. The tadpole can't understand about having legs, no tail and breathing air, even though a frog is exactly what the tadpole would become when it's an adult. I could not express to anyone what it was like to walk over two thousand miles, so I was a frog, surrounded by tadpoles."*

Gosh, I read that comparison and immediately realized that can be my response when people ask me what it is like to paddle 100 miles on the Allagash Wilderness Waterway.

The Voice made me pause and feel Maine-tainer merge with the "AT". I ask myself, hmm, so that is what it is like to have the AT talk to me.

Topo Man made my imagination go wild, and his appearance with Compass was unexpected and appropriate. I could see a person tattooed from head to foot with the map of the AT, and yet this person was always losing his way on the AT.

If you want a book to tell you directions and points of interest on the AT, as most AT books do, then this book is not for you. If you want to "feel" this man's connection to the AT, and would enjoy a more poetic account of an AT thru-hike, then buy Dreaming the Appalachian Trail.

I felt so moved after reading Dreaming the Appalachian Trail I posted a five-star(*****)review on Amazon.com

Purchase *Dreaming the Appalachian Trail*
To buy **Dreaming...** ($10.00 72 pages) go to Amazon.com or Xlibris Online Book Store

Brad's writings include special outdoor enthusiast columns describing his personal exploits. You can read his outdoor pieces by Googling keywords, "Brad Viles Maine".

Enthusiast passes on tips, stories, love of outdoors
In the January 16, 2010 issue of the Bangor Daily news, Brad wrote a book review of **Outdoor Enthusiast** titled, Enthusiast passes on tips, stories, love of outdoors. Click here to read it.

My Maine Connection
In the process of interviewing me for his BDN article, I recalled my Maine adventures - after all, this review is for "Mainers".

Gosh, I am really connected! Not only was my Dad from Maine, I have aunts and cousins throughout Maine, and we are doing a genealogy search to verify my great great grandmother was indeed a Native American Indian.

Moreover, **Outdoor Enthusiast** describes seven of many paddling treks in Maine including my three trips to the Allagash, the Kenduskeag Stream Canoe Race (with my televised flip going over at Six-mile Falls), Kennebunk Fireman Triathlon, Kennebec White Water Rafting, Maine Senior Games Cape Elizabeth Triathlon, and the Androscoggin Trek to the Sea. My Maine club memberships are the Appalachian Mountain Club and the Maine Island Trail Association.

I trust my motivational presentation at the Naval Ship Yard in Kittery, Maine encouraged sailors to enjoy Maine's outdoor opportunities. Both **Outdoor Enthusiast: Never say, 'I wish I had ..."**, and **Outdoor Play Fun 4 4 Seasons** have *Places to Play in Northern New England - the Maine Way.*

Be sure to never say, "I wish I had spent $10.00 to read, Dreaming the Appalachian Trail

> Video Reference Dreaming the Appalachian Trail
> - Blog: Dreaming the Appalachian Trail
>   http://outdooradventurers.blogspot.com/201
>   0/01/dreaming-appalachian-trail.html

Book Review for "Born to Run" by Christopher McDougall

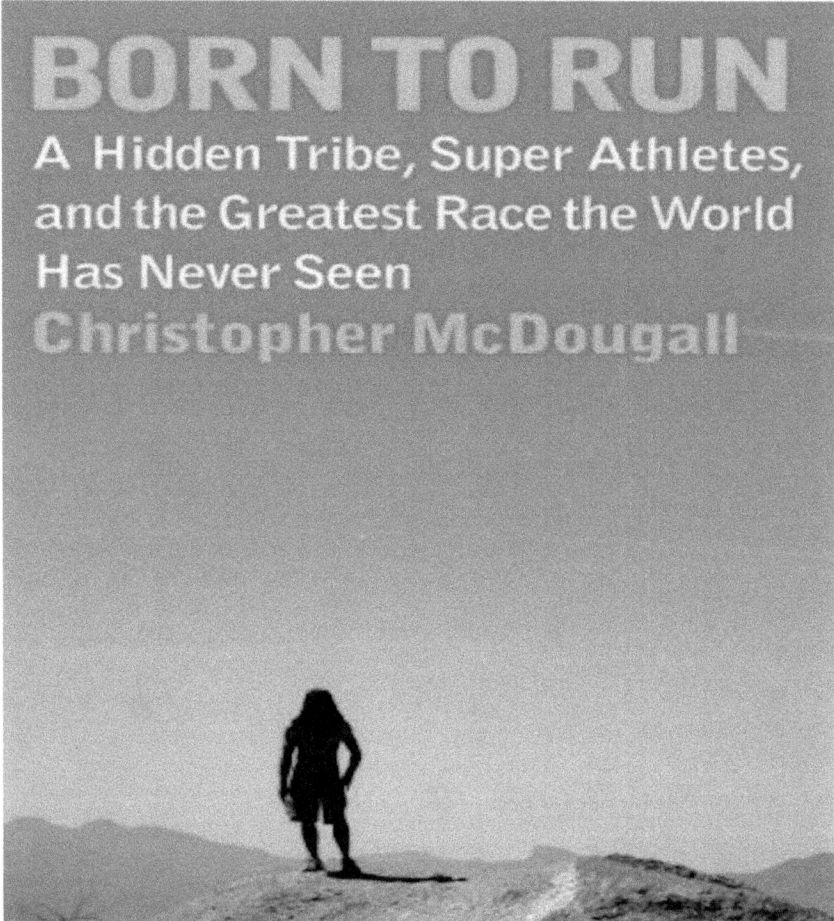

BORN TO RUN

A Hidden Tribe, Super Athletes, and the Greatest Race the World Has Never Seen

Christopher McDougall

Run miles without shoes? Reduce my number of running injuries? My ears perked up when I heard author Christopher McDougall interviewed on national public radio on his new book, Born to Run: A Hidden Tribe, Superathletes, and the Greatest Race the World Has Never Seen. Being a distance runner with chronic heel pain, I just had to read this book (http://chrismcdougall.com/).

McDougall's research and book centered on a Mexican Indian tribe called Tarahumara (pronounced with a silent "h", Tara-oo-mara). The Tarahumara live in the depth of an isolated canyon in Mexico, and run 100 miles or more at a stretch – all miles either barefoot or with crude thin rubber strapped sandals.

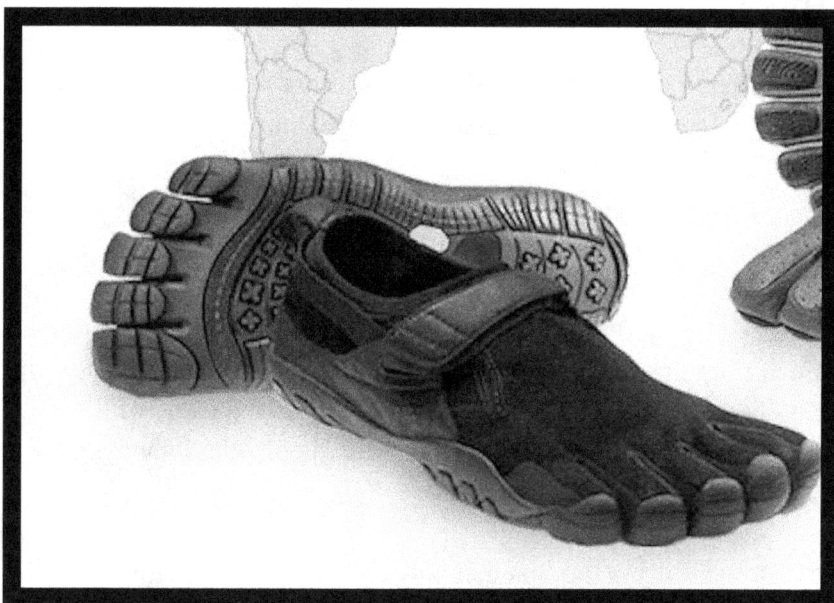

A Five Fingers Running Shoe

Barefoot running brings to mind nasty road stones, sticks and glass that clutter every runner's path. McDougall offers a near barefoot approach with the slim rubber soled Vibram FiveFingers footwear (http://www.vibramfivefingers.com/) that look like a kind of glove for the foot with its articulated toe slots and just enough fabric to keep the thing on one's feet.

Besides the Tarahumara Indians, the book focuses on the sport of ultra marathons (100 or so mile running races on all kinds of terrain).

I write this blog because **Born to Run** goes against the tide of "the more expensive the running shoe, the better it is." My hope is that this blog will generate comments from those who do barefoot running, have worn five fingers, or who have read the book. **Born to Run** suggests an elixir for runners with severe and recurring injuries who refuse to stop. It poses the question for me, "Could barefoot running really help me run without heel pain?"

Writing Style

As a writer, I consciously evaluate how other writers maintain the enjoyment and attention of the reader. McDougall's style was of particular interest to me:

• I enjoyed his chapter lengths. They were generally four to six pages, and focused on one or two areas of the story.

• Each chapter ends with a paragraph or sentence that leads into the next chapter, similar to a TV cliffhanger, where the end of the show entices you to watch the next week's episode. I always wanted to read the next chapter.

• McDougal mixes the Spanish language within his writings, and then gives the interpretation in English. I once worked with Spanish speaking people, and this method brought back to me many Spanish words and phrases.

• While my engineering background shows in my outdoor writings as I take the reader step by step through a story, McDougall assumes the reader will fill in time and people gaps. For instance, my tales might follow a runner's progress throughout a race, whereas McDougall, without an introduction that the place or speaker has changed, jumps into the next paragraph with another runner, and it all makes sense as the reader understands this is a different runner.

Born to Run provides a very well written and unique perspective to distance running. I preach running to my audience as the cardiovascular workout needed for extensive outdoor exercise. Whether paddling, hiking, skiing, or biking, you need a good level of physical health for these endurance sports. Whether the outdoor enthusiast reader agrees or disagrees with the author's assumptions and perspective, the book will surely give you insights to the world of long distance running and a unique view of barefoot running. You also learn a bit about ultra-marathons.

Personal Comment

I ask you to respond with your own thoughts and experience on the topics in **Born to Run**. I must provide my own comment, and confess that while I am intrigued with barefoot running and Vibram shoes, I have not tried them. I continue to wear my expensive running shoes with orthotics. I have not completely given up the idea as **Born to Run** has stimulated my curiosity. I never want to say, "I wish I had tried barefoot running and Vibram Five fingers."

> **Video References Born to Run**
> - **Blog: Born to Run**
>   http://outdooradventurers.blogspot.com/201
>   0/12/book-review-for-born-to-run-by.html

A Volunteer for Running Shoe Development

I received an email from Pedro Rodrigues, a Sports Research Engineer in the New Balance Sports Research Laboratory. New Balance was launching a new research study looking at the effects of running shoes on lower extremity mechanics. Pedro asked if I would be interested in serving as a tester.

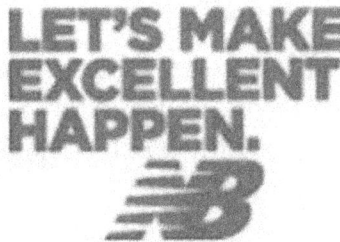

Absolutely! I have been a committed runner for 25 plus years, have experienced a variety of leg and foot injuries, and have run in numerous brands of running shoes to "improve my speed" and avoid injury. In fact, I was currently running in New Balance shoes, and my contribution to this study might provide valuable data and help develop new running shoes and technologies.

Besides, I could had a chance to take part in a running shoe study by an athletic shoe manufacturer making their shoes in the USA.

I drove to the research lab in Lawrence, MA, and signed confidentiality and injury release forms. Pedro explained the goal of the study was to evaluate how a single component of the running shoe affected the mechanics of my leg. Therefore, each shoe was essentially identical other than that single factor, allowing the researchers to understand the specific effects of that one factor. I then ran on a treadmill in ten different pairs of shoes.

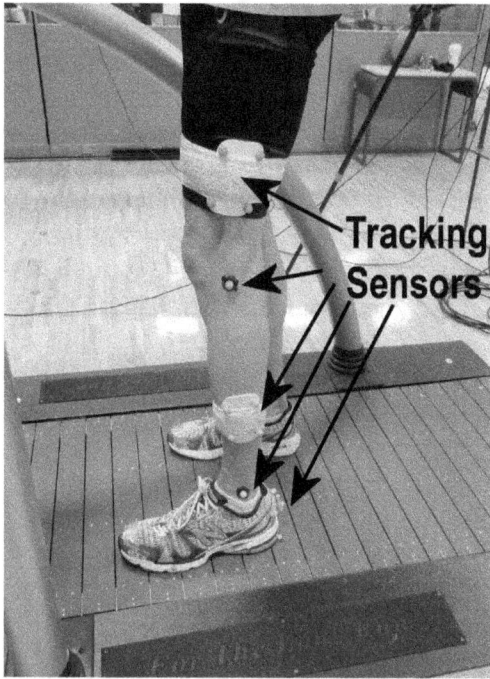

Tracking Sensors on the Leg

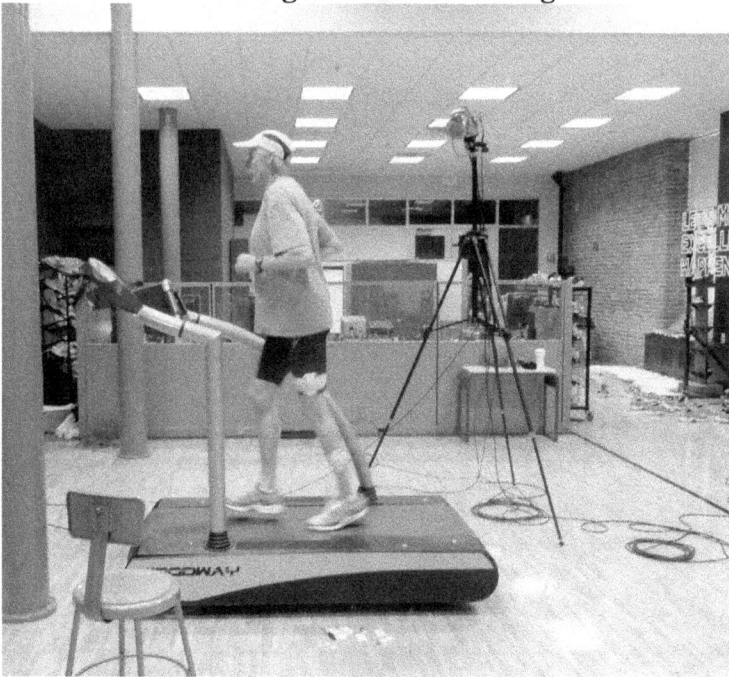

Let the Running Test Begin

Pedro measured my leg and ankle and then placed reflective markers in specific anatomic locations. These reflective markers were then tracked using a motion capture system (Qualisys, Gothenburg, Sweden) as I ran on the treadmill at a constant speed.

This system consisted of 8 cameras, which sent out infrared light that reflected off these markers. Next, by combining the view of each camera, the motion of my leg could be reconstructed in 3-D (see video), allowing the engineers to calculate joint angles, velocities, etc. In this particular case they were interested in the position of my ankle when I first struck the ground, the amount I pronated (foot rolling to the inside), the speed I pronate, etc. They will collect this information on a number of runners and will run statistical analyses to see if the controlled factor had any effect on a runner's lower body mechanics.

Share with me the excitement of running research. New Balance offered me an opportunity related to my dedication to running. Running is a major part of my lifestyle and I firmly believe running helps condition me for the cardiac endurance and fitness levels necessary for me to continue to enjoy my other daily outdoor pursuits. View the below **Video Reference** showing the body marking and reflectors, running on the treadmill, and the 3-D results.

Now, I never have to say, "I wish I had contributed to a running shoe study."

Video References of A Volunteer for Running Shoe Study
- **Blog: New Balance Running Shoe Study**
  http://outdooradventurers.blogspot.com/2011/03/volunteering-in-running-shoe-study.html
- **A Volunteer for Running Shoe Development**
  http://www.youtube.com/watch?feature=player_embedded&v=d-TeUu5UVwE

Places to Play in Northern New England

"Nothing preaches better than the act"
- Benjamin Franklin

*For all sad words of tongue or pen, the saddest of
all are these: "It might have been."*
- Whittier, Maud Muller

The choice of outdoor sports in northern New England is nearly endless--ranging from hiking to biking to running to skiing to snowshoeing, etc. There are literary thousands of mountains, lakes and rivers here. With its four-season weather, an outdoor enthusiast never runs out of a sport to "play".

The Internet is a major tool for locating outdoor sporting events, organizations, instruction and outdoor blogs. Searching on keywords such as, "Hiking in Vermont," "Cross country skiing in New Hampshire", and "Paddling in Maine," reveal hundreds of web sites. Enter "outdoor sports in northern New England" and you will see hundreds of sites to choose from a variety of events in which to participate, learn, and never say, "I wish I had…".

Discussions with other outdoor enthusiasts will reveal personal sports of interest and places to visit and experience.

Outdoor enthusiasts with an interest in triathlons can go to www.trifind.com, pick a state, and find a triathlon club, races, and coaches.

Most organizations, such as the Appalachian Mountain Club (AMC), Catamount Trail Organization, Peabody Mill Environmental Center (PMEC), and Audubon Society have web sites with email lists and e-newsletters routinely announce upcoming events.

Some organizations have diverse group activities. For example, the **Appalachian Mountain Club** (AMC) has an "Over 55 Club", a "Young Members Club", and "Singles Club. The **Peabody Mill Environmental Center** (PMEC) has everyday wooded trail hikes and snowshoeing, and monthly "fireside chats" where experienced outdoor enthusiasts share their knowledge through presentations and demonstrations. The **Catamount Trail Organization** schedules group skis. **The Granite State Wheelmen** and the **Green Mountain Bicycle Club** offer group rides and maintenance workshops.

The New Hampshire Blue Steel Triathlon Club offers a variety of triathlon oriented Clinics and Events for its members to improve performance as well as to encourage teammate camaraderie: bike time trials on summer evenings; winter fun runs for members to enjoy non-competitive group runs; transition clinics for tips and practice to minimize the time from swim to bike, and bike to run; and early morning open water group swims at local lakes.

Join organizations and clubs dedicated to encouraging and providing outdoor sports and recreation, so as to never have to say, "I wish I had...".

Inter-State Opportunities for Outdoor Play

Northern New England has many scenic, relaxing, and simply exciting inter-state outdoor opportunities for all seasons. Certainly waterways, forest trails and mountains have no sense of state boundaries. Here are five non-profit organizations offering unique places to play in northern New England.

The **Northern Forest Canoe Trail, Appalachian Trail, Androscoggin River, Great North Woods,** and **Maine Island Trail** will each be highlighted.

The Northern Forest Canoe Trail (NFCT)

http://www.northernforestcanoetrail.org/ links the waterways of
New York, Vermont, Québec, New Hampshire and Maine.

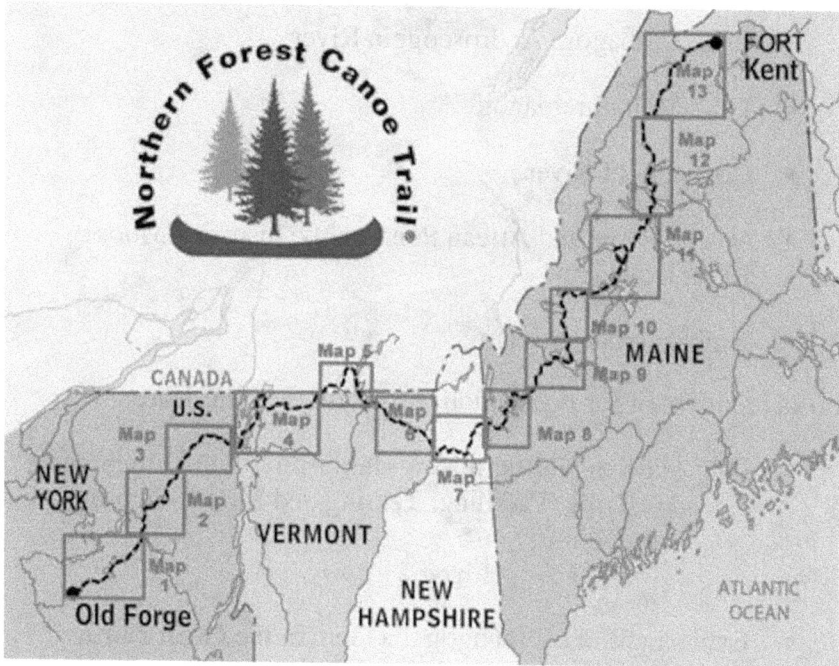

The NFCT is a long-distance paddling trail connecting the major
watersheds across the Adirondacks and Northern New England.
The Trail links communities and wild places offering canoeists and
kayakers a lifetime of paddling destinations within the 740-mile
traverse across New York, Vermont, Quebec, New Hampshire, and
Maine. The NFCT includes flat and whitewater paddling, poling,
lining, and portaging (62 portages totaling 55 miles).

A visit to the NFCT can be a day-trip, an overnight, weeks, or
months. As hikers do sections of the Appalachian Trail, so do
paddlers do the NFCT. You can put-in and take-out at any
appropriate location. The NFCT organization is a great resource
for your trip planning with web links and contact information.

Scheduled regional presentations by NFCT staff can be viewed on
the NFCT web site. See the Planning link at the site for
guidebooks and maps. http://bit.ly/Y3t48h

The sections to date of the NFCT that friends and I have paddled are:

- The Allagash Wilderness Waterway

- Lake Umbagog; Androscoggin River

- Lake Memphremagog

- Connecticut River

- Moose River and Attean Pond on the historic "Moose River Bow Trip"

- Umbazooksus Stream.

Posts on my blog for my section travels on the NFCT are:

- Four Days in Northern New Hampshire with Family and Friends Hiking, Paddling, Tenting and Moose Sighting. http://outdooradventurers.blogspot.com/2012/07/four-days-in-new-hampshire-of-family.html

- Exploring Lake Umbagog – a Gem in the Great North Woods http://outdooradventurers.blogspot.com/2010/09/exploring-lake-umbagog-gem-in-great.html

- Paddling the Allagash Wilderness Waterway http://outdooradventurers.blogspot.com/2009/07/paddling-allagash-wilderness-waterway.html

Appalachian Trail

The AT in northern New England passes through Vermont, New Hampshire and has its northern terminus at the peak of Mt Katahdin in Maine.

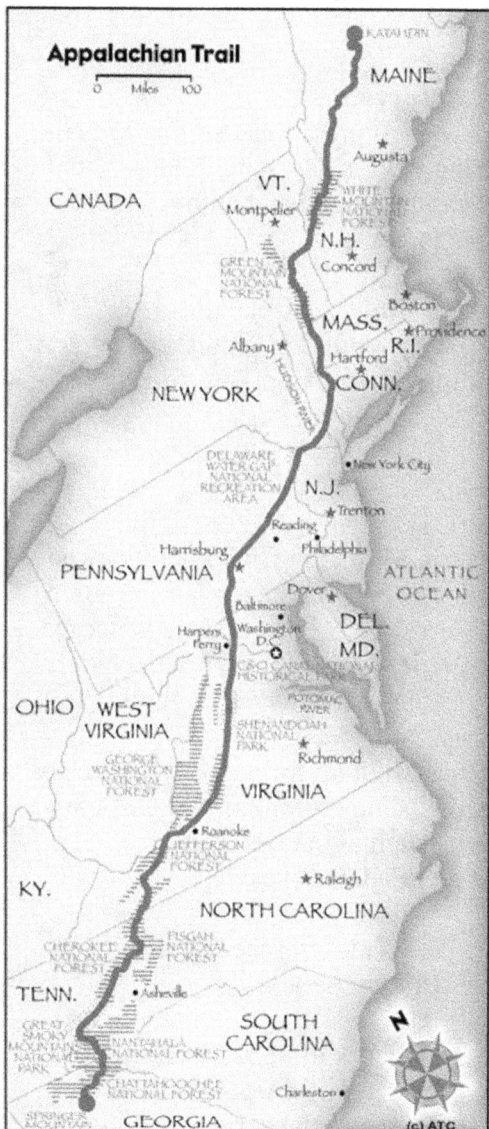

The Appalachian Trail from Maine to Georgia

I recommend two references to get started with understanding the AT:
1) **The Appalachian Trail Conservancy**
(http://www.appalachiantrail.org/)
2) **The Appalachian Mountain Club** (AMC)
(http://www.outdoors.org/)

The Appalachian Trail Conservancy

(http://www.appalachiantrail.org/) preserves and manages the Appalachian Trail – ensuring that its vast natural beauty and priceless cultural heritage can be shared and enjoyed today, tomorrow, and for centuries to come.

The Appalachian Mountain Club (AMC)

(http://www.outdoors.org/) promotes the protection, enjoyment, and understanding of the mountains, forests, waters, and trails of the Appalachian region.

Paddling with the AMC

The New Hampshire Appalachian Mountain Club Paddlers web site (http://www.nhamcpaddlers.org/) is an excellent resource for places to paddle in New Hampshire. The Paddlers welcome beginners, intermediate and experienced paddlers, 16 and older, who are interested in paddling safely while having a great time.

The Paddlers site has a free e-mail sign up for monthly notices of Paddler happenings. The emails include weekend and weekday trips, items for sale by members, such as canoes, kayaks, racks, and other paddling equipment and Paddler events.

The Paddlers web site encourages you to join the Appalachian Mountain Club (http://www.outdoors.org).

The NH AMC Paddlers web site "Places to Paddle" link (http://www.nhamcpaddlers.org/m_content/places.htm) has directions and descriptions to over twenty lake, river and marsh paddling trips, all in New Hampshire. Other links include, "Upcoming Trips" where you can join others for scheduled trips.

The NH AMC Paddlers have canoe and kayak paddles summer weekday evenings.

Four of my Blog posts on the AT:

- **Dreaming the Appalachian Trail**
  http://outdooradventurers.blogspot.com/2010/01/dreaming-appalachian-trail.html
- **Springer Mountain, Georgia - Southern Terminus of the Appalachian Trail**
  http://outdooradventurers.blogspot.com/2009/11/springer-mountain-georgia-southern.html
- **A Mid-week Trek to Tuckerman Ravine**
  http://outdooradventurers.blogspot.com/2009/04/fantastic-mid-week-trek-to-tuckerman.html
- **Hiking Mount Chocorua - White Mountain National Forest**
  http://outdooradventurers.blogspot.com/2011/08/hiking-mount-chocorua-white-mountain.html

Androscoggin River

The Androscoggin River is a major river in northern New England. The Androscoggin headwaters are in Errol, New Hampshire, where the Magalloway River joins the outlet of Umbagog Lake. It is 178 miles long and joins the Kennebec River at Merrymeeting Bay in Maine before its water empty into the Gulf of Maine on the Atlantic Ocean. Its drainage basin is 3,530 square miles (9,100 km2) in area.

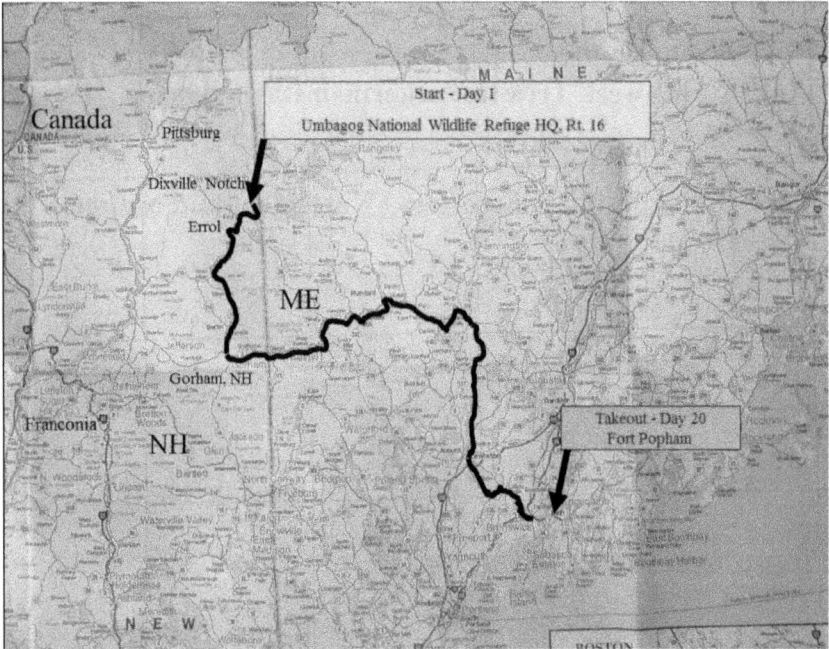

The Androscoggin River Water Shed Council http://arwc.camp7.org/ offers protection, history and paddling of the Androscoggin River. The ARWC sponsors and Source to the Sea Trek http://arwc.camp7.org/trek.

Outdoor Steve has paddled twelve sections of this Trek and you can find numerous descriptions of his fabulous paddle at http://www.outdoorsteve.com/ for articles and other stories such as **Androscoggin River Source to the Sea Canoe and Kayak Trek** http://www.outdoorsteve.com/_pdffiles/8_20Mar05_AndroscogginRiverSourcetotheSea_NewsSentinel.pdf.

Interestingly, 19 miles of the Androscoggin River headwaters are also part of the Northern Forest Canoe Trail (NFCT)!

Great North Woods

Northern New Hampshire, also known as the Great North Woods Region, is the official state tourist region located in Coos County. This area includes Northern New Hampshire, bordering Northeast Kingdom Vermont, and unincorporated townships in the northern and northwestern part of Maine

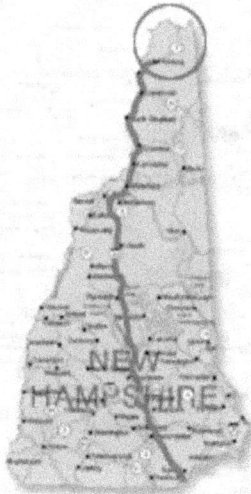

Ten Things to do in the Great North Woods of New Hampshire
(http://www.newhampshire.com/article/99999999/NEWHAMP
SHIRE05/110429465

Great North Woods Online
(http://greatnorthwoodsonline.com/)

Enjoy the Great North Woods
http://www.outdoorsteve.com/_pdffiles/23_21Jun08_Great_No
rth_Woods_NewHampshire.com.pdf

A Hike to Table Rock, Dixville, New Hampshire
http://outdooradventurers.blogspot.com/2010/07/hike-to-table-
rock-dixville-new.html

Maine Island Trail (MIT)

http://www.mita.org/

The MIT begins at Maine's coastal border with New Hampshire and ends in Machias, Maine, with an additional collection of two islands in Passamaquoddy/New Brunswick region of Canada.

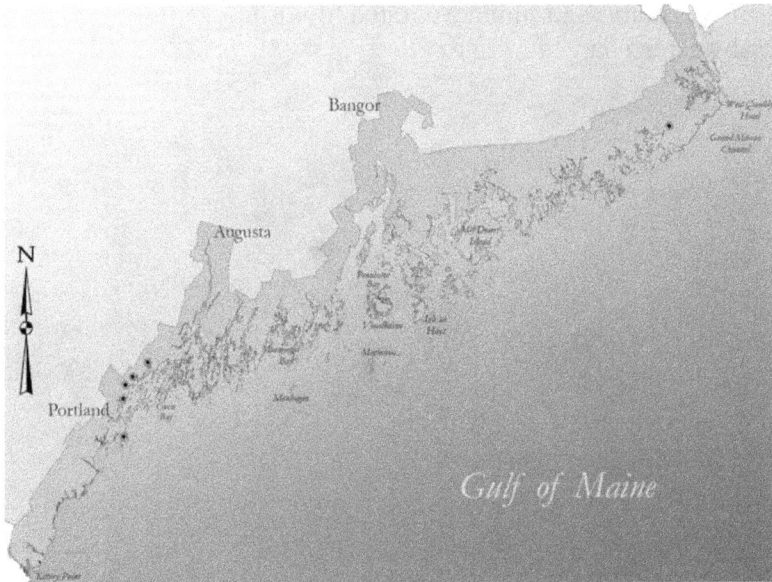

The Maine Island Trail is a 375-mile-long waterway along the coast of Maine that connects approximately 200 islands and mainland sites available for day visits or overnight camping. The trail is operated by the Maine Island Trail Association (MITA).

Through partnerships with the State of Maine, as well as land trusts, non-profit organizations, and generous private property owners, MITA ensures access to these sites for visitors in kayaks, sailboats, motorboats, and other watercraft. In exchange for access, MITA members agree to visitation guidelines set by the island owners and provide a wide range of stewardship services including island monitoring and management by trained volunteers with organized regional island cleanups each year.

FAQ on Site Reservations

The only sites (public or private) on the **Maine Island Trail** that take reservations are Warren Island, Swan Island (Kennebec), Cobscook Bay State Park, and Butter and Burnt Islands. All others are first-come first-served (FCFS). Details are in the member Trail Guide. The MITA advises people to have a backup in mind and arrive with time to spare. However, the fact is that except for peak weekends on smaller most favored islands, people typically do not report difficulties. There are a lot of islands to go around!

See the **Outdoor Enthusiast** blog post on Steve's Maine Island Trail trek.

- **Blog: Places to Play in Northern New England**
  http://outdooradventurers.blogspot.com/2013/02/places-to-play-in-northern-new-england.html
- **Blog: Sea Kayaking and Camping on the Maine Island Trail**
  http://outdooradventurers.blogspot.com/2010/08/sea-kayaking-and-camping-on-maine.html

New Hampshire

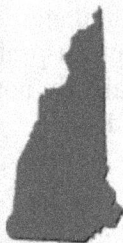

> ## Live Free or Die
>
> ## New Hampshire – Your Own Backyard
>
> ✓New Hampshire AMC Paddlers (www.nhamcpaddlers.org)
> ✓Appalachian Mountain Club (www. outdoors.org)
> ✓Local Hikes (www.localhikes.com)
> ✓The Slackpacker (www.slackpacker.com)
> ✓Granite State Wheelmen (www.granitestatewheelmen.org)
> ✓New Hampshire State Parks (www.nhstateparks.com)
> ✓Outdoor Steve (www.outdoorsteve.com)
> ✓Granite State Senior Games (50+)(www.nhseniorgames.org)

Paddling

Below is but a small sample of paddling opportunities in southern New Hampshire.

- Veterans Park on Naticook Lake in Merrimack NH
  http://bluetoad.com/display_article.php?id=1127713

- Nashua River. A good put-in behind Stellos Stadium.

- Great Turkey Pond, west of Concord NH.

- Lake Massabesic, East of Manchester NH in Auburn. Many put-ins. Try the Auburn Town Beach.

- Hopkinton Lake west of Concord NH. Exit 5 Rte 89 west of Concord NH

- Hoit Road Marsh north of Concord NH

- Glen Lake in Goffstown, NH

- Dubes Pond, in Hooksett, NH. GPS has it at 270 Whitehall Road, Hooksett, NH

- McDaniel's Marsh. Exit 13 from I89 to East Grantham. Route 114 to West Springfield. North on George's Hill Road. At intersection of Bog Road and Georges Hill Road. The Marsh put-in is directly across from Bog Road.

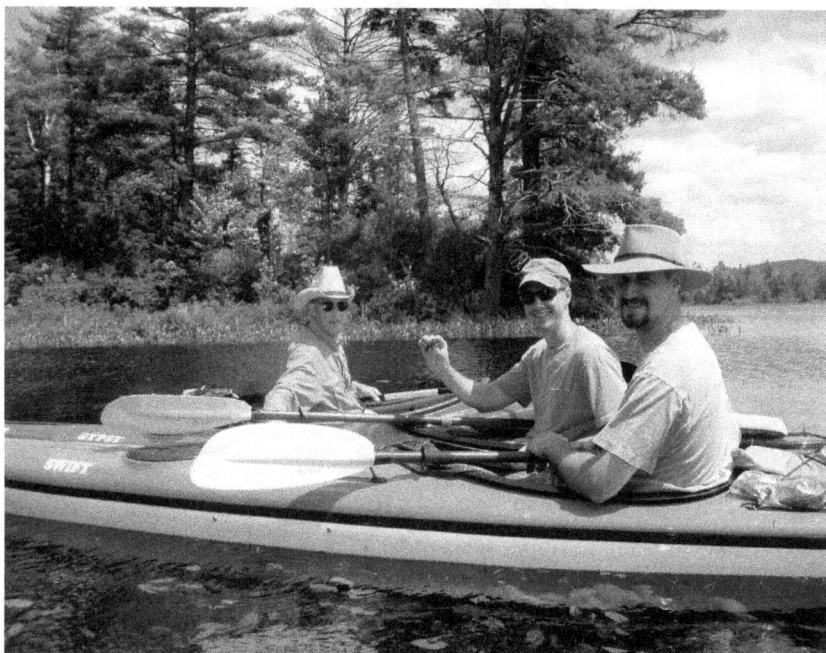

McDaniel Marsh: Dundee, Eric, and Paul

- Merrimack River. Many put-ins and take-outs. One put-in is the boat ramp behind Franklin High School. Paddle 10.5 miles to Boscawen ball fields takes about 4-5 hrs.

Hiking Year Round

o **Welch-Dickey Mountain Trail**
A unique scenic loop over and around the summits of two mountains. Great view of Mad River in Waterville Valley. A 4.5-mile scenic loop. In wet weather the bare rock may be slippery, so this is definitely a summer hike. Located I-93 via Exit 28.
http://tiny.cc/9yoruw

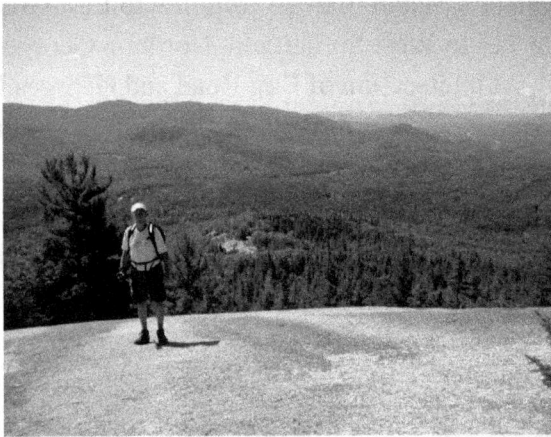
Welch-Dickey Trail

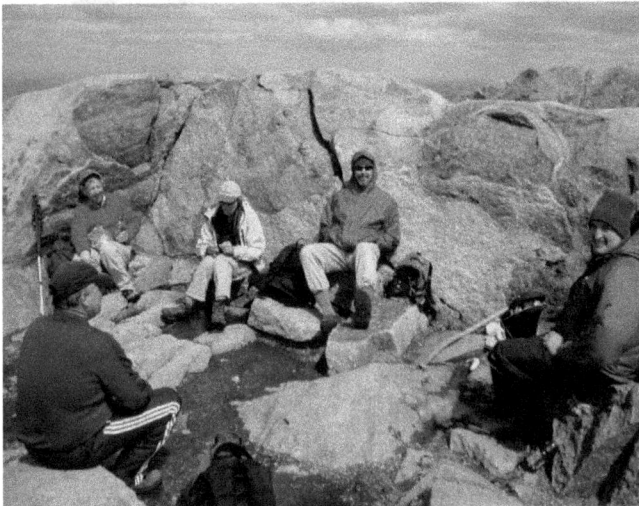
Relaxing Atop Mt Monadnock

- Mount Monadnock Southwestern, NH
  3,165-ft. Mt. 40 mls of maintained foot trails. 100-mile views in all six New England states. Second most frequently climbed mountain in the world, after Mount Fuji in Japan. http://www.nhstateparks.org/state-parks/alphabetical-order/monadnock-state-park/

- Mount Willard Trail, White Mountains, NH
  The Mount Willard Trail leads from the AMC Crawford Notch Visitor Center to scenic ledges overlooking the Crawford Notch. Two hour round trip hike. Just fine for a family day hike. http://tiny.cc/kqoruw

- **Cohos Trail**
  The Cohos Trail is New England's newest long-distance hiking route, extending 162 miles through the woods and mountains of northern New Hampshire. Most likely, you will have a day of absolute solitude.
  http://www.cohostrail.org/

- Mount Kearsarge
  Directions: Wilmot and Warner, New Hampshire. From Route 89 take Route 11. 2,937 feet Summit Length: 2.2 mls
  http://www.nhoutdoors.com/hiking_trails.htm

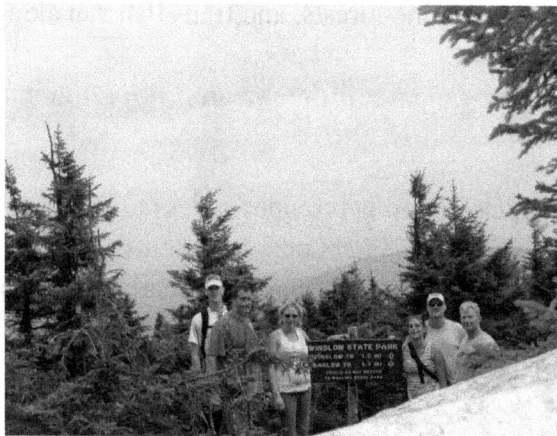

The Peak of Mt Kearsarge

Maine

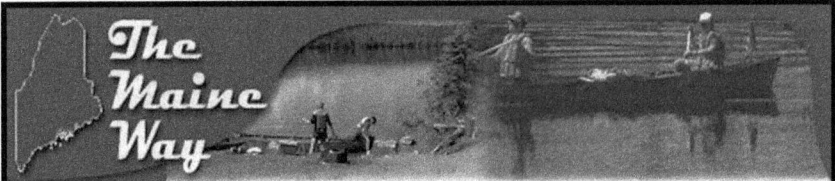

Maine – Your Own Backyard

✓Maine Island Trail (www.mita.org)
✓Maine Outdoors (www.maineoutdoors.com)
✓Local Hikes (www.localhikes.com)
✓The Slackpacker (www.slackpacker.com)
✓The Loonsnest (www.loonsnest.biz)
✓Outdoor Steve (www.outdoorsteve.com)
✓Maine Senior Games (50+) (www.mainesrgames.org)
✓Granite State Senior Games (50+)(www.nhseniorgames.org)

Hiking

- **Hiking in Maine** is a popular reference for hiking trails. Maine has a variety of hiking options available such as difficult trails that are above tree line, trails that meander through cool pine forests, and trails that run along Maine's rugged coast.
  http://www.maineoutdoors.com/hiking/hike_info_trails.shtml

- **Slackpacker.com** is provides access to informative Maine hiking websites. Hikers post comments on their personal hiking experience, thus making research easier to get "an up front and personal" sense of the trails difficulties.
  http://www.slackpacker.com

- **The Local Hikes** provides information on local hiking

opportunities in all areas of the United States. You can find a preferred trail by selecting your metro area, browse the available hikes, or by using the search feature to find the trails closest to your home or office. The hikes reviewed on this site are contributed by volunteer hikers. http://www.localhikes.com

Canoe and Kayaking

- **The Loon's Nest** specializes in wilderness river canoe trips. This site specializes in all forms of outdoor wilderness recreation and is a wealth of information about animals; (hear the four major loon calls); has a fantastic photo gallery of outstanding outdoor pictures taken in all seasons from summer canoeing, sailing, and hiking to winter xc skiing and snowshoeing; as well as many beautiful photographs of Maine's wildlife caught in their natural habitat. http://www.loonsnest.biz

The Maine Island Trail
http://www.mita.org

See the narrative earlier in this section for Maine Island Trail with over 200 islands to "play" on.

Northern Forest Canoe Trail
http://www.northernforestcanoetrail.org/

The NFCT has over 345 miles traversing some of the most scenic, remote, and rugged landscapes the Maine has to offer

Outdoor Enthusiast: Never say, "I wish I had…"

To not duplicate my earlier book, **Outdoor Enthusiast**, I refer you to both the 2009 hardcopy and the updated 2011 e-book version. These books have many more Maine "places to play".

Vermont

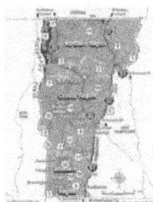

Freedom and Unity

Vermont – Your Own Backyard

✓Vermont Living (www.vtliving.com)
✓Green Mountain Club(www.greenmountainclub.org)
✓Local Hikes (www.localhikes.com)
✓The Slackpacker (www.slackpacker.com)
✓Catamount Trail(www.catamounttrail.org)
✓Frozen Bullet(www.frozenbullet.com)
✓Vermont Senior Games(50+)
(www.seniorgames.org/stategames.htm)

Hiking

- **Vermont Living** and **Trails.com** web sites have trails and backpacking areas
  http://www.vtliving.com/hiking/
  http://www.trails.com/toptrails.aspx?area=10012

- The **Long Trail** was built by the **Green Mountain Club** between 1910 and 1930. The Long Trail is the oldest long-distance trail in the United States. The Long Trail follows the main ridge of the Green Mountains from the Massachusetts-Vermont line to the Canadian border as it crosses Vermont's highest peaks.
  http://www.greenmountainclub.org/

Canoeing and Kayaking

- **Vermont Living** is a good site to locate places in VT for canoeing and kayaking. Some of Vermont's most notable canoeing and kayaking include the Connecticut River that serves as the border between VT and NH, the Batten Kill in southeastern VT, the Lamoille which crosses Vermont's northern region, the Missisquoi in the northwest corner, and the Winooski and White Rivers in north central Vermont http://www.vtliving.com/canoeing/index.shtml.

- **Northern Forest Canoe Trail** has over 170 miles in Vermont Quebec http://www.northernforestcanoetrail.org/

- **Outdoor Enthusiast: Never say, "I wish I had...":** both the 2009 hardcopy and the updated 2011 e-book have more Vermont "places to play".

XC Skiing

- **The Catamount Trail (CAT)**

  The CAT traverses approximately 130 miles of public land including Green Mountain National Forest, Vermont state land, and town-owned parcels. It is divided into 31 section. The CAT is appropriate for a broad range of skiing and snowshoeing abilities.
  http://www.catamounttrail.org

  Biathlon
  - The United States Biathlon site is a good reference to biathlon events and places for instruction and training. http://www.teamusa.org/US-Biathlon.aspx

  - Go to **How Stuff Works** to learn more about the rules and basics of the biathlon. http://adventure.howstuffworks.com/outdoor-activities/snow-sports/biathlon.htm

Senior Games

Encouragement of healthy lifestyles certainly includes outdoor activities for senior athletes. **The National Senior Games Association (NSGA)** is a not-for-profit member of the United States Olympic Committee dedicated to motivating senior men and women to lead a healthy lifestyle through senior athletics.

NSGA is an umbrella for state organizations across the United States that host State Senior Games or Senior Olympics. States have both winter and summer athletic games for female and male athletes over 50 years young. Games may include triathlons, cycling, race walking, track and field events, swimming, road races, pistol shooting, archery, and golf. Some States do paddling, downhill skiing, and cross-country skiing.

New Hampshire, Maine and Vermont are very active both within their states and in national competition.

- o **National Senor Games Association**
  http://www.nsga.com/
- o **Granite State Senior Games**
  http://www.nhseniorgames.org/
- o **Maine Senior Games**
  http://www.smaaa.org/maine_senior_games.php
- o **Vermont Senior Games**
  http://www.vermontseniorgames.org/

So What Do You Do Now?

This Northern New England section is but the tip of the iceberg to locate areas of opportunity, clubs, organizations and fellow outdoor enthusiasts. Local activities are often in our own backyards, and are located by looking in newspaper sections for Outdoor Activities or simply by Internet searching for events in your city or town.

Google key words (such as orienteering, biathlon, bicycle clubs, snowshoe, etc) for locations and sports of interest near you.

Conditioning

The beginning of this book offers **How to be an Outdoor Enthusiast.** It describes a process of physical fitness and how it directly relates to mental preparation and health. Knowing one is not in shape makes it very easy to rationalize postponing an adventure. Moreover, without proper conditioning, we make our companions and ourselves susceptible to injury and failure. Physical fitness complements mental fitness.

The Commitment

A major part of adventure commitment is preparation. The weeks and months before an event are critical. This starts with a mental walk-through of the event itself and working backwards to create a check-off list of things to do and when they are to be done. Do you need campsite reservations? Must you register for the event?

Registration is part of the commitment. When there is a delay in registration, the commitment is not there. A registration commitment can include hotel, campsite or airline reservations.

There must be a plan to reach the required level of physical conditioning. Physical conditioning for a triathlon is much different from white water rafting. Most adventures require stamina, endurance, and quick recovery from cardio exertion. A daily running routine - four to five days a week - provides a baseline conditioning level from which specific conditioning exercises, such as upper body weight training, can support an adventure, such as kayaking and canoeing.

We need to know the extremes of weather we may encounter and plan accordingly. The expected weather conditions may mean gathering specific weather-related clothing, food and medical supplies.

Other preparations, such as for hiking, may include developing skills for map and compass reading. If we work backward from the event, this should provide us a checklist upon which to plan our preparations to scheduling our time, equipment needs, and training. If you are going winter camping, you might practice by sleeping in your backyard to learn what you need for comfort. It is far better to know your sleeping bag does not support cold weather camping when you are in your own backyard rather than to discover this when you are in the middle of the mountains miles away from your car!

Let's continue to play. To enjoy play, one must be physically ready. Hence, exercise is a key enabler of "play." Knowing I have tried, for me, is as important as winning. Regardless of success or failure, my participation provides a never-ending sense of achievement. To me, participation at any level is more advantageous than observation of the highest level.

We need to commit to never say, "I wish I had". Once we have done that - and this could be a financial commitment such as a membership to an outdoor organization such as the YMCA outdoor club or the Appalachian Mountain Club. Then we need to commit to a training program.

We also must recognize it is OK to finish 485th out of 501 entered in a race. It is also OK to finish last! After all, someone has to, why not me! We need to realize that we do not need to go to the other side of the world to achieve a dream. If we simply look around we can see roads for running, lakes for paddling, and woods and mountains for hiking. Even our own backyards can supply the opportunity for the snowcave you might want to build.

A nice thing about being an outdoor enthusiast is most activities cost only our time. A small investment in a canoe, running shoes, bicycle, or cross-country skis will be enough to give us a life time of adventure. We often need to look no further than magazines and newspapers to see these opportunities.

If I have shared my story appropriately, I have both encouraged and supported your enthusiasm for a daily outdoors commitment, made you crave your own "beginnings", and have given insights into new outdoor activities and places to go.

I will thus have achieved my goal of helping others become an "Outdoor Enthusiast" and forever make "Outdoor Play" a component of their daily life.

Never say, "I wish I could find an outdoor activity close to my home."

The Beginning

- o *Give yourself permission to dream* - Randy Pausch
- o *The journey of a thousand miles begins with one step.*
  - Miryamoto Musashi
- o *In the long run one hits only what they aim at.*
  Therefore, though they should fail immediately, they
  had better aim at something high. – Henry David
  Thoreau, Walden

Introduction

This last section of the book is my beginning. I put it here to not take away from the reader's self-motivation. I add it to further encourage individuals and families to make the outdoors a part of their daily lives. And here is my start.

Have you ever thought about sleeping overnight in a snow cave, built by yourself, in the middle of the wilderness? How about running a marathon? What about canoeing through white water, visiting a Shaker museum, or attending a lecture on alternative medicine therapies?

Some folks call these outdoor experiences 'play'. If play is defined as the choice made to take a course of action based on the rewards of participation, and getting a perspective that can only come from 'doing', outdoor adventures are indeed play. Many folks, both adults and children, do not play enough. Play is personal and winning is of no importance. Outdoor play should be a daily component of life.

"I wish I had..." is an expression people often mutter as they rationalize their regret for not having done something. Is it better to have tried and failed than never to have tried at all? Absolutely! Certainly, physical limitations may relate to achievement, but sometimes we erect personal barriers of embarrassment, reluctance, and other self-administrated hurdles.

Try an outdoor trek. Take a chance and peek into a side of outdoor life observed by only the few that do take the chance. How do you describe how beautiful Allagash Falls is at dawn? You can view a thousand pictures, but until you exit your tent at first light, you will never truly know what it is like to experience the sun popping into the sky.

The Opportunity: The Torn Achilles Tendon

Any enthusiast needs to start somewhere. My outdoor emergence began while in an injured state: I had been a couch potato absorbed with the pressures and problems of work, and felt no commitment to outdoor activities other than mowing the grass. Taking time to 'smell the roses' was not a scheduled event, and surely visiting museums was not a part of my lifestyle.

Maybe the outdoor enthusiasm all started with the "good fortune" of tearing my Achilles tendon. Coincidentally, this injury came two years after I had completed my Masters dissertation in Management Engineering with a thesis entitled, The Achilles Tendon as an Indication of Thyroid Function. Years later the anatomy studies required to understand the function of the Achilles tendon helped me to accept my injury.

My injury came as I was playing basketball in a pick-up game. I had positioned myself for a clear outside shot and was in the process of shooting the ball. Suddenly I felt as if someone had hit me in the back of my ankle. I dropped to the floor, and turned around expecting to see who had taken my legs out from under me. Nobody was there. The damage was done – my Achilles tendon had ruptured.

The healing process progressed erratically. A noticeable indentation appeared where the tear had taken place. The medical opinion was that surgical treatment would not necessarily help. Medical professionals told me there was a fifty - fifty chance that the tendon would tear again. I was determined to prove them wrong.

The First Mile

One day, about a year after my injury, I decided I had to do something about my twenty-five pound weight gain, a perpetual "tired feeling", and general lack of exercise. I went down to my cellar and rummaged through old boxes of shoes. I found my ten-year-old ankle-high Army combat boots and reminisced to myself about boot camp and its daily mandate to hit the road running.

The boots were intact, though the leather was a bit stiff and definitely needing a softener. I ignored the tautness, and proceeded to lace them tight in hope of ensuring protection for my "healed" Achilles tendon. Now was the time to determine if exercise would free me from my couch.

I went outside and ran - maybe limped is a better word - a distance of two telephone poles. Even though I was breathing heavily and perspiring profusely, it felt good, despite the sensitivity of a now sore tendon.

The next evening, I climbed into my combat boots and this time with a determination to exceed the previous day's run of two telephone poles. I lumbered, limped, and puffed to achieve the distance of three telephone poles. My quest had begun.

Daily, after work, I continued extending my distances one pole at a time. My Achilles tendon threat to tear again concerned me, but I fervently decided against returning to inactivity.

Initially, my running goals were measured in terms of those ever-present telephone poles. However, after two weeks, I abandoned this strategy, and I reset my goals to reach the end of my street without stopping - about a third of a mile. By the end of the third week, not only had I achieved my objective, but also turned around and began running back home.

I now had a dream that one day I could jog around my neighborhood block. I measured the distance with my car and determined the loop was exactly a mile. Each evening I came closer to completing the neighborhood loop, but exhaustion resulted in walking before I died. Five weeks had elapsed since my emergence from the couch. Each day at work, I would picture myself accomplishing the mile. Every evening I would start, determined to run the one-mile route, only to end up walking.

During week six, I had a feeling that this was to be my time, my day. I saw my house in the distance, and was having no difficulty breathing. I had no thoughts about my Achilles, and until this moment, I was simply concentrating on an issue at work. I suddenly realized I was less than four telephone poles from my quest. With painful joy shared with no one but myself, in what seemed to be mere seconds, my goal was now history. Sucking air with sheer exhaustion, I stumbled into my backyard overjoyed with the thrill of victory.

I ran this one-mile loop - usually six days a week - for nearly two years with no thought of extending my distance. Certainly, other outdoor challenges, such as biking, canoeing, hiking and kayaking, were not even a consideration.

One day I read in the local newspaper about a seven-mile running race. The race was four weeks away. I dared to think that perhaps I could finish this distance. I began extending my daily run, and in one week I was able to do my one-mile loop twice! I had doubled my distance in only one week. I set my next goal at four miles and accomplished it within two weeks. It was now time for me to assess myself against other athletes. I submitted my entry form.

The appropriately named Freedom Trail race was a seven-miler at the University of Massachusetts campus at Dartmouth. My pre-race jitters were compounded by second-guessing myself as to whether I should even be here. I had never participated in any type of official running race before, and I had visions of being elbowed and trampled by a pack of passionate runners.

I overcame this distress by positioning myself at the back of the mass of lightly clad runners who were stretching, jumping up and down, and obviously trying to relieve their nerves while waiting for the start of the race.

I had anticipated all participants to be thin, athletic, and young. Instead, all types, men and women, young and old, and people in various degrees of physical shape - thin, fat, short, tall, and pudgy. Naively, I thought that I surely would finish in front of the older and overweight athletes.

I got a quick education when the official fired the starter gun. After a few hundred feet, not only was I holding up the rear, I was yards behind the last runner. I began to have thoughts of not finishing, and worse, becoming lost as the runners in front of me continued to get further ahead. At the second mile marker, a few runners were still in sight, and I resigned myself simply to completing the race.

At the five-mile marker, I was running side by side with a young woman who appeared to be in her late twenties. We were the last two racers. I was sure she had slowed down to let me catch up, because I knew I was in no condition to speed up. We talked about our jobs and our families - anything to help forget the pain we were both experiencing.

With about a mile to go to the finish line, she suggested we pick up our speed. Unfortunately, I was already at my maximum speed. Off she went, with my blessings, and I was the last runner to cross the finish line. To top things off, there were only two people at the finish line - my wonderful mother and the timer. My mother would not let the timer leave until I had finished!

The immediate aftermath of this seven-mile "triumph" was that I could not sit down! Every time I tried to bend my legs and lower myself to the ground, my hamstrings would begin to cramp. Indeed, I was a "winner", but I now had to pay the price of my personal best distance.

The outcome of this story was I had run seven miles! Little did I know at the time this experience would be the beginning of a lifetime enjoyment of outdoor challenges.

Certainly, a benefit of physical conditioning was my weight loss of nearly forty pounds. I felt different both physically and mentally.

The seat of my pants was floppy and my face lost its fullness. Friends began to ask if I was "sick". I had to buy new suits. It felt great being asked all these personal questions!

A Family Revelation

My outdoor enthusiasm carried forth to my family as we began to participate together in outdoor fun and exercise. My wife and I regularly walk and run together. A summer night can find us kayaking or canoeing on the lakes of New Hampshire.

My two sons and my grandchildren are essential components to my daily outdoor life. As a family, our activities include boating, hiking, canoeing, kayaking, and morning and evening moose sightings.

Let me illustrate a father-son-revelation that occurred while hiking with my son Timothy when he was a teenager. Hiking provides an opportunity to share experiences on an adult level and leave behind the typical parent/child relationship of the home environment. Hiking in the mountains requires reliance upon your partner that breaks down parent/child barriers that develop from the routine of daily life. At home, the parent sets an example and provides the child with an opportunity to learn. This pattern must be adjusted in the wilderness.

Tim and I lumbered along the Appalachian Trail planning to spend the night at the Mizpah Spring hut, one of the eight White Mountain huts maintained by the New Hampshire Chapter of the Appalachian Mountain Club. Just as we reached the peak of Mt. Franklin, the weather quickly changed and it began to rain. The rain became heavy, the sky grew darker, and suddenly we were engulfed in a torrent of rain. Driving rain pelted us, and thunder and lightning roared and crackled all around. It was only three o'clock in the afternoon and yet it was nearly pitch dark. It was a strange and awesome sensation. The top of Mt Franklin is entirely ledge and rock, and we knew immediately we were in a dangerous position - on top of a mountain and without shelter. It was a bizarre scary feeling as we stood there in our rain suits, rain pouring off our faces and our features illuminated sporadically by flashes of light.

An unbelievable sensation of excitement and strength came over me. I felt I united with the earth and the elements and had all their power at my command. At the same time, I feared that this angry and violent deluge would overcome us, and we might not survive this encounter. I suddenly knew before Tim or I died - and it could have happened at any moment - I wanted Tim to know how much a part of me he was. I had an unbelievable urge to hug Tim, kiss him, and tell him how much I loved and admired him - and so I did! It was a moment I still remember today - hugging my teenage son with all my strength and telling him how much he meant to me.

Meanwhile thunder crackled and lightening illuminated the darkness, filling the surrounding countryside with shadows and ghostly sensations. We were in the middle of an enormous storm, terrifying, yet beautiful at the same time.

Tim responded to my hug and kiss with the same embracing closeness and finality that I did. I could feel his strength and our oneness as he embraced me for what could be the last time.

Then, just as suddenly as the storm had come, it was gone. The sun came out as if to say, "Together you have seen the light and felt your courage and unity." We were wet and shivering, but thankful we were without injury. We continued our journey.

Tim had avoided my invitations to learn in the past - that is what it seemed to me. Our stay at Mizpah Spring showed I was wrong. The volunteer naturalist at the hut led an evening tour to learn about the birds, animals, shrubs and trees native to this high altitude habitat. With obvious interest, Tim asked many questions of the naturalist.

A sunrise tour for a different aspect of the habitat was scheduled. Given the previous day's tiring adventures, I never expected to see Tim. We went to bed that night, exhausted.

At 4:45 AM, my watch alarm went off and I quietly whispered to Tim I was getting up for the tour. I left the bunkroom pleased at Tim's delight with the previous evening. To my surprise and much pleasure, who should appear at the morning walk-about but Tim!

Tim and I experienced a bonding on that hike we still discuss today. We depended on each other in a death-defying situation. I saw that he is caring, self-reliant, and levelheaded under pressure. He has a thirst to learn. I have come to recognize these qualities and more as we have shared the joys, challenges and revelation provided by hiking trips along the Appalachian Trail and many other "Outdoor Play" adventures.

If the facts be known, the awakening and growth in maturity was solely mine.

From the Outdoors to Intellectual Pursuits

Interestingly, this curiosity to experience new and different outdoor activities began to carry over to intellectual inquisitiveness and my mantra, "Never say, I wish I had...", I began to visit museums, simply to gain awareness of something new. I became obsessed with the opportunity to learn the unique and interesting worlds of others. I attend lectures with a craving to hear a speaker's insights, and to listen to his or her passion and enthusiasm. Certainly, this curiosity includes presentations on all facets of the outdoors found by simply looking through the local newspapers. Animal tracks, identifying trees, learning about turkeys, Mount Everest climbers, and seafaring presentations are all there, usually for free or a minimal fee.

So, What Do You Do Now?

If tearing my tendon made me recognize the limits of my knowledge and appreciation, the pain and struggle of recuperation was worth it.

This book shares short stories of outdoors and wilderness knowledge gained through personal involvement. It can be a guidebook of places and events to play. It is not a traditional how-to, or you-should kind of book, but life stories for individuals and families to motivate them to make the outdoors a daily part of life.

These stories are meant to stimulate the reader to enjoy the outdoor world and the people around them. The message is it is okay to listen to your inner calling so you will never regret you did not experience the renewal and fulfillment that venturing into the outdoors may provide. Simply being in an audience as others perform and share their views cannot satisfy an eager human being. The motivation is to "get off the couch," and not let others dictate what you know or do.

I do not want to pretend I am a philosopher of what life is about, or a preacher of outdoor activities, nor a non-conformist in life. Henry David Thoreau appears to express my approach to outdoor living. In Walden he said, "I went to the woods because I wished to live deliberately, to front only the essential facts of life, and to see if I could not learn what it had to teach, and not, when I came to die, discover that I had not lived. I wanted to live deep and suck out all the marrow of life…"

My Achilles tendon has never completely regenerated to its former strength. I sometimes have a noticeable limp at the end of a long day on my feet, but the limp has no pain and does not hinder any of my outdoor activities.

I mention my past injury because some people use self-imposed physical and mental barriers, and say, "I wish I could do physical exercise and outdoor adventures similar to yours, but I tore my Achilles tendon" (or whatever physical ailment they have). Other "wish I could" reasons I hear are, "I am too old", "I am way out of shape," and "I do not know where to start." Hmm, guess they did not read the first section in this book, **How to be an Outdoor Enthusiast.**

Be aware - outdoor enthusiasm includes family revelations. As I learned more about myself when hiking with Timothy and Shaun, so did I see my sons become mature and responsible adults. My sons and I have done numerous canoeing and kayaking trips and have sat beside campfires talking about life, ambitions, and family issues.

My wife Cathy and I regularly walk, hike, camp and paddle together. Most important are the conversations we have on our family, finances, and other life issues.

Never say, "I wish I had made the outdoors a part of my daily life."

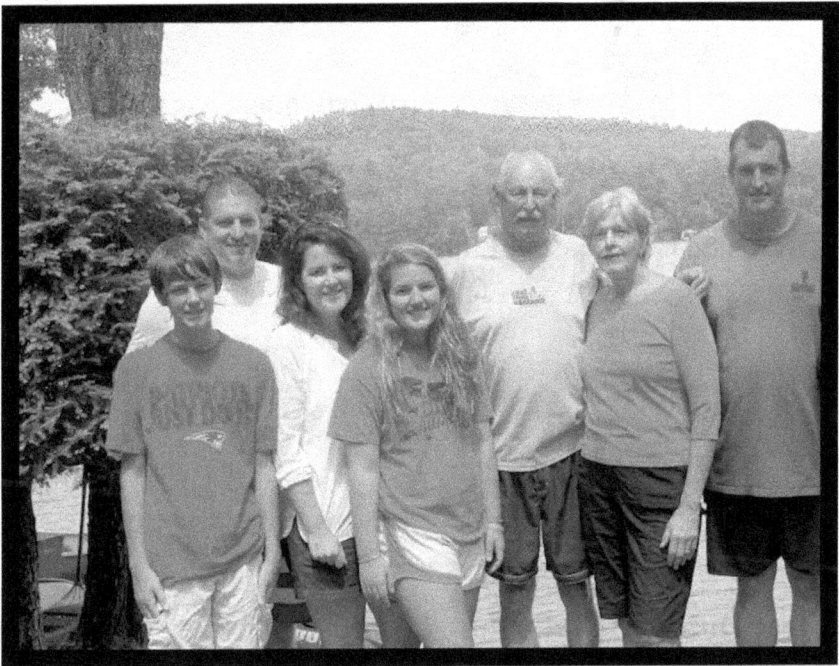

"Everyone must believe in something. I believe I'll go outdoors with my family." – S. Priest

Books by Stephen L. Priest

- **Outdoor Play "Fun 4 4 Seasons"**
  Hard Copy
  https://www.createspace.com/4177334

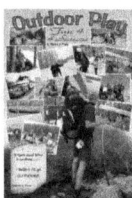

ISBN **978-0-985-03840-3**

- **Outdoor Play "Fun 4 4 Seasons"**
  Hard Copy **Special Edition Full Color**
  https://www.createspace.com/3745716

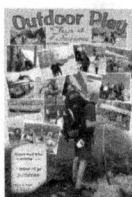

ISBN **978-0-615-22504-3**

- **Outdoor Play "Fun 4 4 Seasons"**
  Amazon.com Kindle e-book
  http://www.amazon.com/dp/B00C2G20HQ

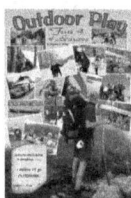

ISBN **978-0-9850384-1-0**

- **Outdoor Enthusiast: Never say, "I wish I had …"**
  Hardcopy
  https://www.createspace.com/3356777

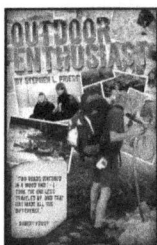

 ISBN 1440438404

- **Outdoor Enthusiast: Never say, "I wish I had…"**
  Amazon.com Kindle e-book
  http://tiny.cc/d2c0t

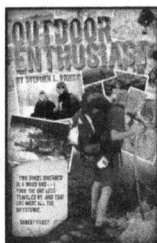

 ISBN 9780615225050

- **Outdoor Enthusiast: Never say I wish I had…"**
  Barnes & Noble Nook e-book
  BN ID: 2940012341037
  http://tiny.cc/85ygs

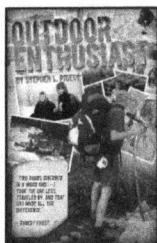

 ISBN 9780615225050

- **Outdoor Enthusiast: Never say, "I wish I had…"**
  Amazon.com Hard Copy
  http://tiny.cc/lli3tw

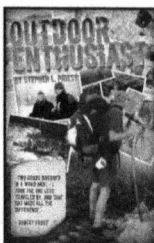

ISBN 1301078331

- **Avoiding Injuries: Great Tips From Master Outdoorsman Steve Priest**
  Create Space Hard Copy
  https://www.createspace.com/3356784

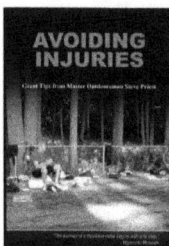

ISBN 9781440438455

Notes

Outdoor Play "Fun 4 4 Seasons"

www.ingramcontent.com/pod-product-compliance
Lightning Source LLC
Chambersburg PA
CBHW052121270326
41930CB00012B/2707